Health Education Teaching Ideas:
ELEMENTARY

Dr. Donna L. Osness and Ms. Karen Thompson, *Editors*

**Sponsored by the
Association for the Advancement
of Health Education**

an association of the

**American Alliance for
Health, Physical Education,
Recreation and Dance**

American Alliance for
Health, Physical Education,
Recreation and Dance
1900 Association Drive
Reston, Virginia 22091

ISBN 0-88314-223-6

Purposes of the American Alliance For Health, Physical Education, Recreation and Dance

The American Alliance is an educational organization, structured for the purposes of supporting, encouraging, and providing assistance to member groups and their personnel throughout the nation as they seek to initiate, develop, and conduct programs in health, leisure, and movement-related activities for the enrichment of human life.

Alliance objectives include:

1. Professional growth and development—to support, encourage, and provide guidance in the development and conduct of programs in health, leisure, and movement-related activities which are based on the needs, interests, and inherent capacities of the individual in today's society.

2. Communication—to facilitate public and professional understanding and appreciation of the importance and value of health, leisure, and movement-related activities as they contribute toward human well-being.

3. Research—to encourage and facilitate research which will enrich the depth and scope of health, leisure, and movement-related activities; and to disseminate the findings to the profession and other interested and concerned publics.

4. Standards and guidelines—to further the continuous development and evaluation of standards within the profession for personnel and programs in health, leisure, and movement-related activities.

5. Public affairs—to coordinate and administer a planned program of professional, public, and governmental relations that will improve education in areas of health, leisure, and movement-related activities.

6. To conduct such other activities as shall be approved by the Board of Governors and the Alliance Assembly, provided that the Alliance shall not engage in any activity which would be inconsistent with the status of an educational and charitable organization as defined in Section 501(c) (3) of the Internal Revenue Code of 1954 or any successor provision thereto, and none of the said purposes shall at any time be deemed or construed to be purposes other than the public benefit purposes and objectives consistent with such educational and charitable status. *Bylaws, Article III*

Foreword

These articles from *Health Education* have been selected and assembled to assist the elementary classroom teacher in the instruction of health education. Some of the articles provide resource information specifically for the teacher while others present examples of activities for students.

The Health Education section consists of general articles covering a variety of topics. Therefore, a short summary of each article is available. The other sections are categorized alphabetically according to specific health topics.

Hopefully, this publication will provide elementary teachers with a wealth of information and ideas to aid them in designing their health instruction. However, most of the articles contain information and/or activities appropriate for the elementary school level.

This collection should provide the elementary classroom teacher with a foundation upon which to build an extended catalog of resources. It is apparent that some of the categories are in need of additional information and activities. However, they are recognized as important areas of a health education program and should be expanded.

Dr. Donna L. Osness,
Director of Health Education and Health Services,
Shawnee Mission Schools
and Ms. Karen Thompson, Elementary Teacher, *Editors*

CONTENTS

Aging

Alcohol Education

Anatomy and Physiology

Cardiovascular Health

Consumer Education

Death Education

Dental Health

Drug Education

Environmental Health

First Aid and Safety

Health Services

Mental Health

Nutrition

Parenting

Sex Education

Smoking

Wellness

Breaking Down Barriers in the Classroom

Boundary breaking is an excellent activity for building rapport, establishing trust and developing listening skills in the classroom. The activity provides structure in allowing students to share their true feelings, opinions and beliefs in a setting where they will not be judged. This process also affords the teacher the opportunity to learn more about students.

When used with health-related subject matter, boundary breaking can give the teacher an idea of what students already know or think about a particular subject while introducing it to class. Used as an evaluation tool, the teacher can determine if knowledge or attitudes have changed as a result of the learning experience.

Additional advantages of boundary breaking include opportunities: 1. for *each* student to be equally involved in classroom activity; 2. for the students to understand their classmates better; 3. for understanding that *different* is o.k.

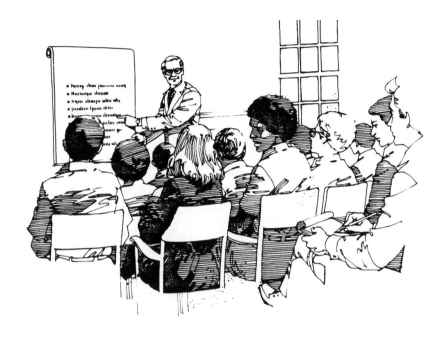

Information Phase

Boundary breaking has two parts: the information phase and the feedback phase. The information phase consists of questions selected on some health topic. For children through fifth grade, eight to ten information questions should suffice. Avoid yes/no questions. For middle school students, ten to fourteen questions are about the right amount, while high school students could sustain interest in the activity for as many as twenty questions. The teacher should be aware of the students' level and try to end the activity while interest is high.

Feedback Phase

The second phase of boundary breaking is the feedback phase. It should be introduced while interest in the activity is still high. It is particularly significant to boundary breaking and the activity should never end without the feedback phase to provide closure and create a sense of cohesiveness among the participants.

Mary Merki is an instructional specialist in health education for the Dallas Independent School District, Dallas, Texas. Don Merki is a professor of health education at Texas Woman's University, Denton, TX 76201.

To begin the activity, the teacher divides the class into groups of six to eight. (The smaller number is recommended through fifth grade). A leader is assigned to each group. No special training or preparation is needed to be a group leader. The leader is responsible for reading the questions, keeping the activity moving and ensuring that the ground rules are followed.

It is important that no non-participants be allowed to observe boundary breaking. Outside observers tend to threaten the desired objectives of boundary breaking. Each person present must participate, including the teacher and all group leaders. The teacher may choose to be a participant in one of the small groups or to lead one of the small groups.

Instructions

Each leader is given a set of questions and the following set of instructions:
1. Sit as close to each other as is comfortable. We are going to engage in an activity to learn more about each other. This activity is called boundary breaking.

2. I will ask the questions.
3. Each person must answer all the questions.
4. Short answers are preferred.
5. If you are not ready to answer, say "pass" and I'll come back to you.
6. Your answer may be the same as someone else's as long as it is your honest response.
7. Watch the other people in the circle as they answer. You can learn a great deal about a person from the way he handles himself in this kind of situation.
8. Listen to the answers from each person and try to understand and accept each person.
9. Remember, the idea is to learn about ourselves and those around us.
10. We are not here to judge others or their answers. The key goal is listen . . . listen . . . listen.
11. There should *not* be any discussion of answers or questioning of responses. Common inappropriate remarks include: That's a good answer. That's kind of strange. I never heard anything like that before. Boy, that's dumb. Are you kidding? Did I hear you right? Do you really mean that? You can't be serious. I wish I'd said that. That's super.

All of these responses are examples of value judgements. The verbal comments are easier to control than non-verbal responses, such as: nodding approval, frowning, looking surprised, etc.

12. We will now begin with the information phase:

Sample information phase questions for health and fitness.

1. What is one thing you do to be physically fit?
2. Name one situation you find stressful.
3. What do you do to relax or unwind?
4. In your opinion what behavior is the most unhealthy?
5. What is your favorite sport?
6. If you could change anything about you, what would it be?
7. What is one nice thing you do for yourself to show you like yourself?
8. In general, I feel _____ . (use a word that describes mood or physical feeling).
9. What percent of the day do you spend being physically active?
10. How would you evaluate your exercise habits?

For Consumer Health

1. What is your favorite commercial?
2. What effect do famous people in ads have on your purchase?
3. What do you think of Ralph Nader?
4. How would you recognize a quack?
5. Who would you tell if you had been "ripped off?"

For Drugs

1. What do you think is the main reason people use drugs on a continual basis?
2. What does "responsible drinking" mean to you?
3. What is the most serious problem related to alcohol abuse?
4. What is one benefit of taking drugs?
5. If you could ban one drug what would it be?

For Sexuality

1. Where is the best place to go on a date?
2. What do you think of trial marriages?
3. What is the best age to get married?
4. What do you think about divorce?
5. Where is the worst place to go on a date?

For Nutrition

1. What is your favorite type of food?
2. What food smells the best/worst?
3. What do you think is the most important nutrient?
4. What do you think is the "all-American" food?
5. What is your favorite outdoor snack?

Feedback Phase

Remember, the feedback phase is the standard closing for all boundary breaking sessions.
1. What person in this group did you learn most about today?
2. What person do you want to learn more about?
3. Who pays the most attention to what is going on around them?
4. Which person do you think you could get along with best over a period of time?
5. Based on today's answers, which person do you feel is the most like you?
6. Based on today's answers, which person do you feel is the least like you?
7. What answer from others pleased you the most?
8. Which answer surprised you the most?

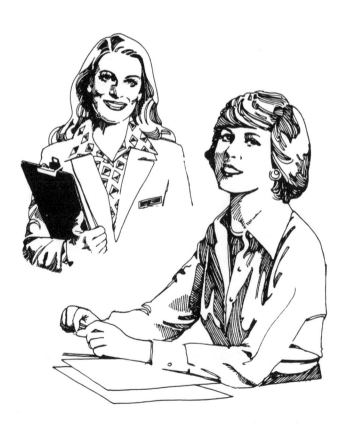

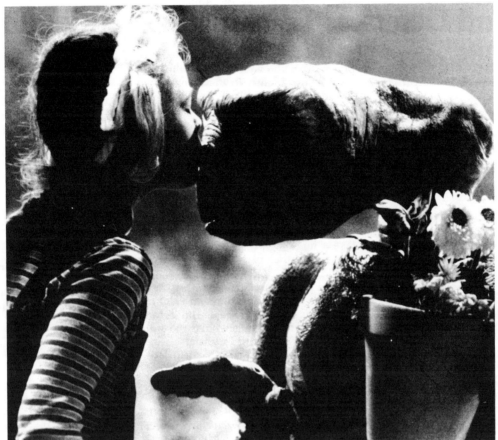

Stellar Pedagogy—H.E. Meets E.T.

Health Education

It is sometimes difficult for students to talk about controversial health topics because they fear personal disclosures, or they are simply "too close" to an issue to be objective about it. If students are provided opportunities to write about, discuss, or react to abstract rather than specific or personal health problems, they will be more likely to experiment with options to current health problems.

David E. Corbin is assistant professor of Health Education in the School of HPER, University of Nebraska at Omaha, Omaha, NE 68182-0216.

Problems can be presented abstractly through the use of music[1], art[2] or through creating hypothetical or science fiction analogies to current health issues. The purpose of this paper is to combine the current fascination and popularity of science fiction movies (*E.T., Star Trek II, Tron, Blade Runner, Firefox,* etc.) with health problems and issues here on Earth today.

Before focusing on specific ways to use science fiction in the classroom, it is worthwhile to emphasize that controversial health issues usually teeter precariously between "pure" science and opinion. In a health classroom "pure" science does not exist, but where possi-

ble the values of science, as published by the Educational Policies Commission of the National Education Association[3], should be ever in mind. These values are:

1. longing to know and understand,
2. questioning of all things,
3. search for data and their meaning,
4. demand for verification,
5. respect for logic,
6. consideration of premises,
7. consideration of consequences.

In addition to and in conjunction with these scientific values, the discussion of controversial health topics requires adherence to the following basic human rights:

1. I have the right to be treated with respect.
2. I have the right to have and express my own feelings and opinions.
3. I have the right to be listened to and taken seriously.
4. I have the right to set my own priorities.
5. I have the right to ask for information.
6. I have the right to change my mind.
7. I have the right to make mistakes— and be responsible for them.
8. I have the right to say, "I don't know."
9. I have the right to say, "I don't understand."

Once these basic values and rights are understood, they will help to focus the students' writings and/or discussions about controversial health topics.

Following are some examples of how a health teacher can use science fiction to inspire interest in and discussion of controversial health topics. 1) Why would health experts on Earth be so concerned about alien creatures coming to this planet? 2) How might it affect the health and lives of the people on Earth? How might it affect the lives and health of the Aliens? 3) If Earthlings who had direct physical contact with the Aliens began to come down with an unexplained illness, what should be done from the Earthlings' point of view? 4) From the Aliens' point of view?

In *E.T.* the alien creature got into a refrigerator and drank several cans of beer. This had a direct affect on both the alien creature and the young boy who befriended him. Assuming you could communicate with the Alien: 5) How would you explain to him the existence of and the effects of alcohol on Earthlings and perhaps on alien beings? 6) Write a brief story or scenario about Aliens whose first glimpse of humans after landing on Earth was a group of teenagers having a "kegger" beer party. 7) What report of human behavior do you think they would send back to their planet? 8) If you were assigned the task of teaching English to the Alien, how would you explain all of the synonyms we have for the word "drunk" (i.e., spaced out, bombed, plowed, plastered, blitzed, polluted, stewed, pickled, smashed, blasted, high, tipsy, etc.)? 9) How would you answer this question asked by the Alien: "Why do you have more synonyms for 'drunk' than you do for 'love' "? 10) If it were discovered that the Aliens got drunk on less alcohol than the average human yet they asked to take a huge supply of alcoholic beverages back to their planet with them, what would you do or advise? 11) If the Aliens offered you some strange looking capsules or tablets that they said would make you feel good, what would your reaction be? Would you take the capsules? 12) If the Aliens were insulted if you declined to join them in taking the capsule, would that change your mind?

For the next question the teacher should have a slide or a poster of E.T. to show to the class. 13) Is it possible to love a creature that looks like this? Why or why not? 14) If you saw the movie, what characteristics either endeared E.T. to you or repulsed you? 15) Did you change your mind about initial impressions you had of E.T.? Why or why not? 16) E.T. could "defy" death under circumstances that would have killed human beings, i.e., freezing. How would you explain the concept of human death to E.T. or another alien?

Following are some related teaching materials:

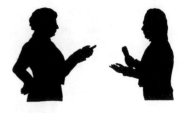

Hall, Jay, "Lost on the Moon Game," reprinted in Greenberg, Jerrold S., *Student-Centered Health Instruction: A Humanistic Approach*, Addison-Wesley, Reading, MA, 1978, p. 36–38.

This is a decision-making exercise whose answers are based on scientific data. It includes health-related problems and survival skills.

Twelker, Paul A. and Layden, Kent, "Humanus," (booklet and cassette), Simile II, P.O. Box 910, Del Mar, CA 92014, 1973.

This is a space travel simulation where students make health, social and survival decisions based upon information given to them by the computer "Humanus."

[1]Corbin, D. E. Ecology and Ecology Songs. *Pennsylvania Journal of Health, Physical Education and Recreation.* 1979, 49, pp. 12–13.

[2]Corbin, D. E. The Art of Health. *Journal of School Health,* in press.

[3]Educational Policies Commission. Education and the Spirit of Science. National Education Association, 1966.

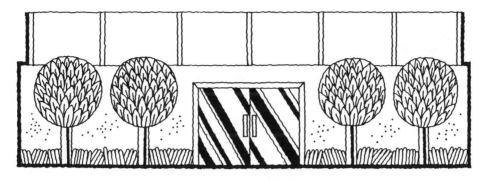

Implementation of a School Based Health Education Project

JOHN R. SEFFRIN is the consultant, CHARLES J. BAER is the project director, and BILL G. KEAFFABER is the project coordinator for the Kokomo-Center Township School Corporation, 100 West Lincoln Drive, Kokomo, Indiana 46901. The project described in this article is being funded by the Division of Addiction Services, Indiana Department of Mental Health.

Innovative school based programs in health education are frequently restricted and fragmentary because of limited and earmarked funds. What is more, many successful efforts at program innovation and revision yield only local benefits, since information regarding their format and development does not reach professionals in other communities throughout the country.

One community has procured federal and local financial support for a comprehensive school-based health education program. The project is now in its second year of implementation, and this report is an update on progress made since the developmental stage, which was described in the January-February 1977 issue of *Health Education*.

During the last year five instructional programs were begun, one for each of five grade levels. These programs were developed and implemented in compliance with the timetable established in the developmental stage. Each program was developed and instituted by a select team of teachers who were also a part of the project staff. While the programs dealt with differing health content

areas, all programs were designed and developed to focus on an identified need or problem for that grade level and be consistent with the overall project goals and objectives. This assured orderly progression toward a well articulated and sequential health education program.

In an effort to establish baseline data in addition to immediate program results, each program was evaluated during the first year. Following is a description of each program and the results of the first-year assessments. It should be pointed out that implementation of programs, evaluation, and revision are all ongoing in this project.

Marshall Monkey

Marshall Monkey is a puppet play on medicine safety which was designed for the third grade reading level. Various mishaps and experiences occurring to jungle animals are used by the central character, Marshall Monkey, as illustrations of good and poor medicine safety habits. Basic concepts regarding the positive use of medicine, not taking medicine prescribed for others, not mistaking drugs for candy, proper medicine storage, and medicinal advertising are stressed.

A take-home flyer is given to parents. This pamphlet includes a home check list and safety tips. Also included is a peel-off sticker for the telephone with the local Poison Control Center location and phone number. Through effective

pupil involvement, the outcome of this unit should be an understanding of the importance of following good medicine safety habits and an attitude of respect for the proper use of medicine.

In an effort to evaluate the Marshall Monkey program, over a thousand third grade children were pre- and posttested with a short cognitive instrument. The instrument was specially designed for the program and was prepared by members of the writing team. Although a slight increase in mean achievement was observed after exposure to the program, the difference was not significant. However, since proficiency is important in the basic safety rules covered in this program, it was gratifying to see that the posttest mean was 9.4 out of a possible 10.0. The distribution of scores was markedly skewed, with a great number of children getting all items correct. Therefore, future attempts to evaluate cognitive achievement will have to rely on the development of more discriminating test items.

Each of the five programs was also evaluated by the classroom teachers who used them. A five-point rating scale was developed which allowed the teacher to react to a series of declarative statements about each program. Several criteria statements dealing with content accuracy, student interest, educational impact, completeness, and utility were used.

A total of 42 teachers used and subsequently evaluated the Marshall Monkey program. Table 1 shows the percentage of teachers responding positively and negatively to the evaluation criteria. Basically the Marshall Monkey program was very well received by teachers as well as by students and parents. Since there was strong endorsement from those elementary teachers using the program, it will not be significantly revised. However, data as well as teacher opinion indicates the program could be used effectively with younger children.

Interview with a Pharmacist

"Interview with a Pharmacist" is a slide and tape presentation dealing with over-the-counter and prescription medicines, aimed at the fifth-grade level. The class systematically identifies a number of questions which the students are interested in getting answered, and then they invite a local pharmacist to visit their classroom. The questions range from what is the difference between over-the-counter and prescription drugs, to why are drugs dangerous and what is drug abuse?

Although this unit does impart some basic facts about drugs, the main emphasis is on making children aware of the resources that are available to them as they assume the responsibility of their own drug use. The overall aim of this program is to help students develop a respect for the power of drugs as they identify the proper reasons to use them.

This unit is designed to be correlated with other subjects besides health, including language arts, social studies, and mathematics. The unit kit includes crossword puzzles, word find, and a self-test.

In keeping with the nature and objectives of this program, approximately 1,400 fifth-grade children were pre- and posttested with a personal-attitude scale regarding their feelings about drugs. The instrument was specifically designed by the writing team for the "Interview with a Pharmacist" program.

Although attitude formation and attitude change is complex and not easy to measure precisely, it was felt that observed shifts could provide valuable feedback as to program impact. For example, on the pretest only 37.1% of the children agreed that "aspirin is dangerous"; however, on the posttest 73.3% agreed with that statement. Similarly, on the pretest 57.3% agreed that "children can take too many vitamins," while on the posttest 76.1% agreed that they could.

Some other types of attitudinal items were used with interesting results. When responding to the statement "if a friend takes drugs, you should *not* like him," 28.8% of the pretest respondents agreed, while only 18.7% of the posttest respondents agreed. The diminution of the percentage from pretest to posttest may have resulted from the positive approach used in this program toward helping friends in need. For example, on the pretest 30.5% agreed that "kids have a responsibility for what their friends get into," while 53.0% agreed with the same statement on the posttest.

As indicated in table 1, the "Interview with a Pharmacist" program was fairly well accepted by the teachers. However, over one fifth (22.9%) disagreed that the program "motivated them to do more teaching" in the area.

Triple S

"Triple S" is a family-relationships program designed for the sixth grade. The basic unit plan is developed around a filmstrip-tape program dealing with concepts of harmonious family interactions and relationships. The presentation is in cartoon form and the setting is a trip to outer space. The main character, Colonel Conners, interviews several families to find out if they are suitable to live on the "Space Wheel." As the program is being used, students complete their own log books which are provided with the instructional kit. In addition to the filmstrip and log books, the program kit includes several student activities, such as puzzles and role playing exercises.

Over 700 sixth graders were pre- and posttested using a self-opinion instrument developed by the project staff. In all, 38 declarative statements were put on the test form for student reaction. In general, posttest results showed small, but favorable, shifts in percentage responses. For example, even though 93.0% agreed on the posttest that "I can keep a secret," 90.7% had already responded in the same way on the pretest. Although the results may reflect a "halo-effect" from students responding as they thought they should respond,

Table 1. Percentage of teachers responding positively and negatively to evaluation criteria

	Marshall Monkey		Interview with a Pharmacist		Triple S		It's Not the Alcohol		The Easy Way Out?	
	1 Positive	2 Negative	1 Positive	2 Negative	1 Positive	2 Negative	1 Positive	2 Negative	1 Positive	2 Negative
Program is complete	85.7	7.1	48.6	20.0	30.7	38.5	77.7	22.2	80.0	10.0
Students were interested	85.7	9.5	65.7	11.4	38.5	34.6	66.6	22.2	50.0	50.0
Program was worthwhile	85.8	9.5	62.8	11.4	42.3	30.8	77.7	22.2	80.0	10.0
Motivates students to act favorably	80.9	11.9	54.3	5.7	30.7	30.8	44.4	33.3	50.0	30.0
Motivated me to do more teaching in the area	71.5	11.9	48.6	22.9	34.6	26.9	55.5	33.3	70.0	10.0
Supplementary material was valuable	78.6	11.9	51.4	11.4	46.2	23.0	88.8	00.0	80.0	10.0
Teacher guidelines were helpful	83.3	11.9	48.6	17.2	53.8	15.4	77.8	00.0	90.0	00.00
Unit plan was helpful	85.7	9.5	51.5	5.7	46.1	23.1	77.8	00.0	90.0	00.00

Key: Column one for each program is the positive responses which includes the summation of those strongly agreeing and agreeing with the criterion statement.
Column two for each program is the negative responses which includes the summation of those strongly disagreeing and disagreeing with the criterion statement.

Percentages do not necessarily add to 100 since an undecided response was possible.

rather than as they actually may behave, other items showed more realistic responses. When responding to the statement "I am always on time," 57.8% of the students agreed on the prettest, while 67.7% agreed to the same statement on the posttest.

Basically these student responses did not yield conclusive results. Further, the teacher evaluations seemed to suggest a need to revise this program. The teachers who used "Triple S" were split in their acceptance, as shown in table 1. In fact, more teachers disagreed with the statement that "the program was complete" than agreed.

It's Not the Alcohol

At the seventh grade level, a two-part filmstrip/tape presentation was developed on ethyl alcohol, its history, use, and abuse. A talking bottle narrates the program with a southern accent which added variety to the normal narrative voice. Through early civilization, colonization of America, Prohibition, and teenage drinking today, the presentation finishes with sources of help for problem drinkers.

The program theme is to encourage teenagers to avoid the abuse of alcohol. Scare techniques are avoided and respect for alcohol is stressed. Discussion questions at the end of the filmstrip help the teacher encourage students to discuss the problem of alcohol abuse among students and adults.

A cognitive test on facts regarding alcohol was developed and used to pre- and posttest approximately 700 seventh grade students. The instrument was comprised of 29 items, although four items failed to discriminate acceptably on either the pre- or posttest. Otherwise, the test analysis showed that the instrument performed acceptably during both administrations.

Although the mean score on the posttest was higher than the pretest mean, the difference was not significant. The posttest mean was 17.6, thus, the average student performance was about 60%. Apparently, a number of the facts were not stressed enough during the presentation.

Most seventh grade teachers were pleased with this program. For instance, as shown in table 1, 77.7% agreed that the program was complete, worthwhile, and helpful. However, one third of the responding teachers disagreed with the statements regarding favorable student behavior and teacher motivation.

The Easy Way Out?

"The Easy Way Out?" is a two-part filmstrip/tape presentation which addresses problems and situations of young people that often lead to drug abuse. The presentation follows several weeks of a young boy's life and the typical problems he encounters. At the end, he is given an opportunity to abuse drugs. The students then discuss the choice they think he will make and write their own ending to the story.

At the end the teacher uses discussion questions to encourage students to voice their own opinions about the problem of drug abuse. The aim of the unit is to help students make decisions on drug use.

Over 800 eighth grade students were tested before and after exposure to "The Easy Way Out?" program. Each student was asked to agree or disagree with a series of 38 declarative statements. Basically, the instrument was designed to assess the students' opinions on various drug facts and issues.

The results showed two definite trends. First, students seemed to learn certain legal facts from this unit of instruction. For instance, in response to the statement "I can be arrested while at a pot party even if I am not smoking marijuana," 65.2% of the students agreed with the statement on the pretest, while 79.5% agreed on the posttest. Similarly, in response to the statement "If I am arrested for possession of marijuana, the amount I have will determine the penalty," 48.7% on the pretest agreed as compared to 70.3% on the posttest.

A second trend seemed to emerge which was most alarming—a tendency toward less trust, especially toward parents. In response to the statement "I would tell my parents if my brother or sister were smoking marijuana," 42.5% agreed on the pretest, while only 36.1% agreed on the posttest. Similarly, "talking to my parents about a serious problem helps me," was agreed to by 57.2% on the pretest, but only 48.2% on the posttest.

It appeared that peer pressure may not have been effectively presented in the program. In response to the statement "I can say no if my friends offer me a marijuana cigarette," 82.7% agreed on the pretest as compared to 77.5% on the posttest.

In spite of the unfavorable results obtained from the student testing, the teacher evaluations of the program were rather favorable overall. However, half of the teachers did feel, as shown in table 1, that the program was not interesting to the students. One third of the evaluating teachers disagreed that the program would "stir the students to act favorably in the areas covered." The results of the student testing phase would tend to corroborate those teachers' impressions. Certainly this program needs to be reviewed carefully before it is used again.

Summary

This school based health education project has now entered the second year of the implementation phase. Several innovative programs have been started and were evaluated in their first year. Although most of the programs showed a great deal of promise, some revision will be needed for each teaching unit. In addition to providing valuable insight for purposive program revision, the student testing phase of the project has provided baseline data for future reference and comparison.

Since any innovative program needs enthusiastic and dedicated professionals to implement them, teacher evaluation was deemed essential to this project. When given the opportunity, the teachers working with these programs were quite helpful in their evaluations. Although all programs were reasonably well received, the criticisms made by the teachers seemed to be corroborated by the evaluative data from the student testing phase.

As with any viable curriculum project, innovation must be followed by evaluation, then by appropriate revision. This project will begin innovation at the secondary level as it begins revision at the elementary and middle school level. We believe that sound and effective programs will be developed which can be used successfully in this school district, as well as others with similar characteristics and needs. For additional information and/or a copy of the complete implementation guide, write to: Charles J. Baer, Project Director, 100 West Lincoln Drive, Kokomo-Center Township Schools, Kokomo, Indiana 46901.

A Story as Health Education

PEGGY J. THOMAS is associate professor in the Health and Education Department, Southwest Missouri State University, 901 South National, Springfield, Missouri 65802.

One way to teach health concepts is through creative writing. The following story originated out of a health class required for those teachers going into elementary education at Southwest Missouri State University, Springfield, Missouri. The story was a way to teach boys and girls about some important bones in the body. A large poster of a scarecrow was placed in front of the room. As the story was read, the boneless scarecrow began to acquire a set of bones. As each bone was mentioned in the story, a name card identifying the bone was placed at the proper location on the scarecrow. The story was entertaining, thought provoking, and motivating.

How the Scarecrow Got His Bones

by Rebecca R. Spencer

Long, long ago there lived a scarecrow who wanted to be a person more than anything else in the world. Every day, as he hung by his limp, lifeless arms on the stick in the garden, he'd dream and wish and dream some more of being a person. Now any other scarecrow might dream of being able to talk or whistle or even sing, but this scarecrow was very ambitious. He not only wanted to do all those things, but he wanted to be able to walk and run about the garden as well. All his dreams and wishes were in vain, however, because we all know that scarecrows can't walk and run, and we all know that the reason they can't walk and run is because they have no bones to make their legs straight and tall. But the scarecrow had no idea how important bones were, so he never bothered to wish for any.

Then one sunny afternoon when the scarecrow was just about convinced that he'd never be able to walk and run, a big brown rabbit came hopping through the garden. He had been nibbling some lettuce two rows over and some carrots three rows over, and now he hopped right up to the scarecrow and looked him right in the eye. The scarecrow would have given his right arm to be able to stomp his foot and chase the rabbit out of the garden, but he was forced to hang by his limp, lifeless arms on the stick and wish until he was blue in the face. The rabbit noticed that the scarecrow's face was turning a beautiful bright blue, and since rabbits are naturally more intelligent than scarecrows, he said, "Sir, may I ask

what is wrong with your face?" Of course the scarecrow couldn't answer, and the rabbit misunderstood his silence for rudeness. He said, just a little louder, "Sir, may I ask what is wrong with your face?" But the scarecrow just hung by his limp, lifeless arms on the stick, wishing he could stomp his foot and chase the rabbit away. "Sir, I'm sure that you can hear me," said the rabbit even louder than before, "for you're looking right at me. Will you at least nod your head to show that you understand?" But the scarecrow, having no bones, couldn't even do that.

Now it was widely known throughout the land, to everyone but the scarecrow, that this particular big brown rabbit possessed wonderful magical powers. But it was also known, to practically everyone except the scarecrow, that the rabbit only used his magic when he became angry. And he was quickly becoming very angry at the scarecrow.

"Sir, in repayment for your rudeness," screamed the rabbit, for he was fairly trembling with rage by now, "I fear I am forced to cast a terrible spell on you." Now the day before, the rabbit had accidentally happened upon a very large book among the old clothes and toys which were to be thrown away by the family who owned the garden. As he thumbed through the pages, he noticed several strange new words that he couldn't quite figure out. They were nice words, however, and so the rabbit made a point to remember them. And they came to mind now as very nice words for a spell.

"Nibbity Nobbity Null—now you have a Skull!" cried the rabbit as he looked toward the sky and hopped three times around an imaginary circle. No sooner had the rabbit uttered these words than the scarecrow felt a strange sensation that covered his whole head. He wanted so badly to reach up and feel his head to see what had happened, but his limp, lifeless arms wouldn't move.

Next the rabbit shouted, "Veeney, Viney Vernum—I'll give you a Sternum!" And just as he said this, the scarecrow felt his chest become straight and firm. "What's going on here?" he thought to himself, "What is this rabbit doing to me?" But even as he was thinking this the rabbit hopped again around his circle crying, "Movicle, Mivicle, Mavicle—give this scarecrow a Clavicle!" This time the scarecrow felt his shoulders become broad and strong. Confused by these strange happenings, the scarecrow began to wish even harder that he could stomp his foot and chase this silly rabbit away. But since he couldn't, he simply hung on his stick.

Now the rabbit chanted, "Bumerus, Fumerus, Klumerus—now you'll have a Humerus." At this the scarecrow's upper arms were filled with strength and power. And now he could raise one shoulder higher

than the other, or both shoulders at the same time. The scarecrow began to be less frightened and more curious as to what was going on. He wanted the rabbit to cast another spell quickly. "Fulna, Fadius, Pulna and Padius—give him now the Ulna and Radius." With these words the scarecrow lifted his hands and touched his head. "This is wonderful," he thought. "More, more!" And once again the rabbit hopped three times in a circle, then chanting, "Fippity, Foppity, Fine, now you have a spine," and "Hippety, Hoppety Hibs—don't leave out the Ribs." Now the whole top half of the scarecrow's body was straight and tall and he could move his head and arms all about. He was so excited he wanted to shout! He clapped his hands and smiled, hoping the rabbit wouldn't stop now. But the rabbit was still angry and was paying no attention whatsoever to the scarecrow. He just kept hopping in circles and thinking of new spells in which to use each one of the strange words. "Milvis, Malvis, Molvis, Melvis—let's give this silly fellow a Pelvis." And the scarecrow's hips and tummy were no longer stuffed with straw! "Lemur, Hemur, Bemur—now you have a Femur," cried the rabbit and just then the scarecrow's legs began to feel almost as though they could run and dance. "Zatella, Fatella, Matella—this fella needs a Patella," cried the rabbit, and the scarecrow bent his knees! "Oh, please don't stop now," thought the scarecrow. But he had no reason to worry. The rabbit still had three more words to use, and even though he was beginning to run low on magic spells, he was determined to use up all his strange new words. So with a burst of fresh energy the rabbit hopped and shouted "Fibula, Tibia and Phalanges—add these three words to our plan, please." And with that the scarecrow felt strength flow all the way down his legs and through his toes. He could even double up his fingers and make a fist! Quickly he jumped down off his stick in the garden and ran up and down every row. "I can run," he thought to himself, "I can walk and run! I must thank the rabbit for what he has done." But when the rabbit realized what his strange new words had done, he ran as fast as he could for home. The scarecrow started to follow him, but thought better of it. "I must protect my garden," he thought, and stomped his foot and waved his arms as three crows flew overhead. And protect the garden he did. In fact, he did such a good job that his was the best garden anywhere around.

Now, you may be thinking that the scarecrow didn't get all of his wish. "He's not really a person," you say, "because he can't talk." Well, now, that's a different story altogether, and if you'd like to hear that one, you'll just have to wait until the big brown rabbit finds another book.

Learning About Health Through Children's Literature

Motivating children in health involves finding the best approach for each particular student in his "culture." Since our country is made up of many groups, our presentations must be sensitive to the child's needs, understandings, and cultural background. Health is the most personal, dealing with the most intimate of matters (*my* eating habits, *my* physical weaknesses), thus requiring the most careful attention to motivation lest all be lost to rejection. With this in mind, let's investigate the potential of children's literature to effectively teach health.

Children demonstrate great interest in learning about children in other lands. Interest, as the prerequisite to effective learning, can be stimulated through children's literature. As children read about other countries many health concepts can be introduced. This is much more productive today than the "name the parts of the body" approach to health.

The third grade class of Franklin School, Kearny, New Jersey, under the guidance of their teacher, Joy Laubach, explored the possibilities of using literature about children of other lands in developing various concepts of nutrition.

They went to the school library and chose books concerning families in other countries. After several visits with planned reading periods and after leisurely reading with a view to discovering the kinds of foods grown and consumed in the

Mildred P. Nugaris is assistant professor of health sciences, Jersey City State College, Jersey City, New Jersey 07305. She is a registered nurse and has an M.A. from Columbia Teachers College with a major in health education and school nursing.

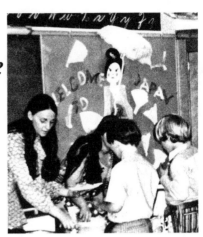

Children enjoy making their selection from various ethnic dishes. An international dinner offers children the opportunity for spontaneous discussion and social interaction about foods eaten in other lands.

country of their choice, the children met in groups to discuss their findings and to share their impressions on the value of these foods. They made notes of the foods consumed in other countries. Having little knowledge on the nutritive value of many of the foods in native diets they invited the school nurse to supplement their background. A discussion on the basic four food groups grew out of this. Then followed several learning activities, such as record keeping of their daily food menus; designing posters on food selections and nutritive values; and further reading to increase the children's basic understandings of simple nutritional concepts.

The children then reviewed the food diets of the country they had chosen, to identify the nutrients that the foods contained and discover any lack of nutrients in that particular diet. They understood that the selection of food and eating patterns is determined by cultural factors and also that the choice of foods determine nutritional balance. Their interest flowed into other concepts, such as the effect of food upon growth in general and in relation to individual members of specific countries.

An international dinner was the culminating activity held in the classroom with invitations to other third graders. The hosts were in native dress to welcome the guests.

In using children's literature, the teacher must help select the particular concepts that apply to the level of the learner. When selecting children's literature for use in this way, the teacher must also be concerned with the scientific accuracy of the information. By using R. R. Bowker's *Best Books for Children* (current edition) as a guide to selection, the chance of error is lessened. The UNICEF Library in New York City has many books on all cultures, and one of its purposes is to help teachers use these resources in various ways.

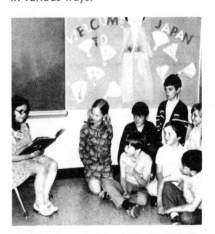

Children are interested in learning about "children in other lands." Oral reading offers the opportunity for practice of verbal expression, and individual contributions to the class. Use it to introduce new health education concepts.

Breaking the Language Barrier

TIMOTHY GLAROS is a physical education and health teacher at Highview Junior High School in the Mounds View School District, 1448 Indian Oaks Trail, Arden Hills, Minnesota 55112.

During our professional preparation we became accustomed to the jargon of our various disciplines. It becomes a part of our working vocabulary. The difficult multisyllabic terms used in anatomy, physiology, and health science become single words that we recognize and understand at a glance. To students who read at the 7th to 9th grade level or lower, however, these health topics make very difficult reading. We should help them understand the language we are speaking and asking them to read, for without this understanding, communication and learning become impossible.

For students to learn the concepts involved in health topics related to the human body, they need not be able to spell and define our jargon by rote. The ability to recognize and understand the basic meaning of these terms in written and spoken form *is* essential, however.

One approach is the use of etymology. Introduction to the many prefixes, suffixes, and roots that appear frequently will give students the tools necessary for putting together the definitions of many terms found in health education. This may be done cooperatively with the language arts department or may be introduced at the beginning of the appropriate health units by the health educator.

The following list may be helpful in providing the parts needed to assemble (or disassemble) the high powered terminology that is commonly found in health textbooks. It is not presented as a complete list, but as a fairly extensive model. Perhaps through this etymological approach we can both facilitate success in health education and contribute to the reading ability of our students.

ab-	*away from*
ad-	*toward*
-algia -algic	*pain*
anti-	*against*
arthr- arthro-	*joint*
arteri- arterio-	*arteries*
-ase	*enzyme*
aud- audio-	*hearing*
aur- auri-	*ear*
bi-	*two*
bio-	*life*
brevis	*short*
carcin- carcino-	*tumor, cancer*
cardi- cardio-	*heart*
-cep -ceps ceph	*head*
chol- chole- cholo-	*bile, gall*
costa costae	*ribs*
cyst- cysti- cysto- -cyst	*bladder, sac*
cyt- -cyte cyto-	*cell*
dent- denti- dento	*tooth, teeth*
derm- derma- dermo- -derm	*skin*
dors, dorsi, dorso,	*back*
duo- di-	*two*
ecto-	*outside*
-ectomy	*surgical removal*
-emia -aemia -hemia	*blood*
endo-	*inside*
gen- geno- gene- -gen -gene	*producer, origin, formation*
-gram	*picture, record*
hemi-	*half*
hemo- hema- hem-	*blood*
hepa- hepar- hepato-	*liver*
hydro- hydr- hydri-	*water*
hyper-	*above, beyond, super, excessive*
hypo-	*under, beneath, less than, lower*
hyster- hystero-	*womb, uterus*
-ia	*pathological condition*
infra-	*beneath*
inter-	*between*
intera-	*within*
iso-	*same*
-itis	*inflammation*
lact- lacti- lacto-	*milk*
lat-	*side*
-logy	*science of*
longus	*long*
medi- medio- medius	*middle*
mono-	*single*
myo- mya- my-	*muscle*
nas- nasi- nasa-	*nose*
nephr- nephro-	*kidneys*

nerv- nervi- nervo-	*nerves*
neur- neuro-	*nerves*
ocul- oculo	*eye*
-oid -oids	*having the form of*
-onomy	*study of*
os- oss- ost- oste- osteo-	*bone*
-ose	*carbohydrate*
-osis	*abnormal or diseased condition, increase or formation*
ophthalm- ophthalmo-	*eye or eyeball*
-otomy	*partial removal by surgery*
ov- ovi- ovo- ovu-	*egg*
ox- oxo-	*oxygen*
para-	*beside, along side*
ped- pede- pedi-	*foot*
peri-	*around, near, enclosing, surrounding*
pil- pilo- pili	*hair*
plexus	*network*
poly-	*many*
post-	*after*
pre-	*before*
pulmo-	*lung*
semi-	*half*
soma-	*body*
sub-	*under*
super- supra-	*above*
therm- thermo-	*heat, temperature*
-tomy	*incision, section, to cut*
trans-	*across*
tri-	*three*
-trophy	*related to nutrition*
-tropic	*attracted to*
uni-	*one*
vas- vaso-	*vessel*
vastus vasta vastum	*extensive, large*
ven- veni- veno-	*vein*
Reference:	*Taber's Cyclopedic Medical Dictionary*

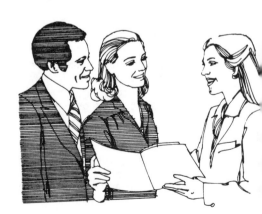

School Health Bee

Bernard S. Krasnow is assistant principal and supervisor of health education at Arturo Toscanini Junior High School in Bronx, New York.

Health education took a dramatic turn last year at Toscanini Junior High School in Bronx, New York. Our school inaugurated its first annual health bee in order to stimulate greater participation and interest in health education and in current health topics.

The project was created out of a desire to change the traditional assembly program so that an atmosphere of excitement would pervade the audience. The health education department held a conference devoted to this idea and it was decided to promote a school-wide health knowledge quiz. This would culminate in a series of grade auditorium programs designed to duplicate the fun and excitement of television quiz programs.

The school's health instructor, Mr. Pluchik, was designated as the teacher-in-charge for the project. He constructed a health knowledge test from our own curriculum which was administered to all the students during their health or science periods. The students who scored highest on this initial survey test were invited to a class winners' run-off. Fifty-five class winners appeared for the run-off test which was held after school. Those with five highest scores in each grade were then designated as finalists and invited to participate in the auditorium quiz programs the following week. They were given extra resources in the form of textbooks, pamphlets, etc., to study from in preparation for the contest.

The auditorium program was modeled after a television panel quiz program. The industrial arts department constructed an electrical response board so that a contestant who knew the answer

was able to press a button to make a light flash in front of him. Mr. Pluchik served as moderator and asked the questions. Three other teachers acted as judges. The questions for the final quiz were selected from among those in the initial survey and the run-off examinations.

There was great anticipation on the part of the contestants and the student body. Publicity had been extensive through public address messages, posters, and class announcements so that most of the students were eagerly awaiting the program. The contests were well received by the audience and seldom has there been more audience enthusiasm. The excitement was, in fact, so great that many times the audience inadvertently shouted out the answer. (We did, in fact, throw the questions to the audience if they were not answered correctly by the contestants.) The scoring was conducted by awarding one point for each question answered correctly. Each contestant had his own personal scoreboard that reflected his current total. This kept the audience posted on the current scores.

Each auditorium program was concluded by awarding a trophy to the health quiz winner of each grade, and the finalists received honor certificates. The school photographer was there to take pictures of all the winners and we plan to display these for publicity purposes.

Our original idea in initiating this project was to focus on health education and current health topics. We are sure that this school-wide program did just that. We are, however, promoting follow-up activities so that our initial efforts are long-lasting. Some of these activities include: establishing a health information reference center in our school library, publicizing the health quiz in the community, establishing a health award for graduation, and promoting health topics to be taught as part of the curriculum in other subjects.

We are also hoping that we can motivate other schools in our district (District 9) to conduct their own Health Bee and, perhaps, even a city-wide contest. We think that it is time to stimulate nationwide excitement for health education. Who knows, a National Health Education Bee may someday stand right alongside our National Spelling Bee.

Promoting Experiential Learning

MICHAEL HAMRICK is associate professor and head, Division of Health Science and Safety Education, Memphis State University and CAROLYN STONE is patient education coordinator, City of Memphis Hospital, 860 Madison Avenue, Memphis, Tennessee 38103.

Getting students involved in health education experiences outside the classroom—experiential learning—continues to be a pressing need in health education. The purpose of this article is to promote experiential learning in health education by providing a list of projects to encourage out-of-the-classroom learning. While this list was developed for use in the personal health course, similar lists can easily be developed and implemented in courses where it is important to broaden students' experiences and to facilitate awareness of attitudes, behaviors, and lifestyles that are difficult to accomplish in the classroom.

These projects are designed for the student, not the teacher. Therefore, we suggest that the list be duplicated and distributed to students. These projects should be structured into course requirements so that points or some kind of credit can be earned. Since the projects vary in the amount of time, effort, and involvement required, possible points/credits should also vary. Some projects require several months to finish while others may be completed in a 30 minute interview. Students should be encouraged to pursue areas of personal interest and to take advantage of their talents. Some projects require skill in journalism, photography, movie production, art, research, etc. Students should be encouraged to select only those projects which offer a new experience for them. Finally, guidelines should be developed which specify how and when projects are to be reported.

Experiential Learning Projects

1. Do a film. Compile either an 8mm film or 35mm slides focusing on some topic. This display can be incorporated into a multimedia presentation using audio-tape or any other appropriate media. For example, you might produce a tape-slide show on eating habits of college students, study habits, recreational habits, dating habits, marriage from the woman's point of view, people trying to make conversation, children's ideas about death, etc.

2. Prepare an audio-tape collage. Tape many songs, poems, readings or sounds around a particular theme. The theme might be aging, drugs, self-identity, or sexuality.

3. Select one of the health habits/behaviors that you are concerned about and would like to work on. Develop a plan of action which focuses on the desired behavioral change. Use a behavioral modification plan as described in class. Keep a log on the success/failure of the plan. Follow up with an analysis of the plan and the behavior and what you learned.

4. Pair up with someone else to form a health "therapy" dyad. The purpose of the partnership is to have someone with whom the health habit/behavior can be discussed. Meet with your partner several hours a week. See if you can develop a plan for achieving desired behavioral change. Keep a log of your meetings. Use your partner both as a sounding board and as a monitor to keep you honest.

5. During the semester, keep a log of the behaviors/habits you change or modify. Examine the circumstances of the changes. Can you identify a pattern to the changes made? What did you learn? Report results.

6. Keep a journal. Record reactions to occurrences related to some topic or activity. The journal could chronicle a physical fitness regime or dietary pattern or an encounter group experience running throughout the semester.

7. Prepare and implement a research proposal. Some of you may have ideas for experiments such as the effects of various quantities of alcoholic beverages on reaction time, food tasting experiment, survey of attitudes.

8. Conduct a health demonstration. Some topics may lend themselves to a demonstration—the effects of smoking on heart rate, blood pressure, body temperature or how a medical test such as EEG or EKG works and what it shows.

9. Go to the Health Department, Venereal Disease Clinic as if you were a client seeking help for V.D. You may use a false name if you prefer. Report what you learned. How were you treated? What did you observe in the waiting room, the treatment rooms? How did you feel? What changes would you suggest to make the experience less negative for those who need their services?

10. Interview a person or persons who smoke heavily (yourself if you fit the category). Get a profile on their smoking habits, when they smoke, for how long, how it affects them, why they think they smoke, comments of family and friends about the smoker. Have they ever quit? Why? Why did they resume smoking?

11. Go to a setting unfamiliar to your lifestyle and report your reactions, feelings, etc. Try a walk through an inner city neighborhood, attend church services of a different religious group, go to an adult movie or bookstore, a gay bar, or shop at a small country store.

12. Spend an evening in a local hospital's intensive care waiting room. Listen, observe. If you feel comfortable, talk with the families waiting. Record your reactions, what you learned medically as well as emotionally.

13. Spend a morning making rounds with a public health nurse, food sanitation inspector, rat control investigator, or environmentalist.

14. Go to a community health center and take a seat in line. Examine the attitudes of the staff who work there. Talk to some of the patients. Find out how adequate they think their health care is, what problems they have getting to see a doctor, etc.

15. Conduct a health campaign. Select a health topic and conduct an educational campaign such as anti-smoking, hypertension, sickle cell anemia, cervical cancer detection, population control, human relations.

16. Visit a health foods store and make a list of what you see. Interview personnel who work there about their philosophies on eating. Compare prices of similar foods in grocery stores or pharmacies.

17. Spend one weekend evening sitting in a public hospital's emergency room waiting area. The same evening, spend the same amount of time in a private hospital's E.R. Compare the two physical surroundings, personal attitudes of the staff, the patients you see, their families. How comfortable/uncomfortable would you be if you were a patient?

18. Write a letter to a newspaper or magazine about a current health-related issue that really gets your dander up. Turn in a carbon copy.

19. Visit a health spa. What practices seem valid? What claims are made which seem unrealistic, unhealthy, deceptive, evasive? What do you get for how much money?

20. Go to a free lecture on transcendental meditation. How do you think it works? What are the benefits claimed? What sort of impression did you get from the whole experience?

21. Talk with relatives who have planned a funeral. What were their impressions of the funeral business and the people who assisted them? What details must be attended to when planning a funeral? What legal problems did they run into?

22. Find out resources for contraceptive information. Make a list and include costs, if any, for the services and/or the contraceptive materials. List at least ten resources.

23. Go to the local Unemployment Offices. Sit in the waiting room and listen to the talk around you. Describe the place. Read the notices on the board. Describe any contact with the employees. Wear old clothes. As a variation two people can go together, one dressed in old clothes and one in really good clothes. Describe how individuals differed in their reactions to you.

24. Go to any of the pregnancy counseling resources and ask to have a free pregnancy test. Describe the place, the people, how they treated you. If you are male, you can carry in a urine sample saying it is for your girl friend.

25. On a given night watch TV programs during prime time hours and count the incidents which exploit sex, race, religion, minority groups, occupations, etc.

26. Look in the want ads for jobs which routinely hire only men or women. Call and inquire about the job if you are of the opposite sex. What attitudes did you perceive? Quote any remarks made about sex requirements for the job. Sex discrimination is now against the law in hiring practices. Variaton: Work with a person of the opposite sex Both call and inquire about the job and record the results.

27. Interview a relative or family friend who is retired. Find out how they spend their time, what they like about being retired, what they dislike. What attitudes about being considered "old" do you pick up on?

28. Arrange for the class to "interview" you about a life crisis you have experienced such as divorce, marriage, childbirth, etc. You do not have to answer any question you don't want to. State any limitations before the interview begins.

29. Read an article in a health journal which interests you. Write a two page typed review of the major points of the article. Include your opinion.

30. Survey 5 "lay" magazines (*McCalls, Ladies Home Journal,* etc.) and write a description of the ads which contradict good health practices. You might want to look at magazines such as *Cosmopolitan, Playboy, Oui,* which emphasize attractiveness and appeal. Include a synopsis of the ads' underlying messages.

31. Attend lecture of guest speakers invited to a local university to discuss their views of health related topics. Example: Life after Life lecture, rape prevention demonstration. Summarize the presentation.

32. Attend health education meetings, fairs, programs sponsored by various community agencies. Summarize presentation.

33. Send in health assessment from back of textbook. Summarize what you learned about your health status, risks and behaviors. Takes about 4–6 weeks to get it back.

34. Get a test for diabetes through the Health Department mobile unit, or get a Pap test. Bring the results to class with a written report of how it was done. Ask questions of the personnel as they perform the tests. Try to find out how many people are detected through this system.

35. Write a summary report on the relationship between personality, emotional state, and cancer (see *Psychology Today,* June 1976).

36. Using a very large map of your city, designate the distribution of doctors in the city. Which areas are heavily populated? Which have only a few? Which are undersupplied? You might want to use colored pins to designate different types of physicians. Do the same with dentists. Write your recommendations.

37. Bring an advertisement to class. List its claims. Analyze it for emotional appeal. Are its claims supported by facts? In what ways is the advertisement misleading? Deceiving?

38. From the list of health products investigated by *Consumer Reports* and published in *The Medicine Show,* select one and summarize the findings of *Consumer Reports.* Does the product render any medical or health benefit? What conditions, if any, must be met in its use? What brands are recommended by Consumer Union?

39. Refer to the magazine, *FDA Papers,* a monthly publication of the Food and Drug Administration and identify an example of quackery. What is the claim of the product? What does the FDA say about the product?

Some examples include Weight-away Belt (Feb. '72); LaVive Body Creme (Nov., '70); Paradise Grapefruit Diet (Aug., '71).

40. Tape a radio or TV commercial and bring to class. What kind of propaganda strategy was used? How is it misleading?

41. Conduct a demonstration to test commercial claims of a health product.

42. Write a company for verification of claims made in advertising. Turn in carbon copy of letter and indicate company's response.

43. Write a brief summary report on the published article on chiropractics (See *Consumer Reports,* Sept., Oct., 1975). Write a report on any other health related article included in the monthly publication of *Consumer Reports.*

44. Tell about the decisions a heart attack victim or cancer victim makes in going through treatment, surgery, rehabilitation. Comment on length of stay, financial aspects, steps in rehabilitation, changes in lifestyles, etc.

45. Write a summary report on an article published during the past calendar year on a disease. Compare the information with that in the text and comment on the differences.

46. Develop a skit or role playing situation illustrating some attitudinal or behavioral aspect of a disease. For example, simulate the typical reaction of a person observing a diabetic in insulin shock; the reaction of someone to the news that he or she has a chronic disease.

47. Write a position statement on some controversial aspect of various diseases and be prepared to read to class. The position does not necessarily have to be your own.
A. Epileptics should have limited driving privileges.
B. Medical science is going too far with heart transplants.
C. Government restrictions in the form of laws, penalties should be imposed on persons with genetically related diseases.
D. Marijuana should be legalized for use by glaucoma victims.
E. The government is restricting distribution of laetrile because of loss of profits and government grants in research.

48. Interview a person who by nature of his/her job observes death and dying (police officer, mortician, war veteran, physician, nurse).

49. Develop a skit or role playing situation illustrating some aspect of death. For example, how people act at a funeral home, a family making funeral arrangements.

50. Write a position statement on some controversial aspect of death and dying.
A. Too much money is spent on funerals.
B. Young children should be taken to funerals.
C. Being dead is more honorable than being invalid.
D. Burying bodies is a waste of good, productive land.
E. There is too much death in movies and on TV.

51. Visit an Alcoholics Anonymous meeting and report your experience.

52. Write one page position statement expressing an extreme point of view on alcohol. The position does not have to be your own. Read to class, time permitting.

53. Conduct a genetic experiment in class demonstrating dominant-recessive traits. For example, obtain small crystals of phenyl-thiocarbamide or PTC test papers. Conduct a taste experiment distinguishing between bitter tasters and non-tasters. What are the expected results?

54. Write a case history or biographical sketch on a person with a genetically related disease or condition. Describe the lifestyle of the person and how it differs from "normality." Describe the effects on the family.

55. Find out what kind of genetic services and counseling are available locally, the conditions for service, prerequisites, costs, location, etc. Report to class.

56. Take a copy of the state penal code from the library and extract the basic criminal statutes relating to sex offenses. Note particularly those describing such acts as rape, seduction, carnal abuse, cohabitation, adultery, indecent exposure, loitering, molesting, and vagrancy. Notice, too, laws relating to marriage, (consent, ceremony, verification) contraceptives, pregnancy, abortion, and venereal disease. Report to class.

57. Develop a skit or role playing situation on some aspect of sexuality or sexually related behavior.

58. Select two newspapers (only one from your city), observe and record for one week the newspapers' statistics on marriages, divorces, and annulment. Graph the results. Include in the graph a breakdown on grounds for divorce.

59. Construct a sample marriage contract for yourself with provisions for facets of marital life you consider particularly important. You may want to consider some of the more common features found in marriage contracts today.
A. division of assets held prior to marriage
B. division of income after marriage
C. to have or not have children
D. responsibilities of partners in child care
E. obligations and rights regarding separate careers

60. Conduct a survey on some aspect of sexuality. For example, married couples of different ages could be asked to answer the following questions.
A. What do you see as the purpose of marriage?
B. Who controls the finances in your family?
C. What effect has the women's movement had on marriage today?
D. What are your views on early marriage?

61. Write a story in the "true confession" style that deals with issues of reproduction, birth control, marriage, parenthood, sex roles, etc. The story may be discussed in class.

62. Write a position paper on one of the following statements.
A. A couple should be encouraged to choose the sex of their baby
B. A single person or gay couple should be allowed to raise a child.
C. Men should assume the responsibility of birth control
D. No one should have more than two children
E. Marriage contracts should become the form of marriage law
F. A couple with hereditary disease should not have children
F. Abortion on demand is a basic human right
H. Unlimited availability of contraceptives encourages promiscuity

63. Conduct an experiment/demonstration in class which focuses on the effects of air pollution, water pollution or noise pollution.

64. Draw a cartoon series which illustrates any health-related topic for example:
A. transmission of venereal disease
B. use of contraceptives
C. access to medical care/physician
D. medical terminology or technology
Design it to get a point across to college level students.

65. Demonstrate in class how to test for blood type; how to test for sugar in urine; pregnancy test; T.B. skin test; test for sickle cell anemia. Be sure you understand the whys and hows of what you are testing for and not just the procedure itself.

66. Interview several women who have experienced menopause. What were their attitudes about it before they experienced it? After they experienced it? What myths about menopause were true/untrue for them? How did it affect their families, their marital relationship? Was any medical treatment given? What were the attitudes of their physicians?

67. Attend a meeting of the LaLeche League, the organization that helps women breast-feed their children. Record what you saw, heard, learned.

68 Compare costs of 15 common prescription drugs among several local pharmacies. Include a chain-owned pharmacy, a small neighborhood one, and a hospital-owned pharmacy. Include the attitudes of those you questioned.

69. Compile a list of local psychiatrists. Call and ask for information on: fee scale, training, group or individual therapy, type of therapy (psychoanalysis, primal therapy, gestalt, electroshock, etc.), hospital affiliation.

70. Contact the local organization for wife abuse. What are their findings regarding wife abuse locally, their services, future plans?

71. Interview someone who lives in what would be considered an alternative lifestyle: communal setting, couple who chooses not to have children, unmarried couple living together, homosexual couple living together. Question each person involved.

72. Collect drawings/paintings from young, preschool children depicting their impressions of sexuality. *Check with parents first!* These could include their concept of anatomy, birth, sex roles, etc. Show these to class with your observations and comments made by children. If you have small children you may use their artwork.

73. Write a report on some new medical "gadget," such as mammography, CAT scanners, fetal monitoring. Include any criticism the technique has received as well as its benefits.

74. Interview a couple who has experienced "natural childbirth" (the Lamaze method).

75. Write a self-help guide to common vaginal infections. Include symptoms, treatment, preventive measures, if any. Alternative topic: insomnia, urinary tract infections.

76. Give blood at one of the hospital blood banks. Bring proof of the donation. Include written report of how community blood donation plan works.

77. Visit a Weight Watchers meeting. Record your experiences along with a description of their program. Include a description of "case histories" you might overhear or learn about. How does their plan work?

78. Write an analysis of migraine headaches: what causes them, what happens when they occur, treatment, new ideas of therapy.

79. Interview an acupuncturist or an osteopath. Thoroughly document their training programs and the usefulness of their skills.

80. Put together a first aid kit designed for a specific purpose (camping, boat, workroom, etc.). Bring to class and explain whys of the contents you chose.

81. Find out and record 20 people's views on raising the mandatory retirement age to 70. Choose a mixture of ages for your subjects.

82. Design a sensitivity exercise to help a group such as a new class break down initial barriers of discomfort. The aims should be to decrease tension about being in a new, strange group and increasing knowledge about each other. Include factors such as: time needed, materials needed, goals, facilitators' roles and responsibilities.

83. Collect at least five health pamphlets from community sources and critique them as to their usefulness, their appeal. Redesign them to make them more "zingy," more appealing.

84. Review filmstrip/tape on one of three consumer products (shampoo, acne treatments, aspirin) and write a critique of it. Include at least five ads for the product which make misleading statements.

85. Take the results of the health knowledge pretest which was administered in class and complete a profile sheet and validation exercise. (See Hamrick, Michael. *Health Education,* Nov.-Dec. 1978, pp. 32-34 for complete instructions).

86. Preview health related films available at local libraries and community agencies. Write a summary report.

87. If none of these projects grab you, think of another. Write a plan of action and turn in for approval. Points will be given after reading project description.

Stress on Reading

ELAINE HALS is a teacher of health education at South Shore High School, Brooklyn, New York 11236.

In the last few years large cities throughout the United States have begun to put pressure on school districts to stress the "three R's"—more reading, more math, and more writing. In New York City, where I teach, all of the principals have been instructed to increase the number of periods per week devoted to reading and other basics in the elementary schools. The high schools have been instructed that all subject areas give reading and written homework several times weekly, and that course curriculum should stress the basics. Employers have also been pressuring the schools to improve the reading ability of their graduates. The push is now on to raise the basic skills level of today's youth.

How does this push for basics affect us as health educators? Do we regress to predominantly cognitive teaching? Do we return to stressing facts, and only those things that can be read, written, and tested? About ten years ago health educators began to realize the importance of humanistic values and behavior modification that could be accomplished in health teaching. Our field has seen positive changes, and we have shifted our emphasis into the affective domain. Health education has truly become learning for living—examination of values, decision making, and behavioral alternatives. If we help young people become better, healthier, and more aware, but do not help them to read better, are we in line with the educational goals of the country? Should we be? The pendulum has swung back to pre-1960s education. Should we as health educators re-evaluate our goals, and fall in line with other subject areas? Reading and writing are important; I do not mean to demean their significance. Young people entering the job market must have basic skills in order to survive.

Because both affective and cognitive education are valuable, I feel that we as health educators must combine them in our teaching. Following you will find a few suggestions.

1. Help students to explore new and controversial health issues by having them read and evaluate current newspaper and magazine articles on various subjects—laetrile, cloning, test tube babies, food additives, new drugs, disease cures.

2. Have students keep a written log (to be checked by the teacher periodically) of feelings about the class, their daily decisions, new material learned, or anything the teacher feels is relevant to the class and the students.

3. Have students keep their own vocabulary list of new words learned in class or from text, pamphlets or other reading sources.

4. Have students write letters requesting information, pamphlets, interviews.

5. Offer reading lists of novels, magazines, etc. for outside projects or just additional information.

6. Give students controversial problems for homework and have them write answers that can later be discussed in class and even made into role playing situations.

> Your parents catch you and your friends smoking grass in your room, what would you do?
>
> You are caught cheating on an exam and the teacher wants to see your parents.
>
> You find that you have venereal disease—your boy or girl friend may have it, too—what do you do?
>
> Do the terminally ill have the right to know they are dying?
>
> You know something that could get your best friend in trouble. You feel what this person did was wrong. You are going to be questioned about the situation. What will you do?

7. Use pamphlets and current publications instead of, or in addition to, text books.

8. Divide class into groups. Have each group research and investigate different aspects of a subject and teach the class.

9. Creative projects that combine reading and writing with other disciplines such as art, photography, music.

10. Have class construct interviews or surveys, then have students survey or interview selected individuals and evaluate results.

Cognitive and affective can be made to work well together. We do not have to forsake our humanistic, affective approach to health education in order to help our students read and write better. Instead of changing the educational goals we have for our students, we should just add one more—a better knowledge of the basics and how they can help our students live better, healthier lives.

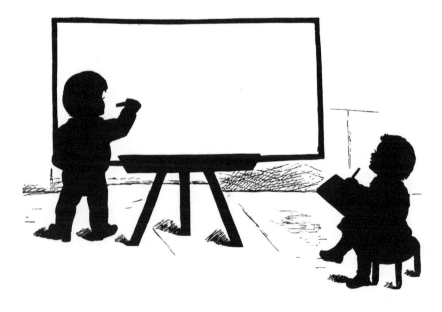

Well-Read and Healthy

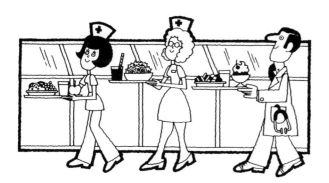

In addition to journalistic exposes of the political chicanery and campaign sordidness of the Watergate Affair, quotes from notables on the current energy crises, photojournalism of royal weddings, and football scores, the press also (believe-it-or-not) spends some time writing on other important, relevant, and worldly issues that confront the general readership—including health education instructors.

With all due respect to the few excellent contemporary American newspapers—like *The Boston Globe, The Washington Post, The St. Louis Post-Dispatch,* and *The Los Angeles Times*—*The New York Times* represents the ne plus ultra in journalism. In his book, *The Making of the President 1972,* Theodore H. White said, "The *Times* is the hometown newspaper of all men of government, all men of great affairs, all men and women who try to think. In the sociology of information it is assumed that any telephone call made between nine and noon anywhere in the executive belt between Boston and Washington is made between two parties both of whom have already read *The New York Times* and are speaking from the same shared body of information. Whether in finance, music, clothing industry, advertising, drama, business or politics, it is accepted that what is important to know has been printed that morning by *The New York Times.*"[1] And that is true in the area of health as well.

JOHN P. ALLEGRANTE is an undergraduate health education major at the State University of New York College, Cortland, New York 13045.

The New York Times has throughout the years published articles of interest, news, and journalistic abstracts of the latest research relating to health. This writer recently conducted a literature review of health related reportage that has appeared in the pages of the *Times* for six months and found the *Times* to be an accurate, concise, and thus, an invaluable and indispensable source of information for the health education instructor.

If one simply picks up almost any daily issue of the *Times,* he will first want to notice that the *Times* is usually indexed for a "Health and Science" article for that particular day. For example:

—Lawrence K. Altman, who is a physician and a member of *The New York Times* staff, writes extensively covering health subjects that would be of interest to all professionally-concerned health education instructors. Altman has written of the effectiveness of health and medical care in Sweden in a three-part series, and recently was still studying the Swedish medical care system as a visiting physician.[2]

—In the area of nutrition and consumer education with respect to the nutritional value of various foods, *Times* columnist Jane E. Brody, in a six-month period has written a three-part series treating the controversial nutritional issues confronting the Food and Drug Administration and nutritionists, the nutritional efficacy of organically grown foods, and fat and vitamins in the diet.[3] She has discussed eggs, cholesterol, and the two in relation to a heart disease risk factor,[4] and reported the recent research findings showing that American women are concerned enough about breast cancer that 1 in 5 women conduct self-administered breast cancer examinations.[5]

—Periodically, articles have appeared in the *Times* that have dealt with alcohol,[6] drugs,[7] and smoking.[8] Physician malpractice,[9] poor infant mortality statistical indices,[10] and the Nixon administration's record on federal health spending[11] have all been documented at one time or another in varying degrees of bias and objectivity by the *Times.*

What does this mean to the health educator? It is a good reason for reading a newspaper like *The New York Times* daily. This is not to suggest that reading the *Times* daily should be substituted for periodic perusal of the scholarly, professional literature. However, in a time when teaching methodology, material resources, and classroom teaching philosophies are often being contested, the well-read instructor—one who is staying abreast of the current events in all aspects of the health scene and is keeping his students similarly informed—is going to be the better instructor. *The New York Times* is an excellent resource material with which the instructor can enhance the health education curriculum for students as well as for himself.

Perspectives in health are changing constantly, so fast, in fact, that textbooks are outdated before they go to press. Monthly journals publish what is new in the field a month after the news happens. A newspaper is, by its nature, the best way in which to know "what's happening" day-to-day.

No other news media commands the unprecedented lines of communication as does the *Times*—direct lines of correspondence that lead to the Department of Health, Education, and Welfare, the National Institutes of Health, the Center For Disease Control, the U.S. Public Health Service, the colleges and universities, and other health and education related agencies—all of which provide the newest health and medical break-throughs and the latest in educational research. Aspects of the secondary health education curriculum like environmental health, first aid and safety, health economics, mental health, nutrition, and sex education invariably surface in the *Times* as part of "All the News That's Fit to Print." That it would behoove the instructor to be well informed in these subject areas if he is to be an effective, competent health educator cannot be stressed enough by this writer.

We must begin somewhere in the never ending effort to improve our scope of knowledge in our chosen profession of health education. So let us begin by taking the time to become well-read individuals of resources like *The New York Times*, lest health educators risk an abysmal reputation as a group of dilettantes, if not Philistines.

[1] Theodore H. White, *The Making of the President 1972*, (New York: Bantam Books, 1973), p. 346. See Chapter 10 for an excellent insight into the power of *The New York Times* and the press media at large in contemporary America.

[2] Lawrence K. Altman, "Swedish Medicine Is Troubled," *The New York Times*, December 23, 1973, p. 1.

[3] Jane E. Brody, "Nutrition Is Now a National Controversy," *The New York Times*, August 27, 1973, p. 1; "Organically Grown Foods: Some Fall Short in Nutrition," *The New York Times*, August 28, 1973, p. 30; "Nutrition: Fats and Vitamins in the Body's Chemistry," *The New York Times*, August 29, 1973, p. 42.

[4] Jane E. Brody, "The Egg Falls Victim to Cholesterol Fears, Industry Ads Defend It," *The New York Times*, November 29, 1973, p. 45.

[5] Jane E. Brody, "Study Finds One in Five Women Check to Detect Breast Cancer," *The New York Times*, November 9, 1973, p. 9.

[6] Lawrence K. Altman, "Alcohol Is Produced in Human Intestine, British Scientist Finds," *The New York Times*, July 16, 1973, p. 11.

[7] M. A. Farber, "Opinion Remains Divided Over Effect of State's New Drug Law," *The New York Times*, August 31, 1973, p. 16.

[8] John D. Morris, "Smoker Rule on Planes in Effect Today," *The New York Times*, July 10, 1973, p. 8; Gerald Gold, "Cigarettes: Why Not a Total Ban?," *The New York Times*, August 26, 1973, The Week In Review, p. 7; "Despite the Warnings, Millions Can't, or Won't Give Up Smoking," *The New York Times*, November 5, 1973, p. 45.

[9] "Doctor and Hospital Are Fined $3-Million for Needless Surgery," *The New York Times*, November 28, 1973, p. 24.

[10] Harold M. Schmeck, Jr., "Infant Deaths Tied to Poor Health Care," *The New York Times*, July 8, 1973, p. 30.

[11] Nancy Hicks, "Economist Scores U.S. Health Budget," *The New York Times*, November 7, 1973, p. 22.

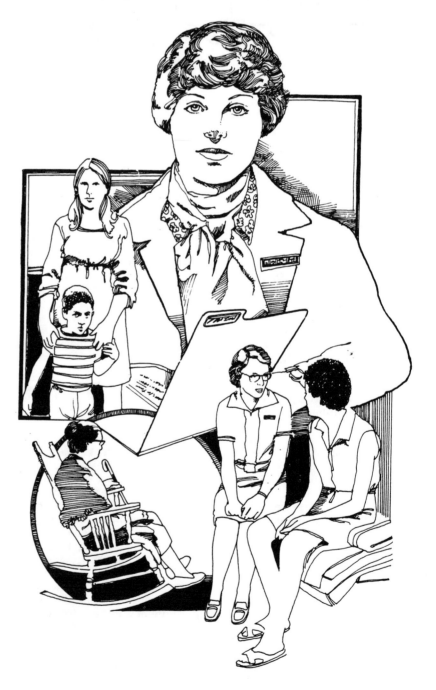

The Health Education Carnival

Giving the Old Health Fair a Facelift

In recent years "health fairs" have become quite popular. Most commonly they are offered as a community service or are held within a school setting. Although health fairs can be organized in many different ways, most of them consist of health education activities combined with various health screening tests.

This paper presents a new approach to the organization and supervision of health fairs. We refer to that new approach as the "Health Education Carnival." In numerous ways it resembles the traditional health fair and uses many of the same kinds of health education methods and materials. However, there are several important differences. First, the health education carnival does not include any health screening tests. Instead it consists exclusively of health education activities in a festive, carnival-like atmosphere. Secondly, although physicians, nurses, dentists and allied health professionals are sometimes used as resources at the carnival, they do not wear their customary "uniforms." Instead they come dressed in costumes similar to those worn by the activity facilitators.

Incidentally, all facilitators are encouraged to create costumes which are as bright and colorful as possible to add to the gala environment. In addition, costumes related directly to the facilitator's experiential learning area, that can also be used in teaching health concepts, are especially encouraged.

Whereas the traditional health fair has been around for a long time, the health education carnival appears new and different to elementary school students, their parents, and even health professionals within the community. This is

Parris R. Watts is an assistant professor of health and physical education at the University of Missouri, Columbia, MO 65201. William J. Stinson is the elementary school health and physical education specialist at Emporia State University, Emporia, KS 66801.

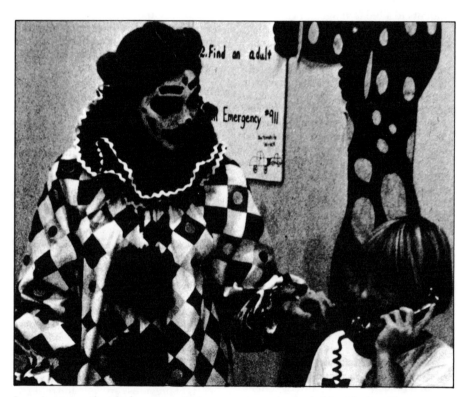

Learning to use the telephone correctly in an emergency is a typical health education carnival activity. Photo courtesy of Parris R. Watts.

seen in the excellent attendance of teachers and parents as well as in their reactions during and after the events.

Teachers and parents have often commented that the carnivals are more structured and health concept-oriented than health fairs that their students and children had previously attended. This is undoubtedly the result of the efforts of the carnival facilitators to assure high educational quality by designing each activity area to meet participants' needs, interests and comprehensive abilities.

Also, teachers and parents have expressed appreciation for the extremely personalized instruction offered at the health education carnival. In developing the carnival activity areas, great care has been taken to provide a one-on-one health education experience in each cen-

ter. Such a personalized learning opportunity is often lacking at health fairs where more emphasis is placed on screening and testing than on health education.

Community health personnel often react negatively to health fairs because of the inclusion of various health "screening tests." Unlike health fairs, the carnivals include neither multiphasic testing nor certain common fragmentary physical examinations. As a result, health service professionals in the community have not expressed the concerns about health education carnivals that we have heard regarding health fairs.

A health education carnival differs from a health fair in that it promotes a greater awareness of and appreciation for health education. This can motivate children to learn more about their health. Teachers have noted more interest in health education subject matter among students who have attended a health education carnival.

A distinctive feature of the health education carnival is its great use of "learning games." The fun-oriented health games are popular with children and certainly accentuate the fact that health education can be an enjoyable experience. The games, which expose the students to a broad range of health education concepts, give the young participants the feeling of being at a carnival.

Many health fairs are "scattered" throughout the facility in which they are held. Our health education carnivals have always been restricted to one location, most often a gymnasium. This has helped tremendously in moving participants through the different experiential learning areas. We have found that this works best when children (and accompanying parents) are clustered in groups of eight to ten people and rotated through all the activity areas. This helps assure that all participants experience every part of the carnival and enables facilitators to plan and teach their material within a predetermined amount of time.

Evolution of the Health Education Carnival

We were initially motivated to plan a health fair in order to expose undergraduate, elementary education majors to the "natural" learning patterns of children outside of a formalized student teaching assignment.

During the next two years, four health fairs emphasizing informal learning experiences and including a few health screening tests were held in selected Emporia, Kansas elementary schools. Each experiential area was developed and facilitated by five or six students at Emporia State University enrolled in courses in health education in the elementary school and physical education for the elementary teacher.

The objectives of the health fairs were the promotion of: (a) personal interaction between the facilitators and children; (b) meaningful health education experiences for the children; (c) cooperative involvement among the facilitators as they planned and implemented the activities; and (d) positive public relations within the university and throughout the community. The first four health fairs (which enjoyed outstanding coverage by the local newspaper and educa-

tional television station) clearly demonstrated that the expected outcomes could be achieved.

During the next two years, a metamorphosis began from the health fair format to the health education carnival. The first true health education carnival was part of the annual convention of the Kansas Association of Health, Physical Education, Recreation and Dance. We realized that the event would have to appear exciting if the elementary students invited from selected Topeka schools were to convince their parents to bring them. Thus, more emphasis was placed on publicity and parental interest and involvement was high.

Organizing a Health Education Carnival

Having coordinated several health education carnivals, we believe we have developed an efficient and effective planning and implementation format. Once a date and location are established, introduce the concept of the carnival to students at the beginning of the semester to enable them to plan to take part.

The introduction to the carnival includes 35 mm slides and video-taped highlights of previous carnivals. The students are then given a list of planned activity areas and they select ones within which they would like to work. Drawing ideas from books such as *Teaching Elementary Health Science*,[6] *Elementary School Health Education: Ecological Perspectives*,[7] *Health in Elementary Schools*,[8] and *Health Education Guide: A Design For Teaching*[9] as well as from summary reports of previous carnivals and other materials, the students begin to develop their experiential activity areas. They determine the area's theme and coordinate all activities to relate to the theme and to other activities. They make decisions about booth design, decorations, and costumes. The lead time we now use to prepare for a carnival is four weeks. That is one-half the time allowed for the first one, but we strongly recommend that two months be allocated for preparation of an initial health education carnival.

Learning Areas

The following experiential learning areas are the most commonly included.

Anatomy and Physiology—human skeleton and torso models, body organ specimens and models, as well as x-rays. For example, a human torso model's organs were taken out one at a time and each of their functions was described. Then the children were asked to help put

the organs back in their proper places. Also, actual body organ specimens were shown for comparative purposes.

Five Body Senses—sensory modality areas represented by facilitators costumed as "Susie Senses and Her Five Children." A "grab bag" of objects enabled the child to reach in and identify objects by touch. An eye-dropper was used to drop a salty, sweet, bitter or sour solution onto each child's tongue. Vision education concepts were presented using a telebinocular device.

Growth and Development—height, weight, and foot measurements, and hand steadiness experiences. Life-sized cut-outs of children representing average heights for every grade were placed on the wall so participants could stand next to them for comparison. Hands traced on a large sheet of paper provided another growth difference comparison.

Personal Appearance—good grooming development and reinforcement. For example, a child could stand in front of a fan to mess up his hair. Then he would be given a comb to comb his hair in front of a mirror. Walking with bean bags on their heads, students illustrated principles of good body carriage and balance.

Environmental Health—dealt with air, water, and solid waste pollution, and emphasized what a student can do personally to improve the environment. Educational materials such as recycled aluminum from cans were obtained from various industries and displayed for handling by the children. Plants grown in various polluted environments emphasized the effects of air pollution on living things.

Disease Prevention and Control—concerned prevention of chronic and degenerative diseases, as well as ways to prevent and control the spread of communicable diseases. Several slides were made from petri dish cultures of "germ sources" such as dirty hands, sneezes, coughs, and unsanitary environments for the children to view under microscopes. Ways to prevent the transmission of diseases were discussed in conjunction with the viewing of the slides.

Nutrition—consisted of games emphasizing accurate knowledge, positive attitudes, and desirable practices related to nutrition. Younger children were asked to place food cartons into the "right" train cars of the "Nutrition Land Express." Each car represented one of the four basic food groups. Older children played games such as Nutrition

Bingo and Nutrition Ring Toss. Nutritious snacks were also provided.

Dental Health—concentrated on correct flossing and brushing techniques, the use of "cleansing food" snacks, the need for a proper diet, and reasons why regular dental check-ups are necessary. Each child was given a graham cracker to eat. Then a solution was administered orally so tooth plaque could be detected under a plaque light. Cleaning foods such as carrot and celery sticks were eaten and then the plaque light test was readministered.

Consumer Health—analyzed various forms of health-related advertising. Unit pricing and identification of quackery were also stressed. The children practiced reading labels and prices of various food items. With bogus money, children were asked to purchase some items from stocked shelves and to explain why they bought those and not other, poor consumer choice items.

Mental/Emotional Health—dealt with values clarification and self-concept development exercises. Each child was told that a shoe box contained a picture of the most important person in the world and could they guess who it was? After several good guesses each, they could look into the box and discover a mirror image of themselves. Faces with different expressions were also shown and discussed during a segment on feelings and emotions.

Physical Fitness—concerned with resting and exercise heart rate comparisons, hand-eye coordination, and strength measurement. Each child was taught how to determine his/her heart rate. A pre and post heart rate count was taken as a part of a stationary bicycle riding test. Such physical activities as standing broad jump, target throwing, and gripping a dynamometer revealed various aspects of body strength and coordination.

Smoking—comprised of human lung specimens and x-rays depicting smoking-related lung damage. Smoking-oriented values clarification activities have also been stressed. Children were shown lungs affected by various smoking-related diseases. A home-made smoking machine collected tar and nicotine from cigarettes. Chest x-rays demonstrated the extent of smoking damage to the lungs.

Alcohol and Other Drugs—consisted of decision-making activities related to alcohol and other drug use, misuse, and abuse. Emphasized were concepts such as understanding that alcohol is a drug with a wide variety of behavioral effects, that drugs are intended to help people and that young persons should not take drugs "on their own."

Safety—focused on bicycle, pedestrian, and fire safety as well as on emergency telephone call practice. A phone system was designed so the children could call a 911 number and describe an "accident" especially created for the carnival. For a fire exit/safety experience, a large poster was used depicting a two-story house with potential fires shown in various rooms.

First Aid—stressed the administration and practice of artificial respiration and how to control bleeding. Each child was given an opportunity to perform mouth-to-mouth artificial respiration with a Resusci-Anne manikin. Direct pressure and pressure point bleeding control were stressed along with prevention and treatment of physiological shock.

Evaluation and Follow-up

We have held our health education carnivals on either Friday or Saturday and conducted the evaluation in classes on the following Mondays. The excitement of the facilitators and their commitment to apply the principles learned in the carnival experience to later instructional work, usually make the evaluations a positive experience.

In evaluating the health education carnivals, we always consider the quality of the entire program as well as each activity within it. The facilitators have often expressed their appreciation for the opportunity to have interacted with the children. Several students have admitted that their apprehension about working with elementary children was replaced with renewed confidence in themselves.

Children also participate in the evaluations. Classroom teachers have older students write a reaction paper about their health education carnival experiences. One child wrote, "It's hard to believe that my body is built just like they showed." Another . . . "liked the smoking area best because it showed what smoking did to your teeth, your lungs, your blood vessels and your fingers." Other children enjoyed "when you rode the bicycle," "when they gave me the toothbrush," "when the lady put my VIP patch on me," "when I got a black eye in the fight against smoking,"

and "when they showed us the heart and the tonsils and the gallstones and appendix." In addition, facilitators visit the schools the week after the carnival and talk with the children about their experiences in an informal learning situation.

During the carnivals work and game sheets prepared by the facilitators and pamphlets from various voluntary health organizations are given to the children. We suggest that the children keep the materials at school for two or three weeks to enable the teachers to use the health information to reinforce some of the carnival experiences. Teachers using this follow-up technique have noticed that the youngsters' recall of the carnival has been remarkable.

The evolution of the health education carnival has been a most rewarding professional and personal experience for both of us, and we are more convinced than ever that it contributes significantly to the professional preparation of undergraduate elementary education majors. However, the real winners in every carnival are the children for whom they are conducted. We would strongly recommend that all college/university health educators who teach elementary school health education courses consider coordinating one. We think that like us, you will be pleasantly surprised with the results.

[1]Blumenthal, D. S. and Kahn, H. S. Planning a community health fair, *Public Health Reports* March-April 1979, *94*:156–161.

[2]Richie, N. D. Some guidelines for conducting a health fair, *Public Health Reports* May-June 1976, *91*:261–264.

[3]Lafferty, J., Guyton, R., and Pratt, L. E. The University of Arkansas health fair as professional preparation, *Health Education*, July-August 1976, pp. 24–26.

[4]Daughtrey, G. The Norfolk public schools health fair, *Health Education*, July-August 1976, pp. 36–37.

[5]Puckett, J. and English, D. Health fair time, *School Health Review*, February 1972, pp. 27–29.

[6]Sorochan, W. D. and Bender, S. J. *Teaching elementary health science* (Second Edition), Reading, Massachusetts: Addison-Wesley Publishing Company, 1978.

[7]Stone, D. B., O'Reilly, L. B. *Elementary school health education: ecological perspectives* (Second Edition), Dubuque, Iowa: William C. Brown Company, 1980.

[8]Cornacchia, H. J. and Staton, W. M. *Health in elementary schools (Fourth Edition)*, St. Louis: C. V. Mosby Company, 1974.

[9]Barrett, M. *Health education guide: a design for teaching* (Second Edition), Philadelphia: Lea and Febiger, 1974.

Validating Health Information

MICHAEL HAMRICK is an associate professor of health education at Memphis State University, Memphis, Tennessee 38152.

Health education has changed considerably in content emphasis and teaching methodologies during the 70s. The emphasis on affective techniques, values clarification activities, decision making exercises, awareness activities, group strategies, facilitating skills, and so on has sparked considerable interest in health education and is, perhaps, responsible for the emergence of one of its most exciting eras. While the humanistic movement appears to have leveled, some serious questions are surfacing. For example, are health educators placing too much emphasis on the affective domain? Is cognition being unduly ignored? Are students learning enough to make wise health behavior decisions? From an instructional point of view, can humanistic approaches be incorporated into health education without compromising knowledge?

The search for a better balance between cognitive and affective learning led to the development and implementation of a health profile/validation learning exercise. Its purpose is to blend the two by promoting health information through student involvement. In a sense it is an exercise, a tool, which promotes confluent learning in health education. While it is designed for the basic personal health course, the principle of the profile/validation exercise can be applied to almost any course.

The exercise consists of two steps: the development of a health knowledge profile and the involvement of students in the validation phase.

Development of Health Knowledge Profile

The purpose of the profile is to identify health knowledge strengths and weaknesses for each student. The first step is to administer a comprehensive health knowledge test, which should be unannounced and given early in the semester. Students should be told that test results will not be used for grading; it is simply a diagnostic tool for revealing health misconceptions.

The test itself need not require too much additional time on the part of the instructor. Administering an old comprehensive final exam or selecting questions at random from a test manual should be sufficient. If computer facilities are available for creating a bank of test questions, your flexibility in developing a variety of tests overnight is unlimited.

Once the test is developed, administered, and scored a health knowledge profile sheet is developed for each student. The profile sheet is a graphic presentation of students' health knowledge strengths and weaknesses according to health content areas. Here are the steps for completing this task.

1. Compute a mean score for the overall test and for each content area. Computer facilities make this a simple task. Without the computer, it may be necessary to use students and about 30 minutes of class time, in which case follow these instructions.

Write the name of each content area from the test on blackboard, poster, transparency, handout, or worksheet. Below each area list the appropriate questions by number. Some questions may relate to more than one content area.

Have students refer to answer sheet and count the number of correct responses for each content area.

Compute an overall percentage score by dividing by the number of questions in each area. Example: Ten questions relate to nutrition—2, 8, 15, 21, 36, 51, 70, 83, 88, and 99. Six correct answers makes a score for nutrition of 60% (6 ÷ 10 = .60).

Repeat this procedure for each content area.

Compute an overall class mean for each content area by adding students' scores for each area and dividing by the number of students.

2. Plot the class mean score for each content area on a sheet of graph paper and duplicate a copy for each student.

3. Instruct students to plot their scores. This will provide a graphic presentation of their strengths and weaknesses in comparison to the class or to a norm established over several semesters.

Once profile sheets have been completed, a packet of materials is prepared and distributed to the students. Contents of the packet include a test booklet, computer printout identifying questions answered incorrectly (if tests are scored by students, answer sheets are returned), health knowledge profile sheet, bibliography of introductory health texts, and validation instructions.

Validation Instructions

Test validation is the most important phase of the health knowledge profile/validation exercise. It consists of correcting answers to the health knowledge pretest according to the following instructions.

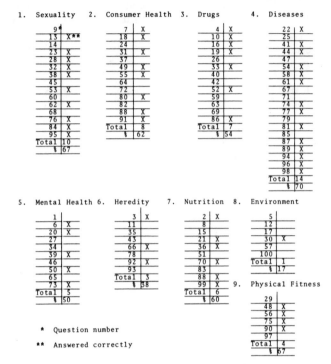

Sample worksheet of questions grouped according to content areas.

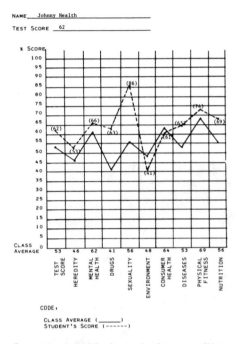

NAME **Johnny Health**

TEST SCORE **62**

CODE:
CLASS AVERAGE (_____)
STUDENT'S SCORE (------)

Sample health knowledge profile sheet.

1. Identify the incorrect answers by referring to the computer printout, answer sheet, or test booklet.

2. Find the correct answer to each question. Validate your answers by indicating the page number of the text from which you find the answer. If a text from the attached bibliography is used, (see sample bibliography) indicate the number of the text and page number beside the answer in the right hand margin. If another source is used, indicate title, authors, date of publication, and page number. Do not use any reference copyrighted over five years ago. Please note that it is possible to find answers which disagree with the master answer sheet.

Examples of validation:
Fertilization usually takes place in the
A. fallopian tubes. (16:160)
B. uterus.
C. cervix.
D. ovaries.
E. stomach.

3. Do all of your work on test booklet.

4. Turn in entire health knowledge profile/validation packet with validated answers on the scheduled date.

5. Work alone and be responsible for searching out your own answers.

Results

Students' evaluations of the Health Knowledge Profile/Validation Packet have generally been positive. Most students like knowing their health knowledge strengths and weaknesses especially when they realize that pretest results don't affect their grades. The profile sheets impress most students and help to motivate them to correct misconceptions.

The validation phase receives mixed reactions initially. It requires much time particularly for students with low pretest scores. However, at the completion of the exercise, students invariably comment on the value of the exercise and strongly recommend it for future students.

Instructors' evaluations of the exercise have also been positive. One of its best features is its versatility as a learning tool. It can be used as a study guide in preparation for a final exam; it can be used as a course project in which a certain number of points are allotted; it can be incorporated into a course contract; or it can serve as a core requirement for an entire course. It can be used equally well by the lecturer who places emphasis on cognitive learning and by the facilitator of affective learning who departs from the traditional practice of giving tests, lectures, etc. Regardless of its use, most instructors agree that the Health Knowledge Profile/Validation Packet is a valuable learning tool for correcting misinformation and learning current facts and concepts in many health science content areas.

Sample Bibliography of Introductory Health Tests

1. Bucher, Charles A., Einar A. Olsen, Carl E. Willgoose. *The Foundations of Health*, 2nd ed., Prentice-Hall, Inc., Englewood Cliffs, NJ, 1976.

2. Burton, Robert A., Barry S. Ramer, Mitchell Thomas, Scott Thurber. *Key Issues in Health*, Harcourt, Brace and Jovanovich, New York, 1978.

3. Carroll, Charles, Dean Miller, John C. Nash. *Health—The Science of Human Adaptation*, Wm. C. Brown, Co., Dubuque, IA, 1976.

4. Corder, Brice W., Ronda Showalter. *Health Science and College Life*, 2nd ed., William C. Brown, Dubuque, IA, 1975.

5. Fitch, Kenneth, Perry Johnson. *Human Life Science*, Holt, Rinehart and Winston, New York, 1977.

6. Gray, Stephen E., Hollis N. Matson. *Health Now*, Macmillan Co., Inc., New York, 1976.

7. Haro, Michael S., Edward S. Hart, Guy S. Parcel, J. Robert Wirag. *Explorations in Personal Health*, Houghton Mifflin Co., Boston, 1977.

8. Henkel, Barbara Osborn, Richard K. Means, Jack Smolensky, James M. Sawrey, *Foundations of Health Science*, 3rd ed., Allyn and Bacon, Inc., Boston, 1977.

9. Hoffman, Norman S. *A New World of Health*, McGraw-Hill Book Co., St. Louis, 1977.

10. Insel, Paul M., Walton T. Roth. *Health in a Changing Society*, Mayfield Publishing Co., Palo Alto, CA, 1976.

11. Johns, Edward B., Wilford C. Sutton, Lloyd E. Webster. *Health for Effective Living*, 6th ed., McGraw-Hill Book Co., New York, 1975.

12. Jones, Kenneth L., Louis W. Shainberg, Curtis O. Byer. *Dimensions III—A Changing Concept of Health*, 3rd ed., Canfield Press, San Francisco, CA, 1976.

13. Jones, Kenneth L., Louis W. Shainberg, Curtis O. Byer. *Health Science*, 4th ed., Harper and Row Publishers, New York, 1974.

14. Kogan, Benjamin. *Health—Man in a Changing Environment*, 2nd ed., Harcourt Brace Jovanovich, Inc., New York, 1974.

15. LaPlace, John. *Health*, 2nd ed., Prentice-Hall, Englewood Cliffs, NJ, 1976.

16. *Life and Health*, 2nd ed., CRM, Random House, Inc., New York, 1972, 1976.

17. Maltz, Stephen, Verne Zellmer, Harold Chandler. *College Health Science*, Wm. C. Brown, Dubuque, IA, 1973.

18. Mayer, Jean. *Health*, D. Van Nostrand Co., New York, 1974.

19. Miller, Benjamin F., John J. Burt. *Good Health—Personal and Community*, 3rd. ed., W. B. Saunders Co., Philadelphia, PA, 1972.

20. Neal, Kenneth. *Knowledge of Health Series*, Eliot Publishing Co., Long Beach, CA, 1975.

21. Read, Donald A., Walter H. Greene. *Health and Modern Man*, Macmillan Inc., New York, 1973.

22. *Readings in Health 76/77*, Annual Editions, Dushkin Publishing Group, Inc., Guilford, CT, 1976.

23. Richardson, Charles E., Fred V. Hein, Jana L. Farnsworth. *Living—Health, Behavior, and Environment*, 6th ed., Scott, Foresman and Co., Dallas, TX, 1975.

24. Schifferes, J. J., Louis Peterson. *Healthier Living Highlights*, 2nd ed., John Wiley & Sons, 1975.

25. Sinacore, John S. *Health—A Quality of Life*, 2nd ed. Macmillan, Inc., New York, 1974.

26. Sinacore, John S., Angela C. Sinacore. *Introductory Health—A Vital Issue*, Macmillan, Inc., New York, 1975.

27. Turner, C. E. *Personal and Community Health*, 14th ed., C. V. Mosby Co., St. Louis, MO, 1976.

Teaching Students to Be Lifelong Peer Educators

Peer education has long been used informally and at times formally in health education courses as a technique for promoting desirable attitudes and behaviors related to health and safety.[1–5] Another goal health educators need to pursue in relation to peer education is to enable students to become effective peer educators outside the classroom so that currently as youngsters and later as adults they can effectively provide accurate information and advice regarding health and safety behavior to their spouses, friends, and coworkers. This article suggests a number of considerations that should be kept in mind in attempting to provide students with this important, lifelong skill.

What is Peer Education?

Peer education involves the sharing of information, attitudes, or behaviors by people who are not professionally trained instructors but whose goal at the moment is nonetheless to educate. Peer educators may have special expertise in a particular subject or skill, or have received training in how to be peer leaders, but they do not have the experience or credentials of professionals in the content or skill areas they are communicating, and their occupation does not involve teaching in these fields. Thus, a physician who talks to a neighbor about the latest developments in cancer treatment is not engaging in peer education, but a roofer who has learned about the prevention of skin cancer because a close friend had a melanoma is engaging in peer education when he or she passes this information on to a coworker. Peer education also needs to be distinguished from peer counseling, which is targeted exclusively to people who need immediate help with a personal problem.

Although structured peer education groups are sometimes established, the informal and usually spontaneous interaction that occurs in the home, on the job, or in social encounters represents

Peter Finn is senior research analyst at Abt Associates Inc., 55 Wheeler Street, Cambridge, Massachusetts 02138.

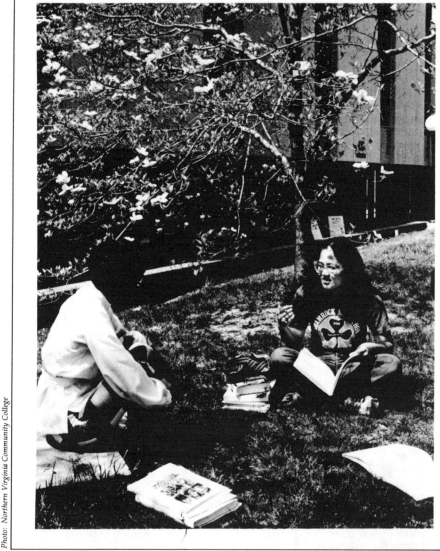

Photo: Northern Virginia Community College

the most common type of peer education. Peer education takes place constantly on an informal basis among most people. Youngsters and adults furnish each other daily with information and advice on how to promote their health and safety, even in highly technical fields. In one survey, for example, 40% of the respondents indicated that friends or relatives provided them with information about hypertension.[6]

A number of studies have established the efficacy of peer education among adults as a powerful technique for modifying health behavior. Support from family members, especially the spouse, has proven to be an effective method for reducing the low compliance rate among patients assigned medical regimens, and for increasing utilization of health services and adherence to preventive health practices. Persistence with diet and smoking cessation programs appears to be strengthened by peer influences. Group discussion approaches have proven effective in nutrition education and breast self-examination and in reducing hospital readmissions of heart patients and encouraging the return of hypertensives for medical care. Peer groups, if properly constituted and guided, are sometimes more effective in promoting proper health behavior than are the individualized, nonpeer exhortations from doctors and nurses.[7-11]

Given this evidence of the ubiquity and power of peer education, it is important that health education instructors capitalize on this learning process in order to help students develop the skills necessary to become effective providers of health information to others and be able to evaluate accurately the information which their peers will always be proffering. Since we all "teach" so much about health to other lay people, and in turn learn so much from them, we ought to purposefully shape this continual peer education so that it constructively furthers important health education goals.

Identifying Opportunities for Peer Education

Educating youngsters explicitly for future peer education involves two goals: (1) identifying what opportunities for peer education students can expect to find as adults and (2) teaching specific peer education strategies they can use when opportunities present themselves.

Students need to learn when to engage in peer education, with whom such education is likely to be most effective, and what health or safety issues to address.

When

There are opportune and inopportune times to engage in peer education, and knowing when a family member, friend, or coworker will be receptive to health and safety information or advice is often an important prerequisite to promoting improved health care behavior in others. Obviously, the ideal time to engage in peer education is when help is requested or when someone expresses a concern about a health or safety problem. A particularly promising occasion often occurs after a health crisis has forced someone to pay strict attention to a health matter. The person who has just had a gingivectomy may suddenly become interested in learning about proper dental care; the woman who has just had a benign lump diagnosed in her breast may for the first

time want to learn how to conduct breast self-examinations. While it may be tempting to leave such matters entirely to the peer's physician in these "traumatic" situations, peer reinforcement of what a doctor has recommended can improve the strikingly low rate of patient compliance with "doctor's orders."

Students need to be sensitive to these promising openings for peer education

---

Given the evidence of the ubiquity and power of peer education, it is important that health education instructors capitalize on this learning process in order to help students develop the skills necessary to become effective providers of health information to others and be able to evaluate accurately the information that their peers will always be proferring.

---

without becoming meddlesome killjoys. It might, for example, merely create resentment to talk about nutrition with a hypertensive, overweight friend just as he orders his fourth beer to wash down his third hot dog in the final minutes of a close football game. Unfortunately, some spouses choose precisely these inappropriate times to rail at their husbands or wives, "What do you want to do, get a heart attack right here in the stands?"

With Whom

Youngsters and adults need to be selective in choosing individuals with whom to engage in peer education. We all know some people who just won't pay heed to us (or to anyone) and others who seem to pay special attention to the things we say. While initially youngsters and adults have to discover who among their family, friends, and coworkers will be receptive to peer education attempts and who will not, nothing will stifle the would-be peer educator more than constant rebuffs from indifferent or even hostile people. Peer education should be reserved for those who we know may benefit from what is offered.

Students should also be aware of how age, sex, occupation, family position, and other factors may enhance or limit

their persuasiveness with others. For example, female heads of households have considerable influence on the attitudes toward health behaviors of other members of their families. Youngsters should be aware of the special advantages they have for engaging in peer education with specific types of peers. Conversely, students should learn to be sensitive to conditions that may make it difficult to engage in peer education with certain peers. A person who works in an alcoholism treatment facility may find that his friends become defensive if he tries to suggest how to avoid a hangover, or points out that mixing drinks does not heighten intoxication. Self-doubts about their own drinking habits may make these peers feel too threatened to be able to benefit from information from someone they assume disapproves of all but the most modest drinking behavior.

What Issues

When it comes to health education, everyone should be sensitive to the special expertise they may have based on their personal health and safety history and their employment, education, and training. Conversely, youngsters should learn to be discreet in their peer education attempts; they should *refrain* from engaging in peer education in areas where they know their knowledge is limited. Many, perhaps most, people disseminate a great deal of misinformation and offer considerable injurious advice about health matters—in part because in this field everyone fancies himself an expert. A major task of the health educator is to help students become aware of when they do *not* have an adequate grasp of an issue, and must exercise restraint in providing peer education.

Learning Peer Education Strategies

Some peer education techniques will be more effective than others depending on the peers, the setting, and the health issues involved. Students should develop a repertoire of approaches from which they can select the most appropriate for each peer education opportunity that presents itself. They should select an approach with which they feel comfortable and competent. Health education teachers can expand each student's options for peer education by helping the class to identify many techniques for peer education and to practice and become proficient at them.

It is beyond the scope of this article to discuss all peer education approaches with which students can experiment, but *role modeling* is one that needs emphasis. It requires no special skills to perform, and in many cases can be more effective in stimulating people to modify harmful health behaviors than any verbal attempts can be. It is also an extremely useful method for reinforcing the effects of verbal forms of peer education.[12,13]

People model health behaviors all the time, whether they want to or not. The goal for health educators is to make youngsters aware that such role modeling is always taking place and, by helping them to become conscious of its prevalence and power, encourage them to put it deliberately to productive use. For example, a host who serves nonalcoholic punch at his party along with alcoholic beverages may stimulate friends to do the same. The example of a man on a hunting trip who brushes his teeth in the stream before crawling into his sleeping bag may serve to nudge a fellow hunter with gum problems into brushing more frequently. Many people have taken up jogging because their spouses did so. One community-based alcohol education program with which this author is familiar provides wine and cheese at every social event it hosts, not only to dissipate any notion that it is attempting to promote abstention, but to set an example of responsible drinking.

In some kinds of role modeling, a peer *must* imitate the behavior of the spouse or friend, or can avoid copying it only at considerable personal inconvenience. If a health-conscious wife, who has been serving noodle casseroles, bread, butter, and apple pie to her overweight husband who has a high cholesterol count, switches to more poultry, vegetables, and fruit, she can help enforce a beneficial health behavior. Furthermore, if, as evidence appears to indicate,[14,15] new attitudes often follow new behavior, rather than the reverse, the husband whose diet changes in this fashion may soon be motivated to alter his lunch and snack habits on the job as well. In an intriguing reversal, a husband who becomes diet-conscious and leaves portions of nutritionally unhealthy food uneaten on his plate may stimulate his wife to prepare more healthful foods, rather than see her culinary efforts go unappreciated. Of course, it is essential that the couple openly and thoroughly discuss dietary or other health differences and expectations, but role modeling in conjunction with frank dialogue can be a potent force in improving one's peers' health habits.

Other approaches to peer education include providing information; referring friends to other people or agencies for information or assistance; teaching skills ("Why don't you keep a record of how much you eat between meals. Here's how I've been doing it. . . ."); promoting decision-making abilities; and humor, sarcasm, expressions of disgust, and a host of other *ad hominem* tactics that can be more or less successful with certain peers.

To be most effective in choosing the

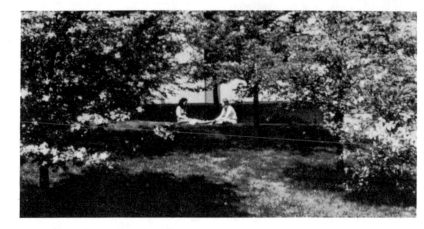

best approach and implementing it correctly, students should become aware of the major principles of learning in the field of health education, including the following:

• Efforts to promote health behavior change are most effective with people who believe the risk involved in their behavior is a serious one, one to which they are personally exposed, and one which cannot be avoided except by behavior change. Furthermore, actions for reducing the danger should be offered that do not conflict seriously with the perceived benefits which the unhealthful behavior provides. Persuasion depends on the credibility of the "educator." Students should practice telling their friends *why* their information is accurate, or their advice reliable (they took a course, read an article, were told about it by an expert).

• A whole literature has developed on the alleged effect and counterutility of "scare tactics," and students should become familiar with the findings of these studies.

• Reinforcement of learning should be an essential ingredient in all health education efforts: a peer education attempt that fails in one instance may become successful if it is repeated under the same or different circumstances, or by different peers.

• Peer education is valuable not only for changing harmful health behavior, but for reinforcing existing healthful behavior so that it is continued.

• Irrational motivations play a large part in every person's decisions about health behavior.

Simply knowing strategies of effective peer education will not enable most youngsters to be effective peer educators. Students must have opportunities to *practice* these strategies, in order to develop the skills needed by effective peer educators. To provide these opportunities, instructors should incorporate peer education teaching methods into current curriculums as much as possible. They should view peer education not only as an instructional strategy for achieving immediate subject area objectives, but also as a *skill building exercise for future use*. Teachers should therefore involve students both in classroom exercises that simulate peer education attempts, and in real-life activities requiring peer education efforts with family, friends, and neighbors. Suggested activities of this nature follow.

• Students are assigned to observe ways in which peer education is already taking place among the adults they encounter. Instances can also be identified from television shows. The illustrations of peer education can then be shared in class and evaluated in terms of how appropriate and effective each one was, and how it could be made more convincing. Pupils can role-play these examples, simulating different and "better" endings, and then compare their own attempts at peer education with those they observed among adults.

• Students identify occasions outside the classroom when peer education should have occurred but didn't, and role-play what might have taken place in class. Drawing on this and the exercise above, students can develop an initial list of opportunities that exist in adult life for engaging in peer education and techniques for doing so effectively.

• Students identify opportunities for engaging in peer education among adults and contemporaries in their own homes, communities, or schools, and discuss in small groups how they could do so appropriately and effectively. The class then "practices" peer education whenever these opportunities arise over the next several days or weeks. Students report the results of their attempts to the other students, who assess whether the effort was appropriate and effective, and suggest how it might be improved.

• Students are assigned in small groups to read a biography, autobiography, or work of fiction, and identify when peer education is taking place, whether the occasion to initiate it is propitious, what peer education techniques are employed, and how effective they appear to be. If every student in a group reads the same source, group members may compare their analyses, and point out to each other what their analyses overlooked. Once again, pupils may role-play their own versions of the peer education attempts, and critique their own performances.

• Students in small groups conduct interviews or polls among classmates or adults, to discover how people learn about health and safety, and when and from whom people feel they are most receptive to peer learning.

Teaching Peer Learning

Attempts to promote peer education among students will be incomplete if they do not help youngsters become wise peer *learners* as well as teachers. Students need to develop skills in evaluating information and advice their peers provide them. They should not uncritically accept information, alter their attitudes, and modify their health behaviors in response to a friend's or family member's erroneous recommendations for healthful living. For example, youngsters need to discriminate between inappropriate change of attitudes and behavior due to peer pressure, and well-advised change motivated by peer education. When students are the object of peer education attempts in the classroom or the community, they need to practice asking themselves the following questions:

• Does my peer have any special expertise in this area that indicates I should

place special confidence in what he has to say? Has this peer provided reliable information about health and safety in the past?

• Where did this person get his information? Are these sources reliable?

• Do I need corroboration or documentation of what this person has told me? If so, how can I get it? Can I test the behavior myself without any risk in order to see if the action is beneficial? Can I ask my physician about it or call a local public health clinic for advice?

• What approaches is the peer using to get me to change my behavior? Fear? Presentation of the facts? Role modeling? Peer pressure? Coercion? Humiliation? What, if anything, do these approaches suggest about how much confidence I should have in the advice?

Students can practice becoming critical peer learners by developing written methods for deciding how much credence to place in a peer's health recommendations and whether verification of the suggestions is desirable. They can then secure this confirmation and report their results to the class. As students identify instances of peer education in the home, the community, literature, and the media, they can observe whether the objects of the peer education accepted the information or advice uncritically, or did so only after careful assessment of its validity.

Conclusion

Instructing students in becoming skilled peer educators will be no panacea for the difficulties in stimulating adults to adopt desirable health behaviors. Some peer education attempts have not proven successful.[16] Peer education can easily become inappropriate peer pressure if students presently or later as adults seek to influence their peers solely on the basis of "superior" age, social standing, experience, or force of personality. Increased use of peer education approaches may also turn some youngsters into presumptuous "know-it-alls" who constantly intrude into the lives of their friends, family members, neighbors, and coworkers under the misconception that they are fully qualified experts in all matters of health and safety.

All of the potential difficulties of peer education fail to negate the fact that this form of learning is going to occur constantly among youngsters and adults regardless of instructional efforts to promote the use of other more "reliable" sources of information and advice. It is

essential that we seek, through formal training, to put the inevitable peer education that will take place to positive use, rather than leave it to the vagaries of chance. As an instructional strategy valuable in and of itself, and as a technique for youngsters to acquire for future use, peer education should be incorporated into nearly every phase of the health education curriculum.

[1]Herold, E., Eastwood, J., Empringham, C., Gall, B., McKendry, S. Human sexuality: a student-taught course. *The Family Coordinator*, 1973, 22:183–186.

[2]Jordheim, A. A comparative study of peer teaching and traditional instruction in venereal disease education. *Journal of the American College Health Association*, 1976, 24:286–289.

[3]Kunkle-Miller, C., Blane, H. T. A small group approach to youth education about alcohol. *Journal of Drug Education*, 1977, 7:381–386.

[4]Larkin, T. Peer teachers: more than equal. *Manpower*, 1973, 5:15–21.

[5]Merki, D. The effects of two educational methods and message themes on rural youth smoking behavior. *Journal of School Health*, 1968, 38:448–454.

[6]Louis Harris and Associates: *The public and high blood pressure: a survey conducted for the national heart and lung institute*. Washington, DC: U.S. Department of Health, Education, and Welfare, 1973.

[7]Green, L. W. *Determining the impact and effectiveness of health education as it relates to federal policy*. Prepared for the U.S. Department of Health, Education, and Welfare, Contract No. SA–7974–75, April 30, 1976.

[8]Hypertension compliance. *Medical World News*, 18:20–44, May 30, 1977.

[9]Caplan, R., Robinson, E. A. R., French, J. R. P., Caldwell, J. R., Shinn, M. *Adhering to medical regimens*, Ann Arbor, Michigan, Institute for Social Research, 1976.

[10]Donabedian, A., Rosenfeld, L. Follow-up study of chronically ill patients discharged from hospitals. *Journal of Chronic Diseases*, 1964, 17:847–862.

[11]Lewin, K. Group decision and social change, in Maccoby, Newcomb, and Hartley (eds.): *Readings in Social Psychology*. New York: Holt, Rinehart & Winston, 1958.

[12]Emrick, J., Peterson, S. *Educational knowledge dissemination and utilization: a synthesis of five recent studies*. San Francisco: Far West Laboratory, 1978.

[13]Simons, H. W.: *Persuasion: understanding, practice, and analysis*. Reading, MA: Addison-Wesley Publishing Company Inc., 1976.

[14]Brehm, J. W., Cohen, A. R. (eds.). *Explorations in cognitive dissonance*. New York: John Wiley, 1962.

[15]Zimbardo, P. G. The effect of effort and improvisation on self-persuasion produced by role-playing. *Journal of Experimental Social Psychology*, 1965, 1:103–120.

[16]Finnish women act to save men. *Health Education Foundation News*, 1978, 2:2.

HORSE RACING IN THE CLASSROOM

PHILLIP HOSSLER is a teacher of health and physical education and trainer for all sports at the Madison Township High School, Old Bridge, New Jersey 08857.

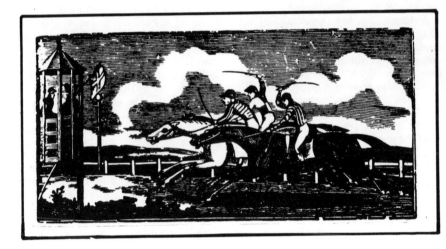

One of the difficult problems faced by high school educators today is motivating their students, especially in required courses. The problem is convincing students that just because they have to be in the class is no reason why they can't enjoy it and learn something at the same time. Giving stars or lollipops for answering a difficult question or solving a problem is not successful in high school, because older students feel their performance deserves a more beneficial reward, such as the improvement of their grade. In many required courses the students may only do that which is required to pass the course. Clearly what is needed is some sort of activity where the older students are able to feel they are properly reimbursed for their endeavors and still learn something in the process.

I initiated an activity in my health classes wherein the students researched, in class, answers to questions and explanations to the notes that I planned to cover that day. This activity took the form of a horse race. To start class when I use the horse race, I blow a whistle or ring a bell. I have signs in the room saying "Stables," "Race Tips," "Cashier," "Grandstand," etc., and have long strings of colored flags hanging in the room to add authenticity and show the class that I too have enthusiasm and enjoy what I am doing.

Each group of four students is a horse, so there are four jockeys to each horse, and each horse has a name. The first day I put on the overhead projector the drawing of the oval track with the grandstands, flags, and finish line drawn in. In the center of the track I wrote "Hossler's Happy Healthy Horse Sweepstakes." Next I showed on the overhead the ideas I planned to cover that day. For example, when the class starts the study of venereal disease, the notes might look like:

Intro to VD
Venus
skin-to-skin contact
pox, clap
cause
damage to infected

Then I give the class 10-15 minutes to look through the books and pamphlets that I have brought to class or ones they have gotten themselves to discover what I mean by each of these short phrases. Each of the horses is questioned to explain my own notes to me. I speak to a different jockey each time so that everyone is involved at some point.

Each of the phrases is worth a certain point value, usually 1 point. If only one horse gives the correct answer, that horse would get the full point; if two horses give me equally correct answers they would each get one-half point and so forth. The points that each horse receives determine its position around the track. It takes a total of 12 points to run the length of the track.

For example, if horse #1, Sugar Daddy, tells me that skin-to-skin contact is the method of transmission when speaking about venereal disease, he would be correct. If no other horse was able to give me this answer Sugar Daddy would receive the full point. If, however, horse #5, Carmel Corn, told me that skin-to-skin contact was the method of transmitting venereal disease and that coitus was the most common form of skin-to-skin contact for transmitting VD, Carmel Corn would receive three-fourths of a point or he might even steal the full point away from Sugar Daddy since Carmel Corn gave me the more complete answer. The students become involved with the race because of the constant advancing and falling behind on each question. After two or three notes, I write the position of the horses on the track. The jockeys then begin to dig a little deeper the next time for that bit of extra information that will give them the edge over the rest of the pack.

I have also found that researching answers develops teamwork and pride among the jockeys on each horse. They must research much material in a short period of time, so the notes are delegated to each of the jockeys on the horse so that one might have the answer to a note that the other jockeys didn't have time to find.

After each horse has given me an answer explaining the note, I write the points awarded on the overhead next to their horse's name amid cheers and groans from the jockeys. Then I tell them exactly what I was looking for and give them time to write it in their notebooks before going on to the next note. The order in which the horses respond varies each time so no one horse gains an advantage by being the last to answer each time.

The race continues until all the horses have finished the course. If horse #1 finished first the jockeys cannot sit back and do nothing; they must still answer questions to ensure that another one of the horses doesn't earn more points and "nose them out at the wire."

If there are six horses running, the jockeys on the winning horse each get six points, the second place jockeys each get five points, and so forth. These bonus points are used at the end of the marking period when grades are determined.

This method of teaching requires more time, because the amount of material covered each day may not be as much as with the lecture method. It requires a teacher who is able to instruct and still maintain control of the class amid mild chaos, much laughter, and student enthusiasm. I have found that the grades on the tests after using this method are the highest grades of the marking period.

I personally enjoy using this method of teaching. I don't use it for the entire marking period; instead I tell the class about it in the beginning and then save it until last. This also helps to build enthusiasm toward the activity.

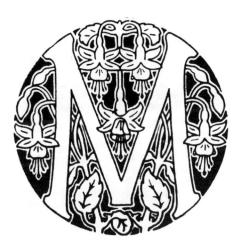

HEALTH ANAGRAMS

KATHLEEN M. SIEGWARTH is instructor, Department of Health and Physical Education, Bowling Green State University, Bowling Green, Ohio 43403.

Health educators realize that the techniques used in teaching can serve as catalysts to the material being presented. One way to help students learn about health care specialists in the community health unit of the health education curriculum is with anagrams. The procedure consists of using handouts containing anagrams, which when properly unscrambled spell out occupations in the health care profession. They are constructed to read as names. Under the caption ''My Name Is'' the anagrams are listed in columns and opposite is a column headed by ''My Occupation Is'' with appropriate blanks. Periods are not to be considered in translation, but all letters must be used.

Example:

My Name Is	My Occupation Is
1. Stu Coil	1. _____

The correct answer is oculist.

Here are several ways this idea might be used in class.

1. Distribute the sheet one week prior to the scheduled lesson day. Make it an individual contest whereby the student with the most correct answers would receive recognition as determined by the teacher. In case of a tie, a ''playoff'' would be held in class. New words would be put forth and a time limit set. When time expires the one with the most correct answers is the winner. Have the other students work the same problems. They then can offer any answers missed by the contestants and rate their own accomplishment.

2. Divide the class into two teams. Have each group elect a captain who is responsible for recording the solution for each anagram and serves as their spokesman. Allow 30 minutes for each team to work. Validate the answers between the two teams at the end of the time limit. The team with the most correct answers is the winner. Should a tie occur a playoff is held immediately, with a five minute time limit.

3. Group anagrams into similar categories. For example, psychiatrist, psy-

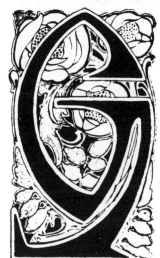

chologist, and analyst. This enables the teacher to distribute them during the unit in which they are pertinent.

4. Release the anagrams in groups of five or ten daily over a one to two week period. Answers to the problems may be turned in the next day and new ones distributed. A winner is declared after all answers have been submitted.

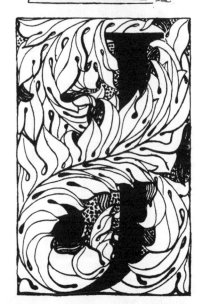

Following is a list of 45 anagrams with the appropriate answers.

	My Name Is	My Occupation Is
1.	Heston Satisgole	Anesthesiologist
2.	Les G. Trail	Allergist
3.	Lenore Vut	Volunteer
4.	Sandie Sure	Nurse's Aide
5.	Togol I. Scadir	Cardiologist
6.	Hope Toast	Osteopath
7.	Lori N. Stouge	Neurologist
8.	Tobias T. Nicer	Obstetrician
9.	Phil O. Mostogoth	Ophthomologist
10.	Patti Goolsh	Pathologist
11.	Nate I. Picidar	Pediatrician
12.	Chris T. Stipay	Psychiatrist
13.	Sol Goitur	Urologist
14.	Gail T. Sodoir	Radiologist
15.	Gib O. Loist	Biologist
16.	Tania M. Torrids	Administrator
17.	Tad I. Porsit	Podiatrist
18.	Seth Doorpit	Orthopedist
19.	G. O. Nurse	Surgeon
20.	Rod Ryle	Orderly
21.	Ted Tins	Dentist
22.	Thor Stondoit	Orthodontist
23.	Ricator Porch	Chiropractor
24.	Gipsy T. School	Psychologist
25.	T. S. Chime	Chemist
26.	Tod Roc	Doctor
27.	Unis T. Tortini	Nutritionist
28.	Patricia Pylsthesh	Physical Therapist
29.	Nyle G. Gostico	Gynecologist
30.	Thom Toilgoes	Hemotologist
31.	Scott Goily	Cytologist
32.	Nat I. Eidic	Dietician
33.	Stanlie Chet Comlodig	Medical Technologist
34.	Caine Y. Xanchirt	X-ray Technician
35.	Peter Lance Grantitoir	General Practitioner
36.	Toni Priceset	Receptionist
37.	Mort G. Sealdito	Dermatologist
38.	Mic A. Prade	Paramedic
39.	Sy A. Lant	Analyst
40.	I. N. Rent	Intern
41.	I. C. Shypain	Physician
42.	R. E. Sun	Nurse
43.	Pam C. H. Stair	Pharmacist
44.	Morie T. Topst	Optometrist
45.	Cher E. Raser	Researcher

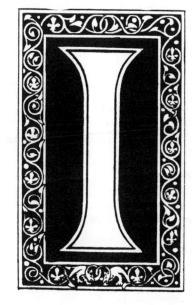

HEALTH GAMES

A recent publication presents learning games in several health education content areas.[1] A drug game and an alcohol game from that source are presented here.

What's On My Back

Slang terms for "street drugs" are commonly used. However, the actual drug, its action, its effect, and correct name are often not known. This game will familiarize students with the names, the type, and the effects of drugs. Index cards, felt tip pen and prizes are used. Place a slang term, correct name, and long term effect on separate cards using the list shown here.

Description for Playing: Pin one card on the back of each student without them seeing it.

Instruct the students that they must go to other students and ask for a clue as to

without a doctor's prescription?

Drinking

Alcohol consumption is a widespread practice among all age groups. Alcohol education is one means of correcting the misconceptions many people currently believe and/or practice. This game is designed to help students discriminate between fact and fallacy about drinking.

Description for Playing: One story is given to each student. Intertwined in this story are misconceptions and/or false statements. Each sentence begins with a number. Circle the number of those statements which are *not* true.

Name	Slang Name	Effect
Amphetamines	bennies, dexies, pep pills, uppers, hearts	Alertness, actively paranoid, loss of appetite, delusions, hallucinations.
Barbiturates	barbs, blue devils, downers	Euphoria, physical dependency with dangerous withdrawal symptoms.
Cocaine	coke, snow, snuff	Excitation, sore nose, paranoia, depressive rebound on withdrawal.
Codeine		Euphoria, physical dependence, constipation, loss of appetite.
Heroin	H., horse, scat, junk, smack, hard stuff	Euphoria, physical dependence, constipation, loss of appetite.
LSD	acid, sugar, sunshine	Insightful experiences, distortion of senses, may intensify existing psychosis, panic reactions, "flashbacks."
Marijuana	pot, grass, tea, MJ, weed	Outside stimuli more vivid, relaxation, euphoria, physical dependence.
Methadone	meth	Constipation, loss of appetite.
Morphine	white stuff, morph	Euphoria, physical dependence, constipation, loss of appetite.

"What's on my back" such as an effect, drug name, or slang term.

After a person correctly guesses what his card says he then finds the other students with the rest of the information pertaining to a certain drug. The first group with the correct cards wins a prize.

Discussion Question: 1. What are the immediate effects of each drug?

2. What are stimulants, depressants or hallucinogens?

3. What is the legal, social, physical danger of many of these drugs taken

[1] Woody, age 20, resides with his parents in Mt. Pleasant where he is a sophomore at the university. [2] The females on campus find him very attractive; 6 feet tall, 175 pounds, blond curly hair, and bright, blue eyes. [3] Final exam week has brought about the usual stress, and anxiety many college students experience. [4] In an effort to alleviate the stress, Woody attended a weekend party. [5] It was the usual kind of party he attended with a lot of women, booze and loud music. [6] Many of the females at the party were in constant pursuit of him because his ability to drink

more than anyone else was viewed as a sign of virility. [7] This is partly due to the fact that the alcohol he consumed affected his muscles first. [8] In Woody's case, the alcohol also acted as an aphrodisiac, as alcohol consumption usually does. [9] With these two factors contributing to his virility, one can plainly see why he was pursued.

[10] Woody is a fairly bright guy and has established guidelines for his drinking behavior. [11] First, he always drinks vodka to prevent rapid absorption. [12] Second, he seldom eats any food before he drinks because it fills his stomach and he cannot hold as many drinks. [13] After all, if it's free booze he wants to get all he can. [14] Third, he drinks slowly instead of gulping his drinks to prevent getting intoxicated.

[15] Since he is physically a big guy, he really can drink as much as he wants because he has more body tissue and fluids to dilute the alcohol.

[16] As the evening progressed (3 hours), Woody consumed six mixed drinks (1½ oz. alcohol per drink) and the only observable sign he showed was a slight intensification of his talkative personality.

[17] As the party continued, he talked with friends, danced and asked Joey, an attractive girl clad in jeans, if he could drive her home. [18] Of course, Joey answered yes, and they left the party.

[19] Should Joey have more carefully considered the possible consequences of leaving with Woody? [20] After all, he was only drinking moderately and there are no risks if he drinks moderately. [21] He wasn't acting "funny;" the alcohol he drank stimulated him—that's the primary effect it has on a person. [22] And because both his parents are alcoholics he probably has inherited alcoholism from them. [23] Oh well, why should she worry?

[24] The simple truth of this story is that Joey is the alcoholic and not Woody. [25] Everyone knows that there are more women alcoholics than men.

Questions: Which statements are false? (6, 7, 8, 11, 12, 15, 16, 20, 21, 22, 25).

Important Considerations: The instructor should carefully explain why the above statements are incorrect. This exercise can be used as a pretest prior to discussion or as an evaluative tool after discussion.

[1] Ruth C. Engs, ed., Eugene Barnes, and Molly Wantz, *Health Games Students Play* (Indiana University: Bloomington, Indiana, 1974), pp. 13-23.

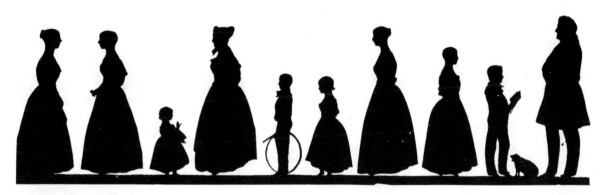

THE MANY FACES OF ROLE PLAYING

LYNN TEPER-SINGER is an assistant professor in the Departments of Health Science, Physical Education, and Guidance and Counseling at Long Island University—The Brooklyn Center, Brooklyn, New York 11201.

Role playing as a classroom technique has provided a marvelous environment for the exploration of health concepts. In the February 1971 issue of *School Health Review* a step by step procedure of the traditional role playing situation was presented in an article entitled, "Role Playing as a Tool in Mental Health Education." Briefly the steps included:

1. *Sensitizing the group*—present a situation where the class discovers that each person perceives a given situation differently based on past experience, assumptions, and expectations
2. *The Warmup*—describe the role playing situation with limited information
3. *The Enactment*—spontaneous dramatization
4. *The Replay*—the same people switching roles
5. *Student Observation*—discussion by the students about their reactions
6. *The Evaluation*—draw conclusions

At this time I would like to present three alternative approaches to role playing. Although any area in mental health can be explored through these procedures, the following are examples for use in drug education.

Example I

Structure: The class is divided into groups of four. Each group sits in a small circle within a large circle that the groups form.

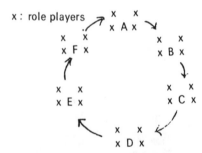

x : role players

Situation: Student arrives home to a family that has discovered a "stash" of drugs hidden away in his/her room.

Roles: Each group will enact the following roles spontaneously without preparation other than deciding on a role. Mother and/or father, brother and/or sister, student.

Procedure: In sequence each group performs their presentation of what they think will happen. (Group A then B then C, etc.) Generally each group has a different approach. The teacher may stop the group and go on to the next group at any point.

Discussion: After all groups have enacted their presentation, the teacher will have several options for proceeding with the discussion depending upon the material presented. Some possibilities include:

1. The class may form new groups based on the behavior displayed by the parents. Students who think their parents would behave as the role was played, would group together with the role players. For example: parent who cries "How could you do this to me"; parent who kicks child out; parent who questions with concern; parent who lectures and does not allow a response, etc.

Discussion questions may include: How do you feel when your parents approach you in this manner when they disapprove of your behavior? For what reasons do you believe your parents respond in this way? How would you approach your child if you were the parent?

2. The class may discuss their reaction to each group's performance.

3. The teacher may present questions for the small groups to discuss based on the diverse material that the teacher has been jotting down during the different presentations. For example:

Describe the ways in which the person caught responded.

For what reason do you believe people would respond in this way?

What information about drugs do you believe was false, which was factual?

What are the penalties for breaking drug laws?

What was your reaction when alcohol was mentioned as alright for the adults but "pot" was put down?

Example II

Structure: Single group performance with stop action directorship by the class. The performing group presents their interpretation of the situation in front of the class (the directors) who are sitting in a semi-circle around the classroom.

x- role players
o- directors

Situation: One student is trying to convince three friends to smoke a joint.

Roles: Person who does the convincing, person who refuses, person who is undecided, person who accepts.

Procedure: The group begins their enactment. At any point any member of the class, as well as the teacher, may stop the action by calling out "Stop Action" and

1. ask a question of a performer about how that performer feels at the moment.

2. assume the role of any of the players with a different approach.

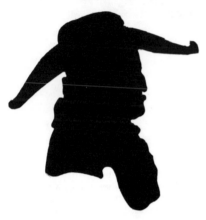

3. ask the present players to switch roles.

Discussion: Questions for discussion may involve aspects dealing with group pressure and the decision-making process.

a. In what ways were the situations realistic or unrealistic?

b. How do you feel when someone tries to convince you to do something that you really don't wish to do?

c. What feelings do you have when you want to convince someone to do something and they refuse?

Example III

Structure: One individual sitting on the edge of the circle who will enact two opposing aspects of himself while the remaining members of the class listen.

x- role player
o- classmates

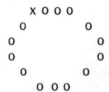

```
        X O O O
      O           O
    O               O
    O               O
      O           O
        O O O
```

Situation: The forces (feelings and attitudes) within the person that motivate him to use drugs versus those that influence him to refrain from using drugs.

Roles: The role is the dichotomy that exists within us that determines our decisions.

Procedure: The student holds up two hands (puppets may be used if appropriate for the age group). One hand is first used for emphasis "On the one hand why shouldn't I use drugs, everyone is doing it?" The other hand is then used "But on the other hand just because others do it doesn't mean I have to follow their example." The alternation of hands is repeated with each feeling and thought for or against the use of drugs.

Discussion: Questions for discussion may include:

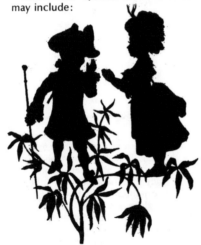

1. In what ways are your feelings similar to and/or different from those presented?

2. What is your response in other situations where a conflict exists between your feelings, thoughts, and attitudes?

When teachers present role playing situations it is most important for them to have a facility for questioning so discussions are meaningful. The teacher's responsibility in role playing is essentially to help students identify and define what they are experiencing, as well as to help them investigate their feelings and reactions. A non-judgmental setting is therefore a must.

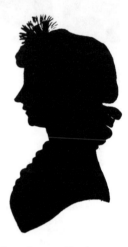

Suggestions for questioning:

1. Avoid questions that merely yield a yes or no response or that call for judgments such as good or bad, should or shouldn't.

2. Explore several ramifications of questions:

Clarify a point: If I understand you, you said. . . .

Seek additional information: Would you tell us more about this?

Evaluate: What do you think this might mean? How does the rest of the class feel about this?

Conclude: What happened? Why is this a problem? How could the outcome be altered?

3. Provide an atmosphere where questions arise from and between students as well as from you.

TEACHING IDEAS

FANTASY GAMES

RALPH BATES is in the Department of Health, Physical Education and Recreation, Ohio State University, Columbus, Ohio 43210.

I have used fantasy games with young children, older children, and adults and have found them to be very successful. Participants become more aware of how they perceive themselves, what they are like as people, their strengths and weaknesses and, most important, they can become aware of emotions and deeper feelings which normally would not be disclosed to individual or group members. I have also found that fantasy is relaxing, helps develop better listening skills, and leads to closer, more meaningful relationships among participants.

In this paper I would like to share several of these games, to use with groups of children as a means of relaxation and to help them learn more about themselves. I will indicate the method I use in presenting these games, and the reader can adapt each one according to individual needs. The books and articles in the bibliography are excellent resources for fantasy games as well as other communication skills for both children and adults.

Make A Person

I have found this game to be effective with children to help you learn what they are like as people.

1. Ask a group of children to think of a person's name and write it on the board.

2. Using the general background of the group as a guide, and the age of the children you are dealing with, establish same criteria for this person. Example: "Billy is 14 and lives at home with his mother, father, brother, and sister."

3. Ask the children the following: With help from each one of you, I would like to find out more about Billy. What is he like as a person? What is he like at home? How does he do in school? What does he like to do? How does he feel about himself? With these general questions as a guide, obtain several responses from each child and write them on the blackboard. If you listen carefully, you will be surprised about how these children feel about themselves, their peers, and their families. Follow this through with a group discussion.

Rosebush and Object Identification

This game is directed more toward older children. You may use the same format for younger children by substituting a flower or animal for the rosebush and object.

1. Ask the participants to close their eyes and get as comfortable as possible. They may sit in their chairs or sit or lie on the floor. Then say the following: I am going to take you on a fantasy trip. I want you to do exactly as I say and be aware of nothing else but my voice.

2. The following questions can be used for the rosebush. You will have to adapt these questions to the other games. What are you like as a rosebush (object)? What are your roots like . . . your stem . . . your leaves . . . your thorns . . . your flowers? What are your surroundings like? What season?

3. Now proceed with the following: In several minutes I will ask you to open your eyes then tell us what you are like as a rosebush. Have each member select a group member after he has described himself to the group. The following questions may be used for discussion.

1. What did you learn about yourself?

2. What did the group learn?

3. How does this relate to disclosure, listening, feedback, communication, and fantasy? (Adapted from Stevens, *Awareness.*)

Ocean Trip

Obtain a record or tape of ocean sounds such as *Environmental Sounds,* or a tape recording from a radio or TV communication center.

1. Have the group relax at their desks or lie on the floor.

2. Tell them the following: I am going to take you on a fantasy ocean trip. I want you to close your eyes, relax, and concentrate on what I say. Imagine yourself approaching a beautiful vacated beach. . . . You begin to walk in the sand. . . . Stop and take off your shoes. As you stand there, feel the sand on the bottom of your feet, the grains of sand sifting through your toes. . . . become aware of that feeling. Begin a stroll toward the water's edge. . . . As you continue your walk, become aware of the sun beating on your face, smell the salty air, hear all the sounds around you. Find a spot ahead of you and sit down in the sand. . . . Hold some sand in your hand. . . . Feel the individual grains of sand sift through your fingers. Stand up and continue your stroll toward the water's edge. . . . Before you reach the water, stand (and sit) in the wet sand. . . . Feel your feet sink into the wet sand. Grab a handful of wet sand. . . . Be aware of the difference between the wet sand and the dry sand. Stand by the water's edge. . . . Feel the water gently flowing under your feet and around your ankles. . . . Stand there and smell the salty air, feel the wind blowing in your face, and be aware of all the sounds around you. . . . (cont'd). . . .

Use your own imagination with this game. After you are through give the group several minutes before they open their eyes and disclose their trip to the group.

The following questions may be used for discussion:

1. How was your fantasy trip?

2. Where were you?

3. What were your surroundings like?

4. What were some of the feelings you experienced?

5. Could you feel the different textures of sand?

Fantasy Dream (This exercise is also directed toward older groups of children.)

Close your eyes and become as relaxed as possible. I am going to take you back to your early childhood to a recurring dream that you used to have then, a dream that you are going to have again.

Don't be afraid. Just concentrate on what I will tell you, and on your experience as my words are spoken. At night, while you are asleep as a small child, the dream would occur over and over again. The dream would begin in the same way. You would get out of bed and walk across the bedroom to the closet. There is now a door behind the closet, a door which you could never find while awake. As you approach the door in your dream it now opens.

As you stand in the door you look down an ancient looking stone staircase. In the dim light you begin to descend the staircase, not at all afraid, down a step at a time. As you approach the bottom of the staircase you stop and hear the gentle sound of water lapping against the rocks below. You approach the water's edge. A small boat is tied to the rocks. Sit in the boat and untie it. Just lie back in the bottom of the boat and let it take you where it wants to go. Sit there, relax, and listen to the water lapping against the boat and rocks, as you gently rock back and forth, back and forth, as the boat drifts down the stream.

As you lie there enjoying your trip you notice a small opening ahead of you. As you approach the opening it becomes larger and larger. You come out of the opening into a new environment which you will now experience. Continue to keep your eyes closed and become aware of the new environment. Where are you? . . . What is it like? . . . What will you do next? . . . What sights, odors, sounds, and movements are you now experiencing? . . . etc. . . . Now open your eyes and disclose your experiences to the group. (Adapted from Masters, *Mind Games.*)

Bibliography

Richard DeMille, *Put Your Mother on the Ceiling* (Addison-Wesley: Reading, Massachusetts, 1974).

Joan Freyberg, "Increasing Children's Fantasies," *Psychology Today,* January 1975.

Lucile Herfat, "The Gut-level Needs of Kids," *Learning,* October 1973.

Edmund Jacobson, *Teaching and Learning: New Methods for Old Arts* (National Foundation for Progressive Relaxation: Chicago, 1973).

Dorothy Jameward, *Born to Win* (Addison-Wesley: Reading, Massachusetts, 1973).

Robert Johnson, *Reaching Out* (Prentice-Hall: Englewood Cliffs, New Jersey, 1972).

Howard Lewis, *Growth Games* (Bantam: New York, 1972).

Robert Masters, *Mind Games* (Delta: Van Nuys, California, 1972).

J. William Pfeiffer, *A Handbook of Structural Experiences for Human Relations Training,* vols. I-IV (University Associates: Iowa City, Iowa, 1972).

John O. Stevens, *Awareness* (Library of Congress: Washington, D.C., 1971).

Health 4 Fun: A Game of Knowledge

RAYMOND NAKAMURA teaches in the programs in physical education, School of Education, DePaul University, 1011 W. Belden Avenue, Chicago, Illinois 60614.

From time to time, as a diversion from standard methods, educational games can be excellent tools for learning. "Health 4 Fun" has been a successful game because it requires a lot of knowledge and provides some fun. It can be cooperative or competitive and can be used to develop research skills in dictionaries, encyclopedias, almanacs, textbooks, journals, etc.

The purpose of the game is to fill in the blanks of a play sheet with words or phrases that fit into pre-selected health categories. The filled-in words must begin with certain letters which are chosen at the beginning of the game.

The health categories chosen must suit the level of the class. Each one is written on a separate 3x5 index card. The cards are shuffled and placed face down; four cards are drawn from the pile. As each selection is read, all players write them down in the four category blanks on the play sheet.

Letters are written on another set of index cards, one per card. These are shuffled and four are drawn from the pile. The chosen letters are written in the appropriate blanks on the play sheet.

The Game

Each player tries to think of a word or phrase in each of the 16 blanks on the play sheet that fits the category at the top of the column and begins with the selected letters. An example of a filled-in play sheet follows. To add excitement, a time limit of 2–5 minutes can be put on the game.

The game can be played as a form of solitaire or by the whole class. Teams can be made for more competitive or cooperative games.

At the end of the game, players should research the answers they could not fill in. Discussions often develop when students come up with words or phrases that the others are not familiar with. Answers may be challenged; then they must be verified by research.

In competitive games the play sheets can be scored by adding up the number of correct answers in each column, horizontally and vertically for a maximum score of 32.

Here are some suggested health categories.

1. Body systems, organs, and glands
2. Bones or muscles
3. Fruits and vegetables
4. Meats, nuts or fish
5. Dairy products
6. Ice cream flavors
7. American foods
8. Foreign foods
9. Diets
10. Fitness: names of sports
11. Fresh and saltwater fish
12. Types of transportation
13. Types of fuel
14. Pollutants: cigarette names
15. Pollutants: automobile names
16. Environmental pollutants
17. Germs or bacteria
18. Medical laboratory apparatus
19. Human diseases
20. Communicable diseases
21. Non-communicable diseases
22. Drugs, medicine tradenames
23. Slang for drugs or medicines
24. Over the counter drugs
25. Pollutants: detergents
26. Wines
27. Beer
28. Soft drink tradenames
29. Hospital names
30. Health related journals
31. Health book titles
32. Health authors
33. Famous health people, past
34. Famous health people, present
35. Health organizations or societies
36. Health agencies, offices or departments
37. Health related professions
38. Environment: mountains
39. Environment: extinct animals or birds
40. Environment: endangered species
41. Environment: rivers and lakes
42. Environment: national parks
43. Bakery products
44. Famous restaurants
45. Kitchen utensils
46. Health related household items
47. Things commonly found in the medicine cabinet
48. Health related words over seven letters
49. Breakfast cereals
50. Famous physicians
51. Chemicals found in the body
52. Articles of clothing
53. Plant names
54. Flower names
55. Category of your choice

The degree of difficulty of these categories should be related to the academic level of the class. Many can be refined to offer greater difficulty. For example, a generalized category like prescription drugs can be limited to barbiturates. However, I have found it necessary to include some easy categories to ensure some success.

Category	Human Disease	Bones and Muscles	Auto Trade Names	Medical Apparatus	
D	Diphtheria	Deltoid	Dodge	Dilator	→4
W	Whooping Cough				→1
F	Fabry's Disease	Fibula	Ford	Forceps	→4
L	Leukemia		Lincoln	Lens	→3
	4	2	3	3	24 Total Score

Pre-selected Letters

Creative Use of a Toy in Health Education

ALYCE SATO is an instructor in the Department of Nursing and LEE NICKELL is a nursing student, both in the College of Health-Related Professions, Idaho State University, Pocatello, Idaho 83209. THOMAS C. TIMMRECK is an assistant professor in the Center for Health Sciences, College of Public and Environmental Service, Northern Arizona University, Flagstaff, Arizona 86011.

Toys used in a creative way can be an intriguing enhancement to a child's education. Familiar experiences seem to be more accepted than the unfamiliar, thus if familiar toys are used in lessons children seem to pay closer attention. Health information given to the elementary student may be retained longer because they identify the toy with the learning experience, making the educational process more meaningful.

As part of the junior year clinical experience, student nurses at Idaho State University serve as health educators to elementary school children. One student centered lessons around the importance of fresh air, sunshine, rest, nutrition, and posture for good health. To visually clarify important points of the lecture, the student nurse health educator showed pictures to third graders that illustrated good or poor health activities. The children identified and shared personal experiences relating to good health. When the presentation focused on posture, students were asked to demonstrate different postures, such as sitting, standing, running, lifting, pushing. After discussing the demonstrations, the toy, "Stretch Armstrong" (manufactured by Kenner Toy Company) was used to evaluate the children's learning. Stretch Armstrong can be molded into different lengths and positions which makes it an excellent visual aid to demonstrate various aberrations in posture. The children were captivated by the poor body mechanics that Stretch Armstrong was put into. They learned to identify poor posture, improper standing and sitting habits, and behaviors that could affect the children's total health.

The children's reaction to the toy model of a human was very positive. Many children owned the same toy and almost all of them had seen the model on television and in the stores. This item

of the children's world brought into the classroom allowed them to learn easily and retain the health education lesson.

The student nurses view this teaching experience as "a lot of fun and rewarding." Perhaps part of the reward comes from the free rein that students are given to use their creativity in developing fun and exciting teaching methods and materials.

It is hoped that this innovative approach to teaching a subject which has been viewed as somewhat dull will stimulate health educators at all levels to explore creative approaches to teaching health education. Familiar items, such as toys, incorporated into health education lessons makes health subjects more meaningful and stimulating. The result of these efforts will be better learning experiences for the children with retention of knowledge and behavior change as the ultimate goal.

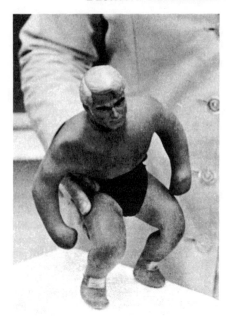

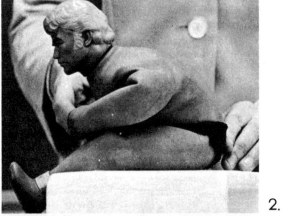

1.

2.   3.

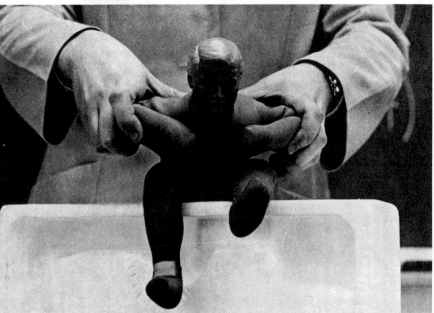

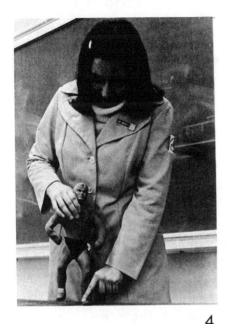

4.

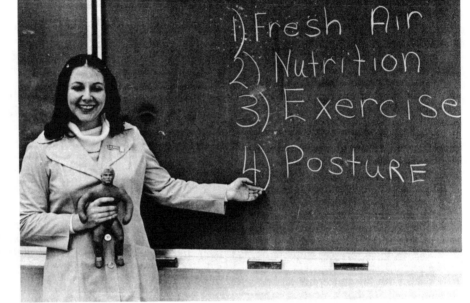

6.

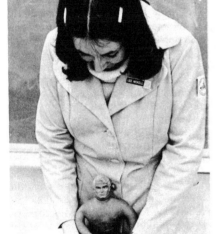

5.

Photos by Ellen Timmreck

1. Stretch Armstrong shows students how they look when they stand with poor posture.
2. Sitting too far forward can also cause poor posture.
3. Stretch Armstrong demonstrates poor posture while sitting.
4. The student nurse asks children to explain why standing on one foot, as Stretch Armstrong is doing, is poor posture.
5. Poor leg alignment can affect the child's overall posture.
6. Student nurse as a health educator teaches about healthy living.

A Kindergarten Health Resource Center

The Ethel K. Fyle Elementary School of the Rush-Henrietta Central School District has developed a kindergarten health education resource center which has proven the effectiveness of learning by doing.

The Center is a concept based on the book *Children's World*, by Wettlaufer, Neeth, Nevry, and Smart, which provides practical suggestions for developing programs for children three to six years of age. It recognizes that each child is an individual. The depth to which a child becomes involved in the program depends on background of experience, language development, and the emotional, social, and physical characteristics of the student.

Physically, the Kindergarten Health Education Resource Center is set up like a miniature health office. It contains a cabinet, cot, scale, waste basket, and various types of medical equipment. To provide interest and stimulation the students have access to pictures of community health helpers, puzzles of health oriented subjects, and books dealing with health topics.

The Center is utilized effectively as an educational setting rather than a play area solely. Pupils are gradually oriented by regularly scheduled visits. The school nurse teacher acquaints the kindergartener with various paraphernalia found in the typical health office and conducts simple demonstrations to help the children comprehend the uses of the many pieces of equipment. Following each scheduled orientation period in the health office the school nurse teacher visits the classroom and assists in the utilization of the Center by the children. She demonstrates procedures, observes the pupils in practice, and works with the classroom teacher in following through on these procedures.

To initiate lessons in first aid, the school nurse teacher demonstrates proper care of simple lacerations and abrasions. In turn, two pupils, one patient and one nurse, carry out the procedure. As each student has an opportunity to practice the procedure his name is checked off on a master list. Knowing the importance of hand-washing before initiating first aid, as well as the complete procedure of applying a band-aid, is rewarding knowledge for a five or six year old.

From such a simple procedure and demonstration more involved first aid is taught, such as: the use and reasons for cold packs on injuries as well as substitutes that can be found in home freezers, how to stop bleeding by use of a direct compress, what to do for a nose bleed, and what procedures to follow in case of a burn or a sunburn.

From the Health Education Guide K-6 that has been developed within the district, areas such as Growth and Development, Mood Modifiers (alcohol, tobacco and drugs), Nutrition, and Mental Health are also covered as part of the Health Education Resource Center.

When students are learning about growth and individual differences in height and weight, the school nurse teacher assists in the weighing and measuring of pupils. She talks about related factors that influence growth, such as the basic four food groups, general health status, individual growth patterns, and diseases. To vary the method of presentation a "tasting party" was used to introduce the food groups.

A model torso from the health office was brought to the Kindergarten Health Education Resource Center, and the pupils were given an opportunity to take it apart and put it back again. The organs of the body were discussed, and the children could see and feel what they would be like for a young person of about ten years of age. As added involvement, the Center is equipped with a stethoscope that creates excitement and motivation in hearing another student's heartbeat.

Drug education was initiated by having the students place various prescription containers (empty and rinsed out) in a special locked section of the cabinet in the Center. The relationship between these and the actual medicines the school nurse teacher has locked in the health office was pointed out, as well as an explanation as to why medicines are kept this way. This naturally leads to a number of questions and explanations: What is a drug? Are drugs good or bad? Where should drugs be stored at home? Why does the doctor sometimes prescribe medicine when we are ill? What can happen if one takes medicine that is not prescribed?

Development of a positive self-concept in the kindergarten children was a definite goal of the school nurse and the classroom teacher.

Evaluative measures of the Kindergarten Health Education Resource Center have been most promising. Observation of the children, checking by simple dittos, and completion sentences verbally indicated students were retaining the basic information. Utilization by the child (that is, his actual ability to develop attitudes and practices) still remains to be seen, but all indications point to the Center as a viable tool promoting health education in the kindergarten.

Authors are all staff in the Rush-Henrietta Central School, Henrietta, New York.
Lorraine Bennigsohn is a school nurse teacher.
Ruth Stanley is a kindergarten teacher (retired 1972).
Eugene C. Kolacki is director of health education for the District.

The Magic of Kindergarten

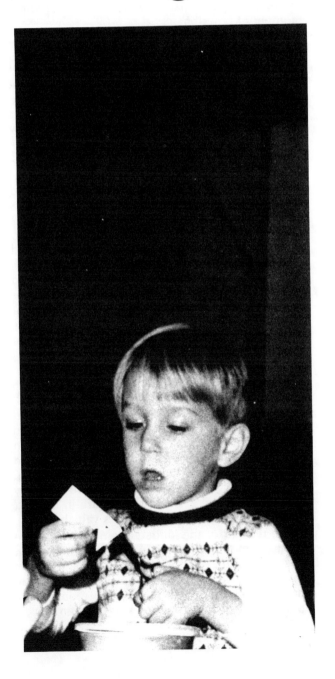

Kindergarten is a magical place which promises five-year-olds all the fun and fantasy that only their age can truly appreciate. It is a land of learning where the discovery of self and others opens a very large door. The children who enter this new world come from a variety of home environments and have been exposed to diversified health habits and attitudes. It is part of the kindergarten teacher's awesome task to carefully cultivate in these children the attitudes necessary for positive, wholesome health care and practices.

It is during this stage of development that the child develops an awareness of self. The child becomes aware that he or she is unique in the scheme of things. The teacher uses various methods to lead the child toward a positive self-concept, extending this awareness to include the responsibilities of caring for the body. From the idea that each person is a unique individual, it follows that it is important to keep the body healthy and clean in order to maintain its best appearance and function. These concepts are basically simple and can be explained without difficulty to the small child.

Activities such as proper washing, brushing of teeth, or preparing and tasting a sample meal are enjoyable ones, while being valuable learning experiences in which each member of the class may participate. Being able to attend to some of the cleansing and grooming procedures, as well as dressing oneself, are all a part of the independence that is an essential ingredient of kindergarten development. The child is proud of accomplishment; there is a feeling of importance when he has mastered a task and knows that he can accept responsibility for himself in these areas. In some cases, progress will be slower than in others, requiring much patience, for often a child is easily frustrated. Some need to be challenged, but never expected to accomplish a feat which presents undue difficulty. Incentives are helpful in the development of good habits and attitudes; praise and encouragement are two that almost never fail.

There are several equally effective ways of incorporating health education into the daily kindergarten curriculum.

One method is through the unit of study. Typical units may include "Washing and Bathing,"

Rosemary Cole is a kindergarten teacher at the Bladensburg Elementary School, Bladensburg, Maryland.

"My Teeth and My Smile," "Good Grooming," and the like. These units may extend for as many days, with as many varied activities, as the teacher or children desire. Activities, such as those mentioned, need to be supplemented with pamphlets, library books, coloring books, and records, to help make the learning experiences both lucid and enjoyable.

A second way to incorporate health education is to plan as part of the daily routine such practices as proper washing before eating and after use of the lavatory, eating slowly, and proper rest. With repetition, these sound practices develop into good health habits which, hopefully, carry over into life outside of school. Health practices become habit through routine.

Incidental learning techniques may also be used as a method of introducing and reinforcing health principles. Invaluable opportunities for the kindergarten teacher are afforded during the course of the school day for inserting a comment or explanation relating to health. Children ask very pertinent and logical questions which may be answered individually or directed to the group. Oftentimes these questions may lead into a "mini-lesson" on the subject, which may be a spontaneous one or prepared for and presented the following day.

Because it is generally beneficial as a teaching technique to capitalize on the real experiences of the child, and since communicable diseases are common at this stage of growth, it is often wise to utilize class time in discussing them as they may occur. For example, the "cold season" can bring on a discussion of preventing communication of the cold or the proper care of a cold. A hospital stay by a member of the class may induce a lesson regarding hospital procedures and benefits, or "How the Doctor Helps Us."

It is essential that the kindergarten teacher consider the child with regard to good mental health. Usually the first broadening experience of any length outside the family unit, kindergarten offers the initial taste of school, and it needs to be a wholesome one for each child! From the first day, when the reactions to school range from open joy to outright fear, and throughout the year, each child must be handled according to his individual physical-emotional makeup. Though there are no formulas, the teacher himself becomes something of a "psychologist" and discovers the personality of each youngster within a relatively short period of time.

For the mental health, as well as the general health, of all the children, the physical environment and the teacher himself should remain attractive, orderly, sanitary, and stimulating. An atmosphere of acceptance, understanding, and flexibility should prevail. Vigorous activities and lively discussions should be balanced with quiet, relaxing ones. Soothing music or voice at a low pitch changes the pace and relaxes the group for rest time or for listening. No activities should be undertaken in a rushed or hurried manner. Enough time must be allotted in the planning of each day to set a leisurely pace, without allowing for a moment of boredom.

The child needs time to discover, to ponder, to lose himself for a moment—all in the wonder of *play*. Play is educational; it is therapeutic. At times, the child should be left to himself without distraction or interruption. The teacher's role is to supply a wide variety of materials and make them available. (She may then very beneficially draw upon her observations.)

As part of fostering good mental health, emotions should be allowed a healthy outlet. Though he unmistakably feels an emotion, the young child has difficulty understanding what it is that he is feeling. This is more subjective than the self-awareness discussed earlier, and now we try to discover "why" together. Facial expressions and inner feelings during various situations which would arouse a particular emotion may be used as part of the discovery. Discuss how a character in a picture feels, with a follow-up discussion of personal feelings that were similar is another way. If there is an incidental classroom experience of anger or fear, stop right then to examine it.

It is imperative that the classroom have an overall tone of security for the children, part of which comes with acceptance and part with careful, consistent planning so that they know "what comes next." The daily or weekly routine need not be rigid, but should have a framework within which to be flexible. Teacher and children should know where they are going. Routine is important for the kindergarten age child; it affords security in itself. Each child should feel secure in the fact that what he offers to the group is valuable.

The teacher of the kindergarten is a key figure in the promotion of health education, and it is an awesome role. Yet the efforts given are greatly rewarded—the grin seen on a childish face or the unrestrained laugh heard at a given moment are indeed part of the magic of kindergarten!

Aging: A Need for Sensitivity

KENNETH A. BRIGGS is an assistant professor of health education at the State University of New York, College at Cortland, Cortland, New York 13045.

With our culture's shift from revering the old to worshipping youth and the breakdown of the extended family into separate nuclear units which usually exclude the elderly, a whole generation of young people are uneducated and insensitive to the elderly and their needs. Comprehensive school health education, which seeks to improve the quality of life through informed choices, is a good place to educate school age children about aging. It not only makes students more aware and sensitive to the needs of the elderly; it also educates them for their own aging.

Following are some suggestions to help create an awareness and caring for the elderly and their problems. These exercises help show students what it is like to be old in a culture that treats senior citizens the way we do.

Sensory Deprivation Simulation Exercises

The following simulation exercises try to bring to the young and healthy a sensitivity to what it must be like to be old and suffering from common sensory insults reported by the elderly.

Arthritis (reported by 33 out of 100 elderly)

Using cellophane tape, tape students' fingers together in various combinations, e.g., tape thumb and index finger together and the 4th and 5th fingers together. Wrap elastic bandages around the knees to simulate stiff knees. Have students perform simple tasks and then share their experiences of what it might be like to be old and have arthritis.

Visual Handicaps (reported by 15 out of 100 elderly)

Take sunglasses or laboratory protective glasses and smear vaseline on them until you get your desired visual loss. Have students wear the glasses and perform everyday things such as reading a

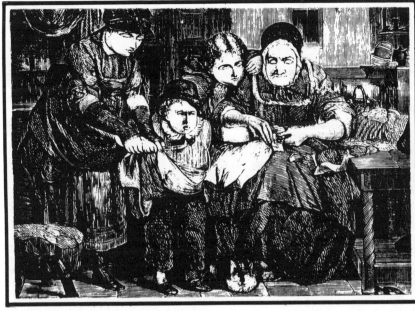

menu or a newspaper, or look up the phone number of a pharmacy that will deliver prescriptions to old people (if there is one). Have students record and share their reactions.

Hearing Loss (reported by 22 out of 100 elderly)

Place a cotton ball in the student's exterior ear canal. For a more pronounced effect, have them also wear headphones or earmuffs. Have students listen to the TV or radio at a low level, or try to carry on a conversation with someone who has no hearing loss and must shout at them to be heard. Again, have students share their feelings.

Loss of Touch

Cover the students' fingers with rubber cement and after it dries, have them try to thread a needle.

Loss of Smell

Have students taste various foods while pinching their nostrils shut.

Multiplicity (polymorbidity)

Certainly many elderly people suffer from many aging insults. They may have a hearing loss, arthritis, and a visual handicap. To help students understand multiplicity and what it might be like, have several students perform tasks with various combinations of the above simulations. For example, one student can simulate finger arthritis, visual loss, and loss of touch and smell then go to the cafeteria and buy a carton of milk. Upon returning, have the stu-

dent share some of his feelings during the experience as an older person with sensory deprivation. Be sure to exercise necessary safety precautions when students perform such simulations.

Songs and the Elderly

A lot of popular songs have been written recently that do a good job of developing a caring sensitivity and awareness of the elderly in listeners. Following are some examples of such songs and their artists.

"Old Man"—Neil Young
"Old Friends" "Voices of Old People"—Simon and Garfunkel
"When I'm Sixty-Four" "Eleanor Rigby"—The Beatles
"Two Lonely Old People"—Wings
"Hello Old Friend"—Eric Clapton
"Lonely People"—America
"Good Company"—Queen
"Hello in There"—Bette Midler
"I Never Thought I'd Live to be 100" "Travelin' Eternity Road"—Moody Blues
"Let Time Go Lightly"—Harry Chapin
"Father and Son" "But I Might Die Tonight"—Cat Stevens

A nice touch to make aging education come alive in the classroom is to add slides of old people to the music. It can be quite powerful in creating sensitivity to aging.

Activities for Application and Discussion

Have students share some of their fears about growing old.

Have students draw pictures of themselves showing what they will be like when they are 100 years old. What losses do they show?

Have students think of or photograph things in a grocery store that demonstrate our insensitivity to the aged such as, unit pricing numbers and prices that are too small to read, bulk packaging, no carry out service.

Have someone in class carry on a conversation with another person in class who has simulated speech problems that follow a stroke by placing a ping pong ball in his/her mouth.

Use the following opinionnaire to generate discussion about the elderly.

Indicate to the right of each statement whether you agree or disagree.

1. Old people are better off living with other old people.
2. Old people need rehabilitation.
3. Rehabilitation is done best in a nursing home.
4. Sixty-five is a good age at which to retire.
5. Old people live happier lives away from the young, competitive world.
6. Old people should be kept active.
7. Old people suffer a sense of loss when their children leave home.
8. Our society encourages old people to be productive and useful.
9. Old people should stay in their own homes, if possible.
10. Old people should be discouraged from dependent relationships with agency personnel.
11. Most older people are ready to rest and don't want to be involved in "doing things."
12. Old people cannot learn as well as young people because of deterioration of the brain associated with aging.

There are two films that are a must to use when trying to create a caring sensitivity of the aged in our young people:

Trigger Films on Aging —This is an excellent film dramatizing five brief situations common to the elderly. The film is excellent in eliciting emotions and a free flow of thoughtful discussion from its viewers. Produced by the University of Michigan Television Center, 400 South 4th St., Ann Arbor, MI 48103.

Peege—A marvelously produced, emotionally charged film of a young man who is successful where others failed in breaking down the communication barrier between his aged grandmother and a family who doesn't understand her. Distributed by Phoenix Films, 470 Park Ave. South, New York, NY 10016.

Take two pictures of, for example, a street corner or the entrance steps to a bus. One picture of your chosen scene should be in focus and the other should purposely be out of focus. This will dramatically demonstrate the problems encountered by those elderly who have a serious vision loss and the insensitivity we have to these people by having such things as "Do Not Walk" signs that are too small to read.

We cannot overlook the most obvious and valuable resource of all—the elderly themselves. Bring the elderly to the students or take the students to the elderly. Allow them to ask questions of each other, spend time together, and most important of all, try to understand each other.

Because of the nature of our modern society and quite often the insensitivity it carries with it for the elderly, health education about and for aging that tries to reintroduce the elderly to those who may be out of touch and insensitive to them is imperative. Such education can be valuable for the aged as well for all those who may better understand the exigencies of the years to come.

Chemically Dependent— But Only for One Week

KATHLEEN FISCHER is a health teacher at the Orono Middle School, Long Lake, Minnesota. She is now in her second year of teaching and participated in the program described here last summer.

Hazelden (Center City, Minnesota), located 40 miles northeast of the Twin Cities, is a treatment center for chemically dependent people. This was the setting for an in-service education program for 80 educators this past summer. The program, in cooperation with the Minnesota Department of Education, was funded by a grant from the Hill Family Foundation. Eight educators per week were provided with a "live in" experience, participating in the full rehabilitation program with patients and staff. The purposes of the program were to develop a "gut level" feeling and attitude toward people with a dependency problem, to become more aware of the causes of chemical dependency problems, and to become aware that patients in treatment share the same basic needs with all men.

"God grant me the serenity to accept the things I cannot change, the courage to change the things I can, and the wisdom to know the difference." These words have taken on a much greater significance for me now after having spent a week at Hazelden. They are words which can be found in every room there, either inscribed on a wall plaque or being verbalized in group sessions. They are one part of the rehabilitation program for the chemically dependent person.[1] But what

---

[1] Chemically dependent refers here to a person who is dependent either on alcohol or drugs. Alcohol is also considered a drug, and it is considered to be the number one drug problem in this country.

does this have to do with rehabilitating chemically dependent people? During my "live in" experience I was able to grasp the impact of that simple verse and its meaning to the entire program, and despite the fact that I am not chemically dependent, my experience was realistic in every other sense.

Eight of us, four women and four men, came to Hazelden as patient-observers. Our backgrounds included public school teachers, high school counselors, and psychiatric clinic personnel. Each of us was assigned a different unit as our home for the week, which would be the essence of our experience. No two of us would have the same situation, and yet we all would have grappled with some intense feelings at the end of our stay.

Hazelden is in a picturesque setting. The long driveway has a way of quieting one's mind with a gentle peacefulness that all works for good here. A patient's first contact with the inside is the detoxification unit. Minimum stay in this area is at least one day, and most patients are eager to move to a unit as there is little to do here.

All of the treatment takes place in the units, which are essentially structured in a home-like atmosphere. There are three units for men and two for women. The only time all of the units are together is at meals and lectures, and then no fraternizing is allowed. The reason behind the no fraternization policy is to prevent patients from building up support groups which will set back their own rehabilitation. Our educator group, though, certainly appreciated the special afternoon sessions we had together. It was the first time I had found myself in an environment where I was the minority. And yet as the week progressed we discovered we were more alike than different.

Surprisingly enough, Hazelden is not harboring a group of skid row alcoholics. There is not a stereotype for a chemically dependent person. All of them are everyday real people—many of the women are housewives and mothers. There were young girls, quite a few older women, and two nuns there at that time. The number of older women surprised me, but it was pointed out that today is as good a day as any to start living a better life.

The day is rigidly scheduled for patients; this is to aid in their treatment, for at some point they must again start meeting these kinds of responsibilities. All three meals must be attended; each patient has a work responsibility such as vacuuming, cleaning the unit kitchen, etc.; morning, afternoon, and evening lectures must be attended; and daily group therapy sessions must be participated in. The rest of the day is spent reading assigned materials, meeting with staff, playing solitaire, sitting around the table drinking coffee and smoking cigarettes. (The cigarette consumption increases during a patient's stay at Hazelden. This could be expected since they are attempting to alleviate one problem at a time. The ever-present smoke, however, can be quite overwhelming to non-smokers.) No recreational pursuits are provided for patients. I found this confining for my usually independent nature, but the patient's purpose for being there is not for having a fun time.

The entire program is based on the Alcoholics Anonymous twelve steps. These steps basically require a person to surrender control of his life to a higher power (belief in God per se is not a requirement), to confess to oneself all one's faults and virtues, and to then confess this to another person. When a patient reaches the fifth step in the program he is then free to return to the outside world. The staff determines when a patient is ready to proceed to the next step, and this can be anxiety-producing for some patients who feel they are further along than the staff thinks.

Upon arrival at Hazelden, patients do not know how long they will be staying there. The normal period of time is approximately three to four weeks, although some patients may go into the extended care unit and remain up to a year. That unknowing fear can be a great stress factor in the rehabilitation. Most of them want to make their confinement as short as possible, but occasionally one will find a patient who has found Hazelden a secure place away from reality and would prefer to stay there. Few patients fully realize the personal depths to which their treatment will take them. Within them are the anxieties, frustrations, worries and resentments which carried them to the chemical escape they so desperately needed. Many of these people for the first time in their lives are having to face feelings they have hidden for years.

Each patient is treated according to his own personal needs. An essential part of recovery is learning to communicate feelings. Informal group therapy sessions aid in this task. In these sessions, patients are forced through questioning by the group to open up about themselves and get their true feelings out. The group can become quite hard on a person, and it is natural for people to avoid making responses that get at their feelings.

Patients do not have a magic formula prescribed for them when they leave so that they will not go back to chemicals. But if treatment has been effective they have much more than magic, for they have gained a self-understanding which can lead to a fuller, happier life. The stresses and difficulties of daily living are always present, and this is where their belief in a higher power must be strong.

The Hazelden experience is extremely worthwhile in a personal and professional sense. All of us should be given the opportunity to look within ourselves. All who are involved in the "helping" professions deal with people every day who are leading themselves to the brink where they only have one other out, and that may be chemicals. Each of us must take responsibility for sharing our own feelings and accepting these feelings as real. In turn, the process of self-acceptance can then go forth to others. This then will become the process we should use in preventing chemical dependency.

Our concern becomes that of the "feeling" life of people. Levi N. Larson, Education Director, North Dakota State Department of Health, says the real hope of drug abuse prevention lies in meeting the emotional needs of people—the need to be loved, to be heard, to be understood, the need to share feelings, the need to have meaningful communication with other people. Responding to these needs is how we get people off drugs. In doing this sooner lies the hope of keeping them from "getting on" drugs.

Alcohol Education

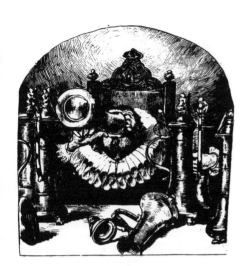

How Much Can I Drink?

H. RICHARD TRAVIS is assistant professor of health science, James Madison University, Harrisonburg, Virginia 22802.

I teach drug education courses and frequently, when discussing alcohol, students will ask how much a person can drink before being considered drunk. I point out that there are many variables that influence the extent to which an individual will be affected by alcohol.

1. Some people are affected more than others because of their biochemical make-up.

2. The attitude or mood of the individual at the time of drinking as well as the environment in which alcohol is drunk influence the effect.

3. Food and liquid in the stomach dilute the alcohol and slow down its absorption.

4. The carbon dioxide in carbonated alcoholic beverages tends to hasten the movement of the alcohol from the stomach through the pylorus to the small intestine where the majority of alcohol is absorbed.

5. The blood alcohol level reached in the body is related to the individual's body weight. A larger person has more body fluids and blood to dilute alcohol than a smaller person. The more alcohol in the blood, the more that can diffuse into the cells of the body. Most states set 0.1% as the blood alcohol level at which a person is considered legally drunk.

A number of charts are available in textbooks or from state divisions of motor vehicles which relate the number of drinks a person consumes to weight

and subsequent blood alcohol level. I use the following chart to have students calculate what their blood alcohol level might be after a certain number of drinks and the number of minutes since they first started drinking. Most students know their body weight, but if not, a scale can be brought into the room for them. They follow these steps to figure their blood alcohol level.

1. Emphasize that this chart is a guide and not a guarantee. Remind the class of the variables that have been listed.

2. If your weight is between two of those shown on the chart, use the lower weight.

3. On the chart, look up the blood alcohol level associated with your weight and the number of drinks that would have been drunk during a certain time period. One drink equals 12 ounces of beer, or 5 ounces of wine, or 1½ ounces of 80–100 proof whiskey.

4. Write down the blood alcohol level from

5. Write down the total number of minutes that would have elapsed between starting to drink and leaving the party, e.g., two hours or 120 minutes.

6. The liver is continuously metabolizing alcohol so we have to make a subtraction from the blood alcohol level from the chart depending upon how long we have been drinking. The correction factor is calculated by first dividing the total number of drinking minutes into 40 minute segments and then multiplying that answer by .01%. This is the correction factor for the alcohol that is metabolized by the liver.

7. Subtract the correction figure from the blood alcohol level that we obtained from the chart in step three. This is the approximate

blood alcohol level after a certain number of drinks in a certain time period.

8. Refer to the chart to see what the effects of this blood alcohol level might be.

The following example illustrates the steps.

A 180-pound person consumes 4 drinks in two hours.

Steps 3 & 4: .083 blood alcohol level from the chart.

Step 5: 2 hours = 120 minutes.

Step 6: (a) $\dfrac{\text{total \# of drinking minutes}}{40 \text{ minutes}} = a$

$a = \dfrac{120 \text{ minutes}}{40} = 3$

(b) $a \times .01\% = $ correction figure for liver metabolism of alcohol
$3 \times .01\% = .03\%$

Step 7:   .083 blood alcohol level from the chart
  − .030 correction for liver metabolism for alcohol

  .053 estimated blood alcohol level for 180-pound person drinking 4 drinks in 2 hours.

Step 8: The chart indicates that at .05 driving becomes increasingly dangerous.

This activity has been used in the classroom and was also set up as a booth for a campus-wide alcohol awareness day. The students found this a meaningful way to estimate how many drinks they could have and the relationship this would have to their blood alcohol level.

Blood alcohol levels (percentage)

Body Weights	Drinks[a]											
	1	2	3	4	5	6	7	8	9	10	11	12
100 lbs.	.038	.075	.113	.150	.188	.225	.263	.300	.338	.375	.413	.450
120 lbs.	.031	.063	.094	.125	.156	.188	.219	.250	.281	.313	.344	.375
140 lbs.	.027	.054	.080	.107	.134	.161	.188	.214	.241	.268	.295	.321
160 lbs.	.023	.047	.070	.094	.117	.141	.164	.188	.211	.234	.258	.281
180 lbs.	.021	.042	.063	.083	.104	.125	.146	.167	.188	.208	.229	.250
200 lbs.	.019	.038	.056	.075	.094	.113	.131	.150	.169	.188	.206	.225
220 lbs.	.017	.034	.051	.068	.085	.102	.119	.136	.153	.170	.188	.205
240 lbs.	.016	.031	.047	.063	.078	.094	.109	.125	.141	.156	.172	.188

Under .05	.05 to 0.10	.10 to .15	Over .15
Driving is not seriously impaired (although some research indicates fine motor skills may be impaired at .02 or .03 level)	Driving becomes increasingly dangerous .08 is legally drunk in Utah	Driving is dangerous Legally drunk in most states	Driving is very dangerous Legally drunk in any state

[a]One drink equals 1 ounce of 80–100 proof liquor or 12 ounces of beer or 5 ounces of wine.
Reference: New Jersey Department of Law and Public Safety, Division of Motor Vehicles, Trenton, New Jersey.

Drinking Myths

Alcohol Education

A guided tour through folklore, fantasy, humbug & hogwash

By Joe Dolan
Senior Program Manager
Operation *Threshold*

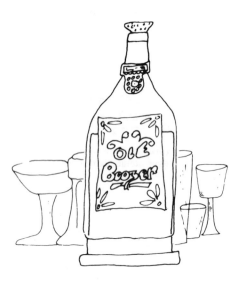

Why bother to de-bunk a bunch of harmless myths about drinking? Because they're not so harmless.

For instance? If a guy thinks it's okay to smash down 8 or 10 beers every night because "it's only beer" . . . he could develop a serious drinking problem without even knowing it.

We have nine million alcoholic Americans. It's become a national plague. Yet in some other societies, where they don't share our misconceptions about drinking, alcoholism is rare.

So the more we know about drinking, the better we can handle it. The better we can decide whether, where, when, why, how much, and with whom to drink.

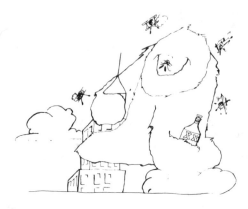

The really serious problem in our society is drug abuse. Right. And our number one drug problem is alcohol abuse. About 300,000 Americans are addicted to heroin. But about 9,000,000 are addicted to alcohol. It's not even close.

"I drive better after a few drinks." In most states, the legal definition of "driving under the influence" is a blood alcohol level of 0.10%. But scientific tests have proven that even professional drivers' abilities diminish sharply at levels as low as 0.03% to 0.05% . . . just a few drinks. Not only that, but judgment is affected, too. So people think they're driving better than ever while they're really driving worse.

All that publicity about drinking and driving is . . . True. At least half the fatal highway accidents involve drinking.

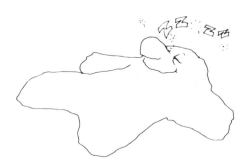

Alcohol is a stimulant. It's about as good a stimulant as ether. Alcohol acts as a depressant on the central nervous system.

Very few women become alcoholic. In the 1950's, there were 5 or 6 alcoholic men to every woman. Now the ratio is about 3 to 1. Evidently this is one area where women's liberation is catching on too well.

People are friendlier when they're drunk. Maybe. But they're also more hostile, more dangerous, more criminal, more homicidal and more suicidal. Half of all murders are alcohol-related. And one third of all suicides.

People get drunk . . . or sick . . . from switching drinks. That shouldn't really make much difference. What usually causes an adverse reaction to alcohol is drinking too much.

It's rude to refuse a drink. Nonsense. What's rude is trying to push a drink on someone who doesn't want it or shouldn't have it .

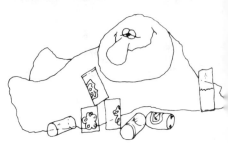

"Ya gotta hand it to Joe. He can really hold his liquor." Don't envy Joe. Often the guy who can hold so much is developing a "tolerance" for alcohol. And tolerance can be a polite word for need.

Your kids will learn what you tell them about drinking. Ha ha. Your kids will learn what you show them about drinking. If you drink heavily; if you get drunk; the chances are your kids will follow the same example.

People who drink too much hurt only themselves. And their families. And their friends, and their employers, and strangers on the highway. And you.

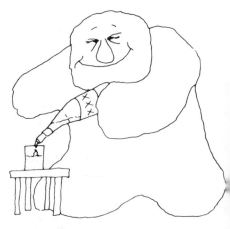

A good host never lets a guest's glass get empty. There's nothing hospitable about pushing alcohol or any other drug. A good host doesn't want his guests to get drunk or sick. He wants them to have a good time . . . and remember it the next day.

It's impolite to tell a friend he's drinking too much. Maybe if we weren't all so "polite," we wouldn't have so many friends with drinking problems.

"What a man! Still on his feet after a whole fifth." When we stop thinking it's manly to drink too much, we have begun to grow up. It's no more manly to over-drink than it is to over-eat.

If the parents don't drink, the children won't drink. Sometimes. But the highest incidence of alcoholism occurs among offspring of parents who are either teetotalers . . . or alcoholic. Perhaps the "extremism" of the parents' attitudes is an important factor.

You're not an alcoholic unless you drink a pint a day. There's no simple rule of thumb. Experts have concluded that how much one drinks may be far less important than when he drinks, how he drinks and why he drinks.

Alcoholism is just a state of mind. It's more than that. It's a very real illness, and there is scientific evidence that physiological dependence is involved.

The "Drunk Tank" is a good cure for alcoholism. Nonsense. Alcoholism is an illness, and can be treated successfully. We don't jail people for other illnesses. Why for alcoholism?

The first round should be a "double" to break the ice. Breaking the ice is a job for a good host or hostess . . . not for a bottle. You must have more to "give" your guests than just alcohol.

Mixing your drinks causes hangovers. The major cause of hangovers is drinking too much. Period.

Most alcoholics are skid row bums. Only 3% to 5% are. Most alcoholic people (about 70%) are married, employed, regular people. All kinds of people.

Operation Threshold

A national major-emphasis program of the United States Jaycees for 1974-75, Operation THRESHOLD is designed to create awareness and understanding about responsible drinking, irresponsible drinking, and the illness of alcoholism. It provides Jaycees and the American people with guidelines about sensible drinking practices, habits, attitudes, and behavior and gives attention to the nature and scope of alcohol misuse and alcoholism in American society. The U.S. Jaycees, in 6,700 chapters across the country, are undertaking a multitude of activities and projects to help create this new understanding about alcohol problems: youth programs and community health seminars are included in this extensive effort. For further information, contact your local Jaycees or the Alcohol Program Manager, U.S. Jaycees, Box 7, Tulsa, Oklahoma 74102.

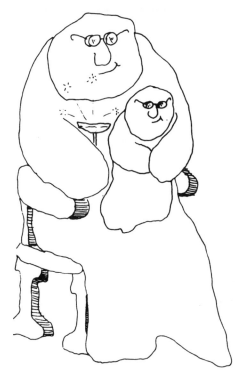

The time to teach kids about drinking is when they reach legal age. By that time, they've long since learned what we can teach them. Like it or not, we teach our kids from birth. And they learn more from what they see us do than from what they hear us tell them.

Give him black coffee. That'll sober him up. Sure, in about five hours. Cold showers don't work either. Only time can get the alcohol out of the system, as the liver metabolizes the alcohol. Slowly. There's no way to hurry it.

Drug? Drug. Alcohol is a drug, all right. It you don't believe it, ask your doctor.

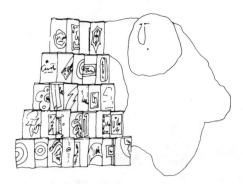

"It's only beer." Sure. Just like it's only bourbon, or vodka or gin. One beer or one glass of wine is about equal to one average "highball." The effect might be a little slower, but you'll get just as drunk on beer or wine as on "hard" liquor.

Today's kids don't drink. Sorry, but the generation gap is greatly exaggerated. The kids' favorite drug is the same as their parents' favorite: alcohol. And drinking problems are rising among the young.

Most alcoholic people are middle-aged or older. A University of California research team has found that the highest proportion of drinking problems is among men in their early twenties. The second highest incidence occurs among men in their 40's and 50's.

Thank God my kid isn't on drugs! If he's hooked on drinking, he's on drugs. With nine million Americans dependent on alcohol, it's time we stopped pretending it isn't a drug.

Most skid row bums are alcoholics. No. See? You just can't count on stereotypes. A recent study found that less than half the derelicts on skid row had drinking problems.

Drinking is a sexual stimulant. Contrary to popular belief, the more you drink, the less your sexual capacity. Alcohol may stimulate interest in sex, but it interferes with the ability to perform.

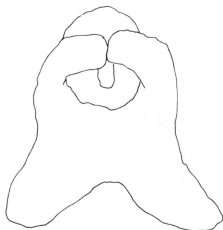

"I don't know any alcoholics." Maybe you just don't know you know any alcoholics. Some of your best friends may have drinking problems. They don't seem "different." And they usually try to hide their illness, even from themselves. About 1 of every 10 executives has a drinking problem.

Getting drunk is funny. Maybe in the old Charlie Chaplin movies . . . but not in real life. Drunkenness is no funnier than any other illness or incapacity.

Never trust a man who never takes a drink. You know that's silly. Yet many of us are a little nervous around people who don't drink.

Alcohol Education and the Pleasures of Drinking

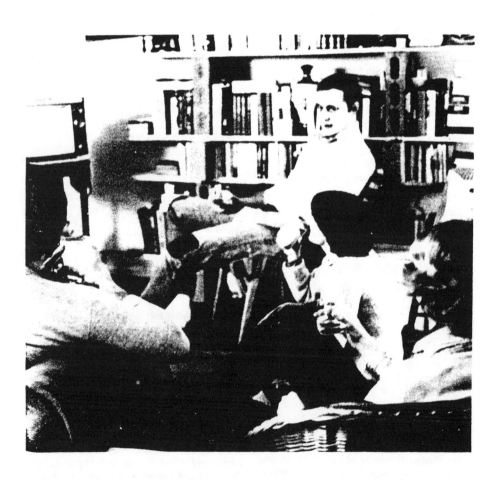

In the past several years numerous pamphlets, books, and curriculum manuals have been developed on alcohol education for use by teachers and students. Several of these resources provide thoroughly objective information about the physical and behavioral effects of alcohol, the uses of alcohol throughout history, and the nature of problem drinking. The best of them recognize that the decision whether to drink or not to drink is up to the individual.

However, most of these materials fail to communicate adequately the significant ways in which alcohol gives pleasure. The introductory or sporadic observations of how alcohol helps people to relax and improves a meal tend to be perfunctory, only pallidly reflecting the enjoyment a majority of Americans experience when they drink.

This imbalance in most of the educational literature between alcohol's pleasures and perils is reflected in how educators commonly teach about drinking. For a variety of reasons, many political as well as educational, teachers focus overwhelmingly on the dangers of alcohol abuse and very little on the satisfactions of alcohol use.

We promote alcohol education because abusive drinking *is* a major problem—certainly one of the most serious half-dozen health problems in America. We naturally, therefore, center most of our attention on the destructive side of drinking, not its troublefree aspects. However, precisely because alcohol abuse is a crisis of astonishing magnitude in this country, we need to

PETER FINN is senior education and training analyst for ABT Associates Inc., 55 Wheeler Street, Cambridge, Massachusetts 02138.

devote more time in our educational literature and classrooms to exploring why and how people enjoy its use.

Rationale for Stressing the Pleasures of Drinking

Most youngsters know very well that a majority of Americans from the age of 14 on find drinking pleasurable. As a result, when educators fail to discuss this enjoyment at some length, they risk losing a student's confidence in the trustworthiness of what they have to say about alcohol *abuse*. If instructors can cavalierly dismiss the delights of drinking, they are liable with equal glibness to exaggerate the dangers. Even if students pursue their study of problem drinking in independent research projects, they may suspect that the persons the teacher encourages them to interview and the suggested literature have been selected to conform to the teacher's apparently negative views about drinking. To ensure that students do believe what they hear, read, and see about the problems of alcohol abuse, teachers must initially secure their pupils' confidence in the objectivity of their curriculum. Gaining this trust requires paying immediate and unequivocal attention to the enjoyment of responsible alcohol use.

The goals of alcohol education are obviously to promote abstinence or responsible drinking. While we may stress the importance of promoting responsible decision making about alcohol use, there are, in fact, only two decisions which we consider responsible: not drinking and drinking in moderation. However, it is clear that most Americans have decided to drink on a fairly regular basis. Given this decision, one potentially effective method to help ensure that this inevitable drinking activity *is* moderate is to deliberately identify and reinforce as acceptable behavior a variety of responsible drinking patterns. Investigating the satisfactions of drinking can provide behavior models for students to emulate if they choose to drink—as 80% of them will.

In the absence of positive role models, many Americans, rather than abstain, will copy the numerous irresponsible drinking behaviors portrayed in many advertisements and in much of the media. These destructive role models associate drinking with masculinity, femininity, sexual prowess, maturity, peer approval, and comic relief. Since these irresponsible drinking behaviors are portrayed to the public in greater abundance and with greater impact than exemplars of responsible alcohol use, we will continue to encourage people to abuse alcohol.

Presenting the Pleasures of Drinking

Honestly presenting the pleasures of drinking means devoting adequate time to discussing and studying them and doing so with a positive attitude. Teachers need to encourage their students to spend a significant amount of time investigating the satisfactions drinking provides compared with the time allocated to exploring alcohol abuse. This "significant" time commitment will vary from class to class, but 20-30% of an entire alcohol unit is a reasonable guideline.

Although a teacher may begin an alcohol education unit by focusing on the enjoyment of drinking, some classes may want to move quickly into a study of alcohol abuse. When this occurs, the instructor can be guided by the students' concerns and switch to a study of alcohol abuse, but suggest that the class might want to resume its investigation of the pleasures of drinking later. What is essential for effective student learning about alcohol abuse is to begin the unit with the clear intention of thoroughly examining the enjoyment of drinking. That way, if students want to study alcohol abuse, the change in focus will occur after the class has realized that the teacher has an open mind about the delights of drinking and will not be presenting biased information about alcohol abuse.

It is also possible—indeed, extremely desirable—to encourage students to investigate both the pleasures and hazards of drinking simultaneously, in addition to focusing exclusively on drinking's gratifications at the beginning of the unit. When students are able to do this, they become better aware that alcohol always presents a double potential for pleasure and suffering, depending on how the drinking is conducted.

Honestly presenting the pleasures of drinking not only requires devoting adequate time to their study, it also presupposes a teacher who approaches the topic with a positive frame of mind. Often instructors discuss the pleasures of drinking begrudgingly or with considerable hedging—"Drinking can help many people to relax, but . . ." Teachers often qualify their descriptions of the pleasures of drinking not necessarily because they do not personally approve of responsible drinking, but they may be concerned about hostile community reactions. They may also feel that their students are too young to be drinking or too suggestible to know how to set limits on an enjoyable activity whose abuse is dangerous.

Another more complex problem from an educational point of view is that presenting drinking as normal and beneficial for a majority of adults may cause some students who are abstainers to assume that something is "wrong" with them and their families for failing to participate in such an apparently desirable activity. There are two educational strategies teachers can adopt which will help avoid potential community repercussions and student alienation resulting from a study of drinking's pleasures.

Teachers can avoid presenting the enjoyment of drinking as if it were a universal experience by using such phrasing as "*Many* people find that drinking . . ." and "Alcohol has the pleasurable effect for *some* drinkers of . . ." After three or four class discussions and other activities, the cumulative effect of such consistently guarded statements can help clarify that drinking is not an enjoyable or acceptable practice to millions of Americans, nor should we expect it to be.

After conducting class activities focusing on the pleasures of drinking, instructors should then discuss why 20-30 million teenagers and adults in America choose *not* to drink. The reasons for not drinking must be presented as being as sensible and acceptable as those given for why most people do drink. In this manner, instructors can provide a series of role models for *abstaining* students to emulate while at the same time clarify to the community that the school is seeking to promote responsible drinking only for those students who choose to drink.

Illustrations of the Pleasures of Drinking

Even when teachers agree that they need to present and have students explore the pleasures drinking gives most Americans, they often have difficulty defining those pleasures precisely and stating them objectively. While the many responsible uses of alcohol in this country preclude descriptions of all of them, instructors can present to students examples such as those shown in the box on page 50 and encourage them to investigate further.

Further Classroom Research

While the examples in the box may prove helpful in indicating what di-

Most people are confronted on a fairly regular basis with a variety of drinking questions, such as: "Care for a drink?"; "How about a beer after work?"; "Cocktails before dinner, sir?"; "Would you care for some wine with your meal?" These are all standard questions which are very much a part of life in America and which tell us a great deal about drinking in our country. Three out of four American adults drink at least a few times a year; many drink several times a week.

Strangely enough, however, many drinkers have to learn to like the taste of alcoholic beverages. When most people swallow their first sip they wonder what everybody who drinks sees in a glass of beer or a shot of hard liquor. Wine and liqueur seem to be the only major alcoholic beverages which are often enjoyed the first time they are tried. Many drinkers continue to delight in the taste of wine and liqueurs. For some families, wine with their meal is a pleasurable habit, like eating bread or dessert.

Once they get used to the taste of beer, countless drinkers also savor what to them is the unique ability of a cold beer to quench a strong thirst on a hot day or after strenuous exercise. These wine, liqueur, and beer tastes are flavors no non-alcoholic beverage can provide.

However, most drinkers never really drink because they like the taste of alcohol. After all, a Bloody Mary can be savored as well without the vodka in it. It's no accident that what has become the most popular hard liquor in America today, vodka, has no flavor at all. Most people drink because they like the effects alcohol has on them after they've swallowed it. Alcohol helps most drinkers relax, forget minor worries, relate to people better, have more fun.

Almost everyone spends part of many days feeling somewhat angry, sad, worried, or tense. People deal with these un-pleasant feelings in many ways, one of which is to have a drink. Many people find a beer or cocktail helps them unwind. At parties or social gatherings people think alcohol helps strangers strike up a conversation, listen to others, and make jokes.

Alcohol is also drunk by many people as part of a variety of special occasions in order to enliven things or to bring out the special importance of the event. Numerous people drink beer at ball games, champagne at weddings, mulled apple cider at Thanksgiving, and hot buttered rum after skiing. They are not drinking to enjoy themselves, they're already having a good time. They drink to heighten their pleasure and have an even better time. Drinking, in short, gives many people another chance to relate to each other in ways that promote and express friendship.

Enjoying alcohol for some people doesn't only mean drinking it. Some people also have fun cooking with alcoholic beverages, bartending at home, and becoming wine connoisseurs.

Marinating a meat in wine or using a liqueur to flavor a dessert can add elegance and festivity to a meal—as when a host places a dish of flaming cherries jubilee before a group of appreciative guests. There are also drinkers who take great pride in their talents as a home bartender. Creating new drinks, mixing "the best Brandy Alexander in town" and stocking "a really fine bar" can be enjoyable pastimes to them.

There are many amateur and true wine connoisseurs who enjoy sampling wine and going through the ritual of wine tasting. The amateurs may settle on a favorite wine for several months and recommend it to their friends until someone introduces them to another wine they like even better. In short, Americans find drinking a pleasant activity. Alcohol helps them feel good.

rections classroom discussions and activities on the enjoyment of drinking can take, there are also several other learning activities students can engage in which will further their understanding of how people find satisfaction in responsible drinking. Students can:

interview wine stewards in restaurants
interview moderate drinkers
attend and observe events at which responsible (as well as, perhaps, abusive) drinking takes place such as, bowling alleys, athletic contests, restaurants, social events
eat dinner with a family which serves wine with its meals
analyze television advertisements for alcoholic beverages
interview people who cook with alcohol, including chefs in restaurants and neighbors
read and analyze descriptions of moderate alcohol use in the Bible, mythology, and contemporary fiction and nonfiction
read and analyze humorous treatments of the enjoyment of drinking in newspaper cartoons and on greeting cards
interview parents or neighbors, asking what kinds of pleasure, if any, alcohol provides them
sample different wines according to cultured wine tasting methods
research the use of alcoholic beverages by different ethnic groups.

The combination of an objective presentation by the teacher and appropriate followup activities on the pleasures of drinking can help ensure that students will move on to study alcohol's dangers, ready to accept open-mindedly whatever negative conclusions the evidence warrants. Students will be much less likely to discount what they learn because it came from a biased instructor who has distorted the facts or who has made available only highly selective followup activities for students.

Alcohol education must begin to face the challenge of presenting alcohol use and abuse in a balanced framework which does not obscure the pervasive reality of responsible and enjoyable drinking in America. Only if we start with an honest recognition and thorough exploration of our culturally approved patterns of responsible drinking will we be able to deal with the enormous social, economic, and health problems alcohol abuse inflicts on problem drinkers and nonproblem drinkers alike.

Alcohol educators have normally attempted to counteract harmful drinking role models by focusing exclusively on the hazards of alcohol abuse. What is needed is a concurrent effort of equal magnitude which presents and reinforces positive drinking role models.

Take the Same Concepts...

If you were to glance through the doorways of our three fourth-grade classrooms at Lincoln Elementary school, you'd probably be unaware that we three teachers were teaching the *same* health unit, with content from the *same* health guide, and using many identical teaching aids.

Children at this age are fascinated by, "What's going on inside me?" Boys and girls alike are interested in building muscles and participating in active sports. Our anatomy and physiology units begin in fourth grade with an overview of the basic body systems and with special emphasis on the muscular and skeletal systems. The fifth and sixth grades follow with in-depth studies of the other systems.

The three of us (fourth grade teachers) do some preliminary planning together and order films and materials which all three classes might use. As we begin teaching this unit we begin with similar introductions. Each student is given an outline of the human body on which to draw anything he knows or thinks about his body. These drawings illustrate a wide variation in knowledge and point out many misconceptions held by the students. Hearts are generally of the heart-shaped valentine variety. With the exception of the stomach, few internal organs appear. The brain is generally somewhere on the drawing, not necessarily near the head. One drawing, I remember, had three separate

JOYCE SWAN is a fourth grade teacher at the Lincoln Elementary School, 200 S. Sampson St., Ellensburg, Washington 98926.

kidney-shaped masses neatly labeled as Brain #1, Brain #2, and Brain #3. These drawings are kept and returned to the student as part of the final evaluation of the unit. They always produce a few laughs from the students and comments like, "Oh, no! Did I really think that?" After this introduction, each teacher follows a distinctly different approach.

The Integrative Approach

Pat Legg, in Room 11, has a strong background in the sciences. She uses an approach which I call "integrative" as she relates the study of anatomy and physiology to all other areas of study. In creative writing the children give names to such things as blood cells, bones, or muscles. They then write imaginative stories telling of the journey of "Red" Corpuscle through the body. They may begin or end the journey wherever they choose as long as they explain what "Red" does at each stop or intersection. A child who may have suffered a broken bone or a torn muscle may choose to use a topic such as, "I am Jim's kneecap, etc." to explain the mending process.

Throughout the day's activities, Pat asks her class to relate their activities to the current study. In gym class during the warm-up activities they examine questions such as: "What are we warming up?" and "Why?" Nutrition is related to the foods which build bones or muscles. Involuntary muscular reaction and stress of muscles are related to an earlier unit on mental health.

For science activities, Pat obtains animal hearts from the local slaughter house. They first identify the functions of the heart as an organ. She dissects the organ in order that the muscle tissue may be examined and, finally, prepares slides so the pupils may look for the individual cells.

Emphasis on Music and Drama

In Room 9 on my left, Lorraine Guthrie approaches the same unit of study with an emphasis on music and dramatic activities. The students learn to sing "Dry Bones" while studying the skeletal system, clarifying *shin* and *chin* in the process. The children write poems using facts which they have learned about the body. These poems are then set to simple musical tunes for their song flutes (another fourth grade activity).

Dramatic play situations are created by Mrs. Guthrie. The pupils choose roles and portray the parts of the body as if the body were a city. The brain is usually the mayor. The student actors

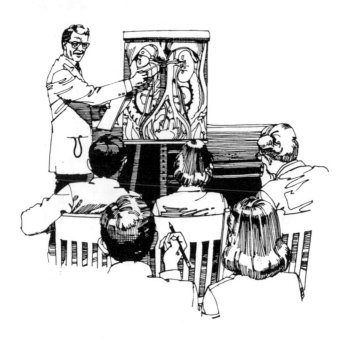

playing blood carry food and oxygen around town. Food is likened to fuel and is dispensed by the service station operator. "Nervy," the local telephone operator, completes your call—unless you have a loose connection.

The Building Block Approach

Now, back in Room 10, my own approach is still different since I'm definitely not musical and do not have a strong science background. I call mine the "building block" approach. The emphasis is upon art activities and visual aids. We compare the body to a machine which has certain specific needs and interdependent parts.

We begin by making our own models, from soft, reusable clay, of a model of the basic cell. Here we note the similarities basic to all cell structures. The differences in shapes and functions are next noted by building individual cells whose functions differ; some build a muscle cell, others blood cells, and still others nerve cells. The child next chooses a particular cell, makes several of one

kind, and joins them, forming a tissue. Next the tissue cells are added to until the child had built a single organ. Each child then makes a large diagram of the system into which his particular organ (the clay model) fits to explain the purpose of the system and the role which the organ plays in the system.

As my pupils examine each system they become aware of the interdependence between systems. The inept floppiness of the skeleton model often inspires warning placards such as, "He should have eaten his spinach" or, with a lunch straw protruding appropriately from his jaws, the warning, "This one smoked a pack a day."

By using the same soft clay to model the various joints, students compare hinge, ball and socket, and gliding joints. They are able to identify joints on their own bodies by observing the clay models.

We use tracing paper and colored pencils to produce overlays illustrating the special protective purposes of skeletal parts. The ribs can surround the lungs with overlays, the brain can be inside the skull, and the spinal cord inside the vertebrae.

As part of a review and evaluation my pupils write riddles. They may choose any part of the body which has been studied. They are considered successful if they give information which produces recognition by most of their classmates. The following is an example in which the child described a nerve cell:

I am a kind of cell.
I never get to have any children.
I could have lived to be 100 years old.
I got cut and killed.
I used to send messages.
It's no fun sitting here dead while all the cells around me are still alive.

We three teachers took the same concepts. Then we each added something of ourselves and our own individual personalities which resulted in three differing approaches. As long as teachers are free, as we obviously were, to approach the subject matter from their special vantage points, teaching will remain enjoyable. And—I believe—so will learning.

Ernie

LILLIAN D. FESPERMAN is a graduate assistant in health and physical education, Miami University, Oxford, Ohio 45056.

Are you tired of teaching digestion, respiration, circulation, the body systems and functions the same way year after year, class after class? Or are you an inexperienced teacher looking for a new approach for old, unchanging yet vital material? In either case, here is a successful, exciting, beneficial solution which can motivate your students.

When I was teaching health at Alexander Graham Junior High School in Charlotte, North Carolina, I was a first year teacher willing to try just about anything that would motivate my students. I had to present a unit on the systems of the body and wanted to try a new, creative approach. After evaluating possibilities, I came up with the idea of constructing a body in class.

Selling my idea to the students was extremely easy and well-received; everyone wanted to "build a body." We first got basic background information on the systems of the body and gathered our ideas and materials for building a body. We included five systems—digestive, skeletal, respiratory, circulatory, and nervous—on our body. Since there were five seventh grade health classes, each class contributed one system to the body.

Information about systems was covered in class by a series of handouts, lectures, discussions, pictures, and films. Students were required to keep a notebook related to the systems which they handed in at the end of the unit. To further instill interest in the students, as we discussed the systems I mentioned ideas and suggestions about the body that we could try. We all knew we were working to gather enough information to construct a life-size body out of a variety of "raw" materials.

After completing the general background information, a system was assigned to each class and that class was responsible for bringing in any materials related to their system. They were also required to read books and study pictures and charts related to their systems. Specific tasks were assigned to small groups, who worked together to make their particular system fit into the body.

The skeletal system included the pelvic bone, upper and lower bones of the arms, finger bones, upper and lower leg bones, the kneecap, the sternum, collarbone, and back vertebrae. The nervous system had the brain and spinal cord, and nerves. Our digestive system was made up of the tongue and esophagus, spleen, liver, stomach, small intestine, large intestine, and the rectum. The nasal cavity, trachea, bronchial tubes, and lungs (one open and one closed) with alveoli were the

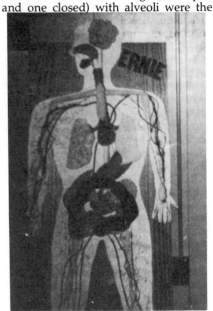

"Ernie", created by seventh grade students.

parts of the respiratory system. The circulatory system consisted of the heart, aorta, large and small veins, and arteries.

We needed a base on which to mount our body parts. After considering the possibilities of cardboard, wood and other hard material, we decided to use a big sheet of plywood so we could attach the organs and have them stay in place. The plywood (about 5' by 3') was supplied by one student's parents. We cut out a body frame from paper, glued it onto the plywood and started assembling organs and parts.

The materials brought in by the classes for use included chicken bones, styrofoam of all sizes and shapes, sponges, thread of assorted colors, wire and plastic-coated wires of various colors and sizes, clay, newspaper, paints, cardboard cylinders, empty thread spools, balloons, nails, cloth scrap, glue, and toothpicks.

We made some of our bones out of sticks covered with papier maché, and others with styrofoam cut into the shapes of the bones we wanted. The bones were attached to the body frame first along with the trachea, which we made from a cardboard cylinder wrapped in yarn for the cartilage, and the bronchial tubes, which were made from clay. The digestive system was then attached. The tongue was a small, semi-inflated balloon; the esophagus was a small cardboard tube fitted inside the trachea. The stomach and large intestines were papier maché wrapped over blown up balloons. The balloons were then deflated and the papier maché organs cut in half to make a flat surface to mount on the plywood body. The small intestine, liver, and spleen were made out of clay which was dried and painted, then nailed or glued onto the frame. The nasal cavity was cardboard cut into shape, the bronchial tubes were clay, and the lungs were styrofoam. One lung was painted as if it were closed, the other lung was constructed as if it were open. The capillaries were drawn with magic marker and little pieces of sponge glued on it to show the alveoli.

The heart was made by cutting the shape out of a thick sponge, with veins and arteries drawn into it. The pulmonary vein and artery and the aorta were inserted into the sponge with big red and blue wires. From the heart came red and blue arteries and veins made from wire and thread. Veins and arteries not made of wire or thread were drawn on the body with red and blue pens. The nervous system was done with various colored wires for the nerves leading all through the body to the fingers and feet. The spinal cord was made of yellow yarn leading from the brain, which was a piece of plastic cauliflower since the bumps and shape were similar. We cut the cauliflower to make a flat back surface to fit onto the frame. It was definitely an authentic-looking part of the body.

All of the parts were either glued, taped, or nailed into place on the body frame. The bones were mounted first with the trachea, esophagus, and bronchial tubes. Then the lungs, heart, and digestive system was fitted into place. The veins, arteries, and nerves were intertwined into place last, making our body complete. The classes then named our project body "Ernie."

Other suggestions for materials that we did not include in our project that could be added to yours are a mop for hair, or maybe garden hose for intestines. Or how about bottle caps or ping-pong balls for eyes? Other ideas may be to use false teeth or plastic ears to make your body more complete.

The project was stimulating and interesting to the students. The students responsible for making system parts and placing them onto the body also had to explain the operations of the organ or part. They benefited greatly from this project by learning about the human body and working together and had fun doing it. It is an excellent idea to try in your own classroom. Why not create your own "Ernie"?

AN ELEMENTARY FITNESS PROGRAM THAT WORKS

Running for Life is designed to increase childrens' fitness while improving their knowledge of academic subjects. The fitness components most affected are cardiovascular efficiency and body composition. The major cognitive component is geography, although math, reading, and science can be incorporated into the program.

The most popular approach to Running for Life is to organize it as a low level competition between teams. The teams provide motivation for the exercise component. Competition can be conducted within a particular grade level or the entire student population. The latter can be accomplished by organizing each class into three or more color teams, e.g., red, white, and blue. Each team will have children from every grade level. The mixed grade team approach, however, does not provide as much motivation as the intragrade competition.

Whichever method is used, however, the exercise is the same. After a preconditioning period of at least three weeks, children are supervised by the classroom teacher for daily 20-minute periods in which they attempt to see how many laps they can complete by running, walking or a combination of the two. Wheelchair-bound students can wheel themselves or be pushed by a classmate with both pusher and wheeler getting credit for each lap. To count laps, give a token to the child as he or she crosses the start/finish line. The distance around the track can be any length as long as it remains constant for every child. After 20 minutes, each child records his laps. The class's total laps are used to calculate the distance traveled.

The laps are converted to meters and used to plot progress on a map. To convert to meters, divide the total team laps by a number selected by the program director. The size of the number determines how fast the team will progress. The same number must be applied to all teams. For example, the total weekly laps for three teams are: red—345,

Robert G. Davis is an associate professor of physical education at Virginia Commonwealth University.

white—283, blue—240. Using a conversion number of 15, each team total is divided with the following results: red—23 meters, white—19 meters, blue—16 meters. Progress would then be marked on a map. If the director wished to move the teams more quickly, a lower conversion number would be used. The same divisor must always be used in recording any weekly total but can be changed from week to week during the program to speed up or slow down all teams' progress.

Although the program director is usually a physical educator, the program is conducted by the classroom teacher, but not during physical education time. Since the program requires a minimum of three workouts per week and physical educators traditionally see children only once a week, it would not be possible for the specialist to supervise the running. It should also be emphasized that fitness is only one aspect of physical education and other appropriate physical education activities should be taught by both the specialist and the classroom teacher.

Geography is the classroom focus of Running for Life. A 4' × 6' map of the United States is displayed in a prominent area of the school. The starting point for the race can be the childrens' hometown or they can begin on one side of the country and progress across it. Map tape is used to mark progress (determined by converting laps to meters). As teams cross into states or time zones, various subjects such as terraine, weather, or information about a particular state can be discussed. Math can also be integrated into the discussion by having the children calculate average speed, distance traveled, or other math problems. If Running for Life is a schoolwide program, a K–5 geography curriculum should be developed to avoid redundancy over the years.

Some innovative ideas have been generated by those who have already participated in Running for Life. At one school, children got pen pals from their ultimate destination and discussed their progress through an exchange of letters.

In another instance, teachers shared vacation slides from various states. In another program children ran to states famous for various fruits, e.g., the Georgia peach. No matter which team arrived in the state first, everyone went to the cafeteria to have a piece of the fruit.

The activity can also be varied by using maps of the world or perhaps the universe, creating opportunities for discussions about oceans, tides, rivers, cities of the world, etc. Music, art and dance, could be incorporated by discussing and participating in the cultural activities of other countries. Program variety would keep childrens' interest over the years.

Running laps can get boring, so to keep interest, goals must not be too long term. Around Thanksgiving children can run to Massachusetts and have their Thanksgiving meal. From Thanksgiving to Christmas children can run to the North Pole. The cross country run seems to work best in the spring and can last six to eight weeks (not including the three weeks of preconditioning) without losing participants' interest.

As an alternative to lap running, credit can be given for a certain amount of aerobic activity such as aerobic dance, rope jumping, and/or continuous running or vigorous walking anywhere around the playground. Progress then can be determined by converting aerobic points to meters as with laps. The program might be called The Lifetime Aerobics Program or Aerobicing Along.

No matter which organization pattern is selected, the goal is to improve childrens' fitness. Developing positive attitudes toward and participation in aerobic activities is essential to the health of all youth. Research results are quite clear on the positive effects of reasonable exercise on the growth and development of children, but the attitudinal effects of individual exercise programs must be evaluated. Running for Life has been studied to determine the participants' attitudes toward the various components. A researcher, using an anonymous questionnaire, found that children, teachers and administrators expressed very positive attitudes toward all aspects of the program.

STORYTELLING: AN AID TO INTRODUCING CPR IN THE ELEMENTARY GRADES

Storytelling has been used for centuries as a pedagogical technique. It provides elementary school children an opportunity to experience living language. The teacher can relate experience or knowledge which creates a picture in the mind of the student. Since students are listening, and not reading, they may focus better on the content of the story.

The following story can be used to introduce the topic of cardiopulmonary resuscitation (CPR) to elementary students. While reading the story, the teacher needs to be simple and direct, change his/her voice, and use gestures to express a point. The teacher should know the story well enough to tell it in his/her own language and make sure he/she is talking on the children's level. As with all learning experiences, an opportunity should be provided for follow-up activities emanating from the story. This particular story should stimulate many questions which can be used to initiate a unit on CPR. A glossary and references are provided for the teacher.

The Story

Once upon a time a little Indian girl was born in Aneurysm, Oklahoma. When she was born her heartbeat was so strong and healthy she was called Little Red Flowing Blood. One day Li'l Red ventured out on her very first shopping trip. First she had to stop off at the neighborhood blood bank to cash a check. As she pushed her way through the revolving valves, who should she see but her fat neighbor, Mr. O.B. Sity. Lo and behold, he was carrying a large sack of coins with his blubbery biceps. Li'l Red just could not believe her eyes and cried out, "Mr. Sity! Fat men like you

Vicki Cleaver is an assistant professor in the HPER Department, 119 Huston Huffman Center, University of Oklahoma, Norman, Oklahoma 73019.

should not be doing such hard work. Your heart has enough strain on it already without carrying such a heavy load." All of a sudden Mr. O.B. Sity broke out into a cold sweat and started getting pains in his chest and left shoulder. The pain was too much for him and he fell to the floor. A passing policeman entered and shouted, "You're under cardiac arrest!" "Oh, poor Mr. Sity! I knew he should have been watching his weight and exercising. He just wasn't in good enough shape."

Li'l Red Flowing Blood cashed her check and wished all the people a hearty farewell. As she was walking down the sidewalk she thought to herself, "Just last week I was reading in the *Daily Aneurysm* that 650,000 people die from heart attacks each year and 350,000 of them occur outside the hospital." As she approached the corner, the light turned red and she stopped next to a man smoking one cigarette after another. His name was Nic O. Tine. Li'l Red thought to herself, "If only Mr. Tine realized that smoking doubles the chance of him having a heart attack and besides he just celebrated his fifty-fifth birthday which is the prime age for having a heart attack!" As the light turned green, Nic said something to Li'l Red but she could not understand him because of his shortness of breath. So she moved closer and asked him to repeat himself, but before he could speak he became very sick. Li'l Red was afraid because she liked Mr. Tine and wanted him to be well. Suddenly she remembered her first aid class at school. "I should remain calm and send someone for help. While I am waiting for the ambulance to come, I will keep Mr. Tine in a comfortable semi-reclining position." Mr. Tine kept saying that he was not having a heart attack, but Li'l Red expected him to say that.

"I was not a bit surprised that he would deny it because the teacher said we should expect this from a person having a heart attack." The ambulance soon arrived and because of her quick action and first aid training, Li'l Red helped Mr. Nic O. Tine survive.

Li'l Red walked around the corner and climbed on her red bicycle. As she started riding down the street she heard a yell from Sue Crose, a diabetic friend. She asked Li'l Red if she could have a ride to the corner Candy Store. "Why, Sue, don't you know that sugar isn't good for your diabetic condition? And besides, don't you know walking is the best exercise for your heart—you should walk at least three times a week! I'm sorry, I won't give you a ride!"

As Li'l Red started to leave she noticed Sue had fallen onto the sidewalk. Li'l Red jumped off the bike and ran to her. "What's wrong! What's wrong!" She said, "I feel very weak and my chest hurts." Then she fainted and stopped breathing and her heart wasn't beating. Li'l Red remembered cardiopulmonary resuscitation (CPR). "First, I'll shake Sue and see if I can wake her up. If I can't, I'll open her mouth, tilt her head back, and see if she's breathing. If not, I'll give her four quick breaths. Then I'll check again to see if this helped her start breathing and heart start beating again. Since I am alone, I will give her fifteen chest compressions to every two breaths. If someone comes by, I will get them to help me by giving her five chest compressions to every one breath I give her."

Little Red Flowing Blood did the right thing and saved Sue's life. Later, Li'l Red's tribe rewarded her quick actions and agreed that heart attack knowledge was strong medicine.

Resources

Note: The following materials are available through the American Heart Association.

Cardiopulmonary Resuscitation—Self Instructional Program (9 workbooks/sets) 70-025-A, B, C, D

Cardiopulmonary Resuscitation—Basic Life Support Slide/Tape Series (383 slides and 5 cassette tapes) 70-026-A, E, H

CPR in Basic Life Support 70-023-E

CPR in Basic Life Support—Wall Chart 77-006-A

Heart Attack: Signals and Actions for Survival (Booklet) 70-039-A

Manual for Instructor-Trainers and Instructors of Basic Cardiac Life Support (100 pages) 70-024-B

First Aid for Choking (leaflet)-70-051-A

First Aid for Choking (poster)-77-005-A

Take Care of Yourself

The Grade 6 of the School Health Curriculum Project titled *Our Health and Our Hearts* uses the heart as a focus for health education activities. The unit is approximately 13 weeks long and involves a complete teacher training component. The activities described below are part of that unit. The "Take Care of Yourself" lesson is conducted after students have experienced other activities aimed at helping them understand risk factors related to the heart and circulation. This lesson is designed to be positive, emphasizing prevention. The major concept and instructional objective relating to the lesson have also been indicated.

Major Concept

Problems concerning the heart and circulatory system may be lessened with preventive methods and proper health care.

Objective

The student identifies reliable resources concerning prevention, care and information about heart and circulatory problems and diseases.

Lesson

1. DISCUSSION: Where Can You Get Help?

Conduct a short discussion concerning the need to know where to get reliable help and care when problems of the heart and arteries arise. Also, explain the importance of finding someone to talk to concerning these problems.

Kathleen Middleton is Director of Curriculum for the School Health Education Project, National Center for Health Education, 901 Sneath Lane, Suite 215, San Bruno, California 94066. The Project is funded by the Center for Health Promotion and Education under Contract No. 200-81-0610 Centers for Disease Control, Public Health Serivce. Project Officers are Mr. Roy Davis and Ms. Beth Layson.

QUESTIONS:

a. What are some of the ways people obtain information about problems of the heart and circulatory system? (They might find out from their doctor, from family and friends, from reading about these things in newspapers, magazines and books, from informational programs on TV or from health agencies.)

b. Who are some people that could be consulted if someone wants help or information about health problems? (doctors, nurses, health educators, pharmacists, counselors, health agency personnel)

c. Who should be contacted in case of an emergency such as chest pain and other signs of possible heart attack? (Call the fire department or paramedics first, then call the doctor.)

Teacher Resource Materials: Pamphlet—*Heart Attack* from the American Heart Association

2. ROLE PLAY: Take Care of Yourself

a. Set up a role play situation concerning high blood pressure. Choose 7 students to participate. This participation should be *voluntary*. Give each of the students a card that indicates the role to play. The roles are explained on the teacher reference, *Role Playing Cards: Take Care of Yourself*. (See Figure 1) Each role can be pasted onto or written on cards.

b. Briefly explain the roles of each individual using the *Role Playing Cards: Take Care of Yourself*.
    Man with high blood pressure
    Wife
    Son/Daughter
    Doctor
    Nurse
    Pharmacist
    Health Educator
Explain that the players are to act the way they think *that* person would act in a real life situation. Players do *not* use a script in role playing situations.

c. Give the players a few minutes to get organized, then present the play.

d. After the play, conduct a short critique. Ask if any important points were left out. Ask what might be different had the disease been a heart attack or stroke. (Students may want to put on other plays using other heart and circulatory related diseases if time allows.)

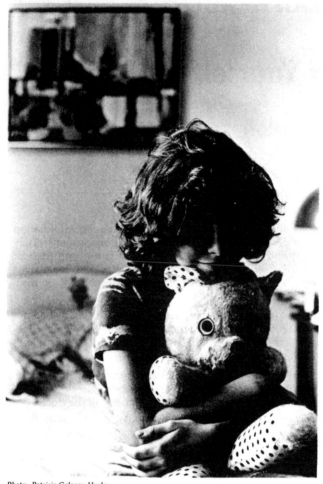

Photo: Patricia Galagan Hurley

3. EVALUATION ACTIVITY: I Can Take Care of Myself

To evaluate students' ability to find reliable health information and care have them complete the duplicated, *I Can Take Care of Myself.* (See Figure 2)

Using the following as example, evaluate students on their ability to identify:

a. Information about the heart and health can be obtained at:
   • health departments
   • health agencies
   • school
   • physician's office
   • books and magazines

b. People to talk to about the heart and health:
   • health educator
   • school nurse
   • physician
   • counselor
   • other health professional

c. In emergency situations, contact first:
   • fire department
   • paramedics

d. To help prevent problems of the heart:
   • exercise
   • use very little salt
   • control weight
   • don't smoke
   • practice stress management
   • keep a check on blood pressure

Figure 1. Role Playing Cards: Take Care of Yourself

Note: Cut and paste on cards

YOUR ROLE—Child Age 12

You have just heard that your dad has high blood pressure. He doesn't seem to be worried about it because it doesn't hurt. He has complained about the cost of the medicine and thinks he'll stop taking it.

You heard about high blood pressure in your health class. You are concerned about your dad and feel you should tell him what you know about treatment and prevention of this disease and where to get more information.

YOUR ROLE—Pharmacist

One of your customers has just been prescribed medicine for high blood pressure.

He doesn't think he needs the medicine because he feels no pain.

You need to explain the importance of the medicine.

YOUR ROLE—Nurse

You take the blood pressure of someone who has come in for a routine check-up.

You find out it is high.

What do you do?

YOUR ROLE—Man About 40 Years Old

You are a middle-aged adult who has to go into the doctor's office for a routine check-up.

They find high blood pressure.

You're not worried, however, because you feel no pain. But you do mention it to your wife.

You are concerned at the cost of the medicine prescribed. You think to yourself that you really don't need it.

YOUR ROLE—Woman About 40 Years Old

Your husband has just come back from a routine check-up at the doctor's office.

He says he has high blood pressure but he is not worried because he feels no pain.

Your husband does smoke and he is overweight. You have heard these may be problems for people with high blood pressure.

What do you say to him?

What can *you* do for him?

YOUR ROLE—Doctor

You have just discovered high blood pressure in one of your patients.

He is overweight and a smoker with a stressful job.

You have to explain the disease to him.

YOUR ROLE—Health Educator

You are teaching your students about problems related to the heart and circulatory system.

You explain to your class about high blood pressure.

If you don't feel sick, what should you do to find out if you have it?

You explain *HOW* you might prevent high blood pressure and what to do if you have high blood pressure. Then give information on *where* to get more information on high blood pressure like the American Heart Association.

Figure 2. I Can Take Care of Myself

Name _____

If I need information about my heart and my health, I can find it. . . .(list 2 places)

1. _____
2. _____

If I need to talk to someone about my heart and my health, I can talk to a . . .(list 2 people)

3. _____
4. _____

If I have an *emergency* regarding my heart, I can call . . . (list one place)

5. _____

If I want to prevent problems for my heart, I can . . . (list 4 things you can do)

6. _____
7. _____
8. _____
9. _____

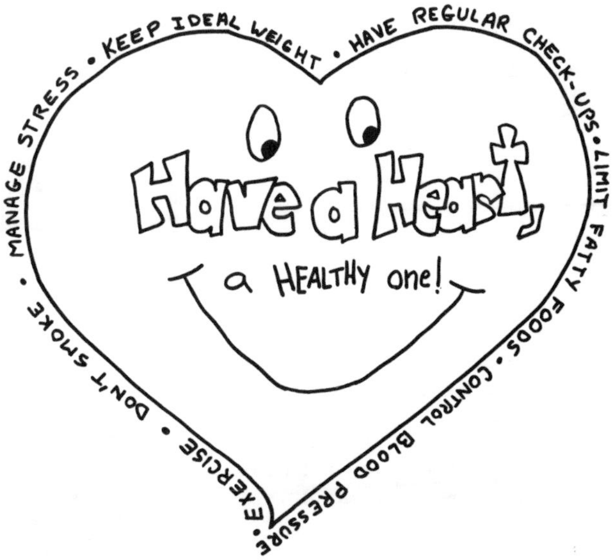

Taken from Grade 6 of the School Health Curriculum Project. Funding provided by the Center for Health Promotion and Education under Contract NO. 200-81-0616 Centers for Disease Control, Public Health Service.

59

Strategy for Consumer Education

MOON S. CHEN, JR. is an assistant professor of health education, 215 Pomerene Hall, Ohio State University, 1760 Neil Avenue, Columbus, Ohio 43210.

The popularity of daily newspaper features such as the "Dear Abby" column is indicative of the tremendous interest in seeking answers to personal problems. Students also want to know about certain consumer health products or services, for example, "Can you give me some advice in choosing a health center or health spa?" "What are steroids and could I benefit my weight training program by taking them?" "Do food supplements really help?"

Based on the "Dear Abby" letter is the classroom-tested "Dear Connie" letter that has been successfully employed in consumer health classes at Texas Tech University. "Connie" is just a fictitious name for the Abby of consumer health education. The idea is for students to generate their own questions and problems in an area of consumer health that interests them. A short letter describes their dilemma and appeals for a solution from "Connie." Inquirers do not sign their real name; they concoct an appropriate pen name such as "Frustrated," "Overweight," or "Anxious." (To receive credit for writing these letters students can write their social security numbers at the bottom of the letter.)

There are many ways in which the teacher can use the "Dear Connie" letter in a unit or course in consumer health. It allows students to express any particular concerns about consumer health products or services. If the student's concerns as expressed in this letter can be satisfactorily answered, the unit or course in consumer health has met a real need.

If the "Dear Connie" letter is assigned prior to the formal instruction in consumer health, the teacher can collect the letters, read them, and make a rough assessment of students interests and needs. This should be extremely beneficial in organizing the consumer health unit or course.

Students can share or extend their expertise by writing replies to other students' letters. After everyone has written a "Dear Connie" letter, all letters are put into a pot. Students draw a letter from this pot to answer. They have a week to write a reply based on library research, interviews with health practitioners, or personal experiences. The objective of the reply is to satisfy the original author of the letter. The letter and reply are returned to the original author, who grades the reply according to his or her satisfaction with it.

Student response to the "Dear Connie" letter has been good. Students are creative and realistic in their requests and have compiled excellent replies to complicated questions.

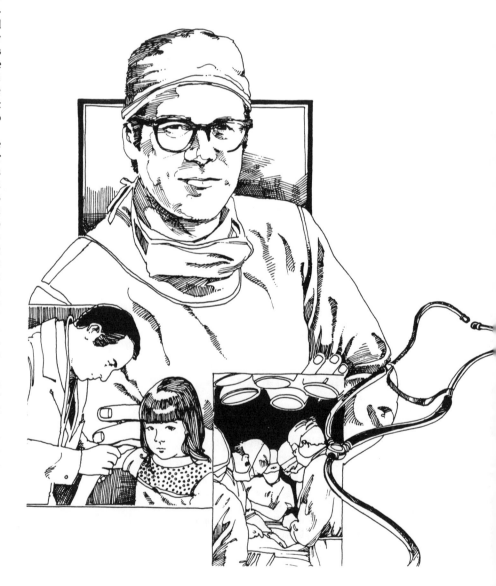

Consumer Education

Consumer Wellness, One School's Approach

JON W. HISGEN is a health instructor in Pewaukee Public Schools, 210 Main Street, Pewaukee, Wisconsin 53072 and an instructor of consumer health for the University of Wisconsin, Milwaukee.

Every year I instruct my consumer health units at the seventh and ninth grade levels I am made acutely aware of people's trusting nature. In this "credit card culture" where we exist, instant pleasures are a signature away. There is no better example of this approach to consumer decisions than in the world of health products and services. We blindly use hit or miss tactics in everything from wiping out those unsightly blemishes with steam to strengthening our rectus abdominus muscle with electric belts.

The condition of wellness is a combination of many interacting forces, including the individuals' environment, their reaction to it, associations, psychological background, and ability to accept attitudinal change. Today's health consumer is more likely to face these forces after his/her health has been threatened in some way. Consumer wellness is not an easily acquired status but must be learned.

My initial seventh grade consumer health activity is to sell each student a bottle of Dr. Lemke's Stomachic Drops using a stereotypical medicine man approach. The following is an example of the pitch I use to convince the class the product works.

1. I tell students about a college assignment to recreate a medicine from an old medical text.
2. I chose Dr. Lemke's drops because of its advertised ability to cure both acne problems and split ends (7th grade concerns).
3. The mysterious ingredient is capsicum that must be imported from Africa and grown hydroponically.
4. I finished making the product in two months and successfully field tested it on my friends and myself.
5. I unsuccessfully asked for support from the AMA and Bristol Meyers.
6. I decided to market the product through magazines after receiving a patent on the product.
7. I bought a factory to grow capsicum and produce Dr. Lemke's drops.

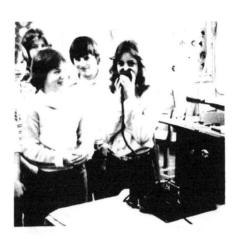

8. Sales have increased each year for the last three years.
9. Famous people have endorsed the product (the Osmonds, the Jackson Five).
10. A local newspaper is coming to take advertising pictures of students holding the product.
11. If the students bring the money next time we meet, I'll give them a special offer of two bottles for the price of one.

Over the past five years around 91% of the students have agreed to bring the cost of the product the next day while in fact 70% actually did. When I tell the students that a cruel hoax was played upon them the following responses can be heard: "I'll never trust you again." "We thought you were above that." "Well, you certainly made me look foolish." "I was just playing along with your little game."

The alarmingly high number of gullible consumers pointed out the need for

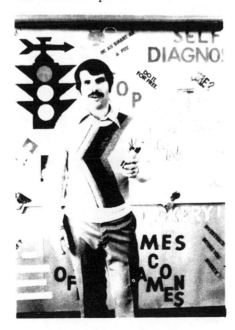

some direction in our consumer health program. Out of this we instituted a consumer health program entitled WISE MAN.

W ise
I independent M otivate
S afe/effective A ware
E valuate N otable

Each of the letters represented a competency we wanted our students to have by the time they left our health program.
1. The student will be able to make *wise* and careful decisions about the consumer products and services he/she uses (consumer health protection).
2. The student will be able to make decisions *independent* of outside influences (e.g. advertising, pseudo-science, etc.).
3. The student will be able to choose products and services that are both *safe* and *effective*.

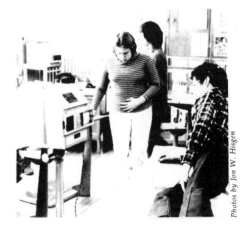

Photos by Jon W. Hisgen

4. The student will be able to *evaluate* new and existing health products and services (the work of government agencies, insurance programs, alternative medical practices, etc.).
5. The students will be able to *motivate* others in their present or future family to make wise consumer health decisions (well-thought out family medicine chests and first aid kits).
6. The student will be *aware* of pitfalls facing the consumer of health products and services (quackery, superstitions, fads, and fallacies).
7. The students will be able to make *notable* savings in their consumer health budget and notable improvement in their overall wellness.

Our school's consumer health program is based on these competencies. A copy of our consumer health curriculum and methods guide can be obtained by writing the author.

Consumer Education

Students Can Have a Say

JOAN L. BERGY, *formerly a consumer specialist with the U.S. Food and Drug Administration in Seattle, Washington, became on September 4, 1973 the director of the Seattle Area Office of the U.S. Consumer Product Safety Commission. BARNEY HANTUNEN is the regional public information officer, Public Health Service, Department of Health, Education, and Welfare, Region X, Seattle.*

A student voice in government rule-making? A consumer voice in government rule-making? Impossible, you say?

Not really, if you look into a little known publication—the *Federal Register*. Students—consumers—can have an impact on, for example, the selection of the route for the proposed Pacific Crest National Trail, the labeling of cosmetics, and a whole host of planned federal actions which affect all aspects of our daily lives, if they learn about this publication and are willing to take action.

The *Federal Register* is a legal document published Monday through Friday by the Office of the Federal Register, National Archives and Records Service, GSA, Washington, D.C. 20402.

The *Federal Register* provides a uniform system for making available to the general public regulations and legal notices issued by the Executive Branch of the federal government. Also included are Presidential proclamations and Executive Orders as well as various federal documents required to be published by Act of Congress.

The format used to present regulations in the *Federal Register* includes:

. . . A preamble which reviews the background of the proposal

. . . A statement of the proposal

. . . Information on the procedure for submitting comments

. . . Where comments should be forwarded

. . . The deadline date for receipt of comments

Following the expiration date the federal agency considers all comments and takes action. The action may be in the form of a "final order" printed

in the *Federal Register,* including the effective date for the regulation.

A new requirement now makes it mandatory that every "final order" is to include a summary of the types of comments received and whether the "final order" includes, rejects, or modifies comments received. In any case the "final order" must include the information on which the decision was based.

The process of rule-making begins after Congress passes a law and the President signs it into law. Then, it is the responsibility of the federal agency charged with carrying out the law to prepare appropriate regulations to implement the law. Preparation of regulations is a complex and time-consuming task. However, once that job is done, the regulations are printed in the *Federal Register.*

This is the critical point. Usually 60 days are allowed for comment. This is the time when the student—the consumer—will have the opportunity for reacting to and commenting on the proposed set of regulations. It is also possible to change current regulations by the rule-making process. An individual or any group may petition a federal agency to propose a change in regulations.

The system falls short, however, when consumers do not participate. More often than not the number of comments received in response to *Federal Register* proposals is very limited.

In March 1973, as an example, FDA published in the *Federal Register* a proposed change in regulations that would require cosmetic ingredients to be listed in descending order of predominance on labels attached to each cosmetic product. The proposal specified details about the label design, language to be used, size of print, as well as fragrances, coloring, and flavoring used in the product. As of May 1973, the sources of comments were as follows:

. . . Cosmetic industry and associations—19

. . . Professional organizations—1

. . . Universities—3

. . . Other federal agencies—1

... Organizations—5

... Individual consumers—267

A second example is the proposal to require a warning statement on the labeling of aerosol containers, which was published in the *Federal Register* during March 1973. One of the several proposed warning statements was: "Warning: Do not inhale directly; deliberate inhalation of contents can cause death." As of May 1973, the following summarizes comments received:

... Aerosol industry and associations—21

... Organizations—2

... Universities—5

... Consumers—1

It should be pointed out that the *Federal Register* is not the easiest document for the student or the consumer to locate. It is available from the Superintendent of Documents, Government Printing Office, Washington, D.C. 20202 at a cost of $25.00 per year, or single copies at twenty cents. Most libraries stock the publication. It is also generally available through libraries maintained by federal agencies in the Regional Office cities of Boston, New York, Philadelphia, Atlanta, Chicago, Dallas, Kansas City, Denver, San Francisco, and Seattle.

From time to time proposals published in the *Federal Register* are included as news items in local daily newspapers. However, more often than not very little information is included to guide the student or consumer in submitting timely comments to the appropriate place.

So how can students become involved? How can they gain access to the "system" of federal rule-making? How can they gain a perception of the process which will stand them in good stead as they move from academic community into the community at large?

A prerequisite, of course, is availability of the *Federal Register* in the classroom or the school library. A committee of students might review the *Federal Register* for a period of time in order to select a proposal for class consideration.

Once the proposal is selected, the committee might develop information and perhaps a demonstration project to illustrate to the class what the present regulations are and what changes are contemplated in the proposal. In addition, the students might analyze proposed changes in the regulations and their effect upon industry, the consumers, and others concerned with the subject under consideration.

Upon reaching a consensus and having reconciled various points of view, the comments could be submitted to the agency, as indicated in the *Federal Register,* which has responsibility for preparing the "final order."

The students would then need to develop a follow-up plan to assure continuity in their efforts to observe the final outcome of the process. When the "final order" does appear in the *Federal Register* the students will be in the unique position of comparing their own experience and accumulated materials to the final outcome.

Most important of all, they would have seen, and shared in, the rule-making process. They would, hopefully, have developed a heightened concept of their rights and responsibilities in the American rule-making process.

About Aging and Death

JAMES TERHUNE is in the Department of Health Science, California State University at Chico, Chico, California 95926.

Aging consciousness is finally becoming vogue. Newspapers, periodicals, and newscasts are increasingly reporting about the problems and needs of the elderly. The war against discrimination toward older persons is slowly and effectively being waged. Government agencies including the Administration on Aging and the many state offices on aging, as well as nonprofit public organizations such as the Gray Panthers and the National Council on Aging, are wielding more political power. Universities throughout the country are developing new programs in gerontology, and the word "gerontologist" is beginning to be more than a word. It is time for the elementary and secondary schools to get into the act and include aging, death, and grief education as a part of the comprehensive school health program.

Shown here is a scope and sequence chart for aging, death, and grief education in grades K-12. The chart also includes ideas for integrating these gerontology issues into the common subjects taught in the schools.

Many of these areas could easily be integrated into a comprehensive health program without developing entirely separate units. Teachers should set up a school committee to determine the extent of the program and the personnel who should handle various responsibilities. The health teacher, or person responsible for health in the school, might be the logical chairperson of such a committee. Other good choices for chairpersons are teachers of social studies, English, history, psychology, and American problems. These people seem to have the most flexible subjects to incorporate studies in aging. The chairperson would be responsible for coordinating the various disciplines so

SCOPE AND SEQUENCE CHART FOR

AGING, DEATH AND GRIEF EDUCATION

Key for Integrating Aging Issues into School Curriculum

1. Economics	6. Industrial Arts	11. Science
2. American Problems	7. Math	12. Physical Education
3. Political Science	8. English—reading	13. Health
4. History	and grammar	14. Social Studies
5. Fine Arts	9. Music	15. Speech
	10. Psychology	

Grades K-3	**Integration Ideas** (See key)
Death and Separation—animal deaths, all living things die	9,11,13,14
Grief—okay to cry	2,8,10,13
What Is Old	4,8,13,14
Loneliness—dependency, aloneness	13,14
Discrimination—jobs, put out to pasture, no authority, sexism (hags, witches, old maids)	8,13,14
How to Call for Help in Emergencies	13
Communication with Grandparents—hearing and vision problems	8,13,14,15
Safety—falling on toys	13
Services by Elderly—foster grandparent programs, senior-student aids	13,14

Grades 4-6	
Grandparents Living at Home—contributions, obligations, social, spiritual, and financial needs	7,8,13,14
Health problems—affecting communication, sensitivity, mobility	13,8
Emergency Care—treating for shock, sensitivity to temperature, ABCs of first aid, falls	13
Preventive Health Measures	8,12,13
Necessary Diets—diabetes, hypoglycemia, low cholesterol, low sodium, obesity	11,13
Economics—food stamps, social security, medicare and medicaid basics	1,2,3,4,7,14
Transportation—buses, senior services, wheelchair	3,4,13,14
How to Show You Care	8,10,13
General Statistics—number of elderly nationally, statewide, locally	7,13,14
Disorders—vision, hearing, smell, taste, balance, touch, speech	8,9,10,11,12,13,15
Life Long Physical Fitness	12,13,14
Services by Elderly—senior-student aides, hospital volunteers, home health aids	3,4,13,14
Physical Changes with Age—bones, muscles, pigment, hair, digestion, fatigue, etc.	11,13

Grades 7-9	
Diseases—arthritis, diabetes, strokes, heart attacks, alcoholism, etc.	4,11,12,13
Drug Dependencies—barbiturates, antidepressants, amphetamines, aspirin, cortisone	8,10,11,13,14
Depression and Anxiety	2,4,8,10,13,14
Death and Dying—funerals, what to say and do for dying and family	2,4,8,10,13,14
Miscellaneous Conditions—forgetfulness, hostility, fault-finding, authoritarianism	8,10,13,14

Bedridden and Handicapped—bedsores, clothing, type of bed, chairs, feeding	13
General Statistics—numbers of men and women, minorities, wage earners, physically handicapped, income levels, marital status, geographical distribution	1,2,3,4,7,13,14
Economic Benefits—low cost transportation, meals, movies, special discounts	1,2,3,4,7,8,13,14
Safety—handrails, tacked down rugs, lighting, clearly marked temperature settings on stoves, chain-pull sockets vs. wall outlets, storage of medicines	10,13,14
Grief—stages of grief, needs for others, to be alone, helping others grieve	2,4,10,13,14
Discrimination—sexism, racism, poverty, widowhood, retirement	1,2,3,4,10,13,14
Preventive Health Measures—diet, attitudes, exercise, hygiene, checkups, etc.	10,11,12,13,14,15

Grades 10-12

Crime and Consumer Fraud	2,4,10,13,14
Nursing Homes—conditions, what to look for, costs, alternatives	1,2,3,4,7,8,13,14
Home Health Care—when to call a doctor, what families can do, where to get services	2,4,13,14
Grandparents Living at Home—organizing household, who's boss and when, arranging living quarters, medical preparation	2,8,10,13,14
Legal Aspects—wills, estates, taxes	2,3,13,14
Death and Dying—discussing deaths of friends, living wills, donating body parts, funeral costs, postmortems, signs and symptoms, what to do if a doctor isn't present, hospices, philosophies, cultural differences	1,2,3,4,7,8,10,13,14
Diseases—symptoms of heart and lung, digestive, urinary, and skin conditions; how acute illness affects older persons, senility, mental illness, incontinence	4,10,11,13,14
Surgery—risks	2,11,13
Rehabilitation—what's possible	2,10,11,13,14
Recreation—life long activities such as crafts, dancing, art, golf, lawn bowling	5,6,9,10,11,12,13,15
Sexuality—myths, capabilities, desires	10,11,13,14
Marriage and Alternatives	2,4,8,10,13,14
Bedridden—help in sitting, standing and walking	13,14
Economics—budget planning, social security, retirement planning, hospital costs	1,2,3,4,13,14
Specific statistics—numbers voting over 85 or 95 years, causes of death and infirmity, types of housing, numbers using food stamps, health, sources of income, education, etc.	2,7,13,14
Meaningful Employment	1,2,3,4,8,10,13,14
Health and Life Insurance	1,2,4,7,13,14
Drug Therapies	2,4,10,13
Political Potential and Activities	2,3,4,14
Educational Opportunities	1,4,13,14
Retirement Communities	2,4,10,13,14
Services for the Elderly—taxi, buses, information and referral, classes, hearing aids, magazines, medical	1,2,3,4,13,14

that overlap is minimized and important points are seen from a variety of perspectives. If each discipline in the school agreed to integrate a few of the learning experiences during the school year, a child could get a substantial education in gerontology, grief, and death education.

Printed here is a list of references that might be useful in determining curriculum content, objectives, and evaluation methodologies. Included are some of the content areas that have been explored quite thoroughly in each of the publications. The references cover many issues and problems related to the elderly, but specific emphasis was placed upon health aspects of aging. These publications were used to develop the scope and sequence chart.

A third listing includes some of the agencies and societies that could be used as resources for developing a gerontology curriculum. The chart on page 16 explains which ones are national, state, or local agencies.

SELECTED RESOURCES FOR GERONTOLOGY STUDIES

Books	Major Areas Covered
Birchenall, Joan and Streight, Mary Eileen. *Care of the Older Adult.* Philadelphia: J. P. Lippincott Co., 1973.	Normal aging, illnesses, restorative nursing care for cancer, circulatory-respiratory, nervous, and skeletal systems, death and dying.
Birren, James E., et al., eds. *Human Aging: A Biological and Behavioral Study.* DHEW-NIMH Pub. # (HSM) 71–9051.	Research on health and health concerns of elderly including: cerebral circulation, metabolism, brain waves, mental abilities, auditory perception, personality, etc.
Brantl, Virginia M. and Brown, Sister Marie Raymond, eds. *Readings in Gerontology.* St. Louis: Mosby, 1973.	Issues and problems of elderly, assessment of elderly, aging as it relates to activities, attitudes, grief, suicide, nutrition, etc.
Butler, Robert N. and Lewis, Myrna I. *Aging and Mental Health.* St. Louis: Mosby, 1973.	Overview: mental health problems, statistics, evaluation, treatment, and prevention, diagnostic evaluation forms, home care.
Caldwell, Esther and Hegner, Barbara R. *Geriatrics: A Study of Maturity.* Albany, N.Y.: Delmar Pub., 1975.	Health problems, care, rehabilitation, special needs: drugs, hygiene, diets, safety.
Field, Minna. *The Aged, the Family, & the Community.* New York: Columbia U. Press, 1972.	Families, living accomodations, economics, ill health, leisure, social work.
Lowenthal, Marjorie Fisk and Berkman, Paul L. and associates. *Aging and Mental Disorder in San Francisco.* San Francisco: Jossey-Bass Inc., Pub. 1967.	Research and evaluation of the effects of illness, time, and deprivations upon mental health. Detailed study.
Martin, William C. and Wilson, Albert J. E. III. *Aging and Total Health.* St. Petersburg: Eckerd College Gerontology Center, 1976.	Proceedings of a conference sponsored by Eckerd College Gerontology Center, St. Petersburg, Florida. Quality of life community support systems, social medicine.
Hickey, Tom. *Grief—Its Recognition and Resolution.* Proceedings of a National Invitational Conference. Gerontology Center. College of Human Development, Pennsylvania State University, University Park, PA, November, 1973.	Intervention and the helping professional. Recognition and resolution of grief. Death and dying. Pastoral role in grief resolution. Collaborative roles of clergy and funeral director. Grief and the family.
Poe, William D. *The Older Person in Your Home.* New York: Charles Scribner's Sons, 1969.	Considerations involved in moving an elderly person into your home. Conflicts and resolutions of problems in the home. General health considerations. Resources for the aged.
Simpson, Ida Harper and McKinney, John C., eds. *Social Aspects of Aging.* Durham, N.C.: Duke University Press, 1966.	Many chapters with individual authors—work, family, and community in retirement. Disorientation and orientation by the elderly.
Townsend, Claire. *Old Age: The Last Segregation.* New York: Bantam Books. 1971.	Ralph Nader's study group report on nursing homes. Written in narrative form. Lots of good examples of problems.
Vernick, Joel J. *Selected Bibliography on Death and Dying.* National Institute of Child Health and Human Development. DHEW, Bethesda, MD.	Author-Subject index and bibliography from 1920s–1960s.
Woodruff, Diane S. and Birren, James E., eds. *Aging: Scientific Perspectives and Social Issues.* New York: D. Van Nostrand Co. 1975.	History of gerontology. Sociological, psychological, and biological perspectives. Environmental planning. Politics and economics. Many authors wrote individual chapters.

Periodicals	Major Areas Covered
Age and Aging ($33 subscription). Official Journal of the British Geriatrics Society and of the British Society for Research on Aging. Williams & Wilkins Co. 428 E. Preston St. Baltimore, MD, 21202.	General
Aging. U.S. DHEW Office of Human Development. Administration on Aging. National Clearinghouse on Aging.	General
Current Literature on Aging. National Council on Aging.	General
Dynamic Maturity. AIM, Division of AARP. Have to be 50 yrs. old to join. $3. AIM Membership Processing Department, P.O. Box 199, Long Beach, CA, 90801.	General. Written to a lay audience.
Educational Gerontology, An International Quarterly 4 issues/yr. $19.50. Hemisphere Publishing Corp. 1025 Vermont Ave., NW Washington, DC, 20005.	General. Educational orientation.
Excerpta Medica. "Gerontology and Geriatrics." Vol. 19.5, Sect. 20. Abstracts, Book Order Dept. Associated Scientific Publishers. P.O. Box 211, Amsterdam, The Netherlands.	Medical orientation.
Geriatrics. Lancet Publications. 4015 W. 65th St. Minneapolis, MN, 55435. $15.	Nursing and health problems.
International Journal of Aging and Human Development. Robert J. Kastenaum, ed. Baywood Publishing Co. 43 Central Drive, Farmingdale, NY	General
Journal of the American Geriatric Society. 10 Columbus Circle, NY., NY 10019. $25/yr.	Nursing and health problems.
The Journal of the American Society for Geriatric Dentistry. American Society for Geriatric Dentistry, 11 E. Adams St., Chicago, IL 60603.	Dental problems.
Modern Geriatrics. (Free to general practitioners.) Annual $9. Modern Medicine of Great Britain, 20 Southampton Place, London, WCIA 2BP.	Nursing and health problems.
Omega, Journal of Death and Dying. Baywood Publishing Co., 43 Central Drive, Farmingdale, NY 11735. $35.	Research in death and dying.

RESOURCES FOR A GERONTOLOGY CURRICULUM

Name of Agency or Society	Special Services
Administration on Aging, Social Security Administration DHEW, Washington, DC	Grants of money to public and private agencies including state offices on aging and research projects.
American Association of Homes for the Aging, 529 14th St., N.W, Washington, DC 20004.	Directory of nonprofit homes. Accrediting agency to protect residents.
American Association of Retired Persons National Hdqts. (Includes National Retired Teachers Assoc. and The Institute of Lifetime Learning) 1225 Connecticut Ave., NW Washington, DC, 20036.	Publish *Modern Maturity*, AARP News Bulletin of Lifetime Learning. For 55 years and older.
American Geriatrics Society, 10 Columbus Circle, New York, NY, 10019.	Yearly meeting made up of physicians.
American Nursing Home Assoc. Suite 607, 1025 Connecticut Ave., NW, Washington, DC, 20036.	Accrediting agency for nursing homes. Has a directory.
Family Services Assoc. of American, 44 E. 23rd Street, New York, NY, 10010.	Figurehead of over 400 local agencies.
The Gerontological Society, 1 Dupont Circle, Washington, DC, 20036.	Research and comments in biological sciences, clinical medicine, social and psychological services. Does social research. Annual meeting. International meeting every 3 years.
Gray Panthers, 6342 Greene St., Philadelphia, PA, 19144.	Reference and political action group made up of older people.
The Institute of Retired Persons, The New School of Social Research, 60 W. 12th St., New York, NY.	Educational advantages for older people.
International Senior Citizens Assoc., Inc., 11753 Wilshire Blvd., Los Angeles, CA, 90025.	Attempts to consider older people of various ethnic groups.
National Assoc. of Jewish Homes for the Aged, 2525 Centerville Road, Dallas, TX.	Information on homes, nursing homes, geriatric hospitals for Jewish aged.
National Assoc. of Retired Federal Employees, 1909 Q St., NW, Washington, DC, 20009.	Lobbies for retired federal employees.
National Council on the Aging, Inc., 1828 L St., NW, Suite 504, Washington, DC, 20036.	Information and consulting. Local offices.
National Council of Health Care Services, 407 N St., SW, Washington, DC	Represents commercial nursing home groups.
National Council of Homemakers Services, 1790 Broadway, New York, NY, 10019.	Supplies trained and professional supervisorial women to help families during periods of stress and illness.
National Council of Senior Citizens, 1911 K Street, NW, Room 202, Washington, DC, 20005.	Educational and action group for 2000 autonomous senior citizens' clubs and other groups. Has lobby group.
National Legal Aid and Defender Assoc., 1155 E. 60th St., Chicago, IL, 60637.	Provides referral service for those who can't pay for legal aid. Advice about lawyers, education, speakers. Local bar assoc.
National Tenants Organization, Inc., Suite 548, 425 13th St., NW, Washington, DC, 20004.	Aid for all people with public housing problems.
United Community Funds and Councils of America, 345 E. 46th St., New York, NY 10017.	Coordination of local community grant monies.
U.S. Dept. of Health, Education, and Welfare, I-Social Security Administration.	700 district offices; Medicare, Home Health Benefits. Medicare handbook.
OTHERS: State offices on Aging, City or Regional Councils on Aging.	May coordinate use of federal and state funds for aged.

Bibliography on Agencies and Societies

Birchenall, Joan and Streight, Mary Eileen. *Care of the Older Adult.* Philadelphia: J. P. Lippincott Co. 1973.

Butler, Robert N. and Lewis, Myrna I. *Aging and Mental Health.* St. Louis: C. V. Mosby, Co. 1973.

Poe, William D. *The Old Person in Your Home.* New York: Charles Scribner's Sons. 1969.

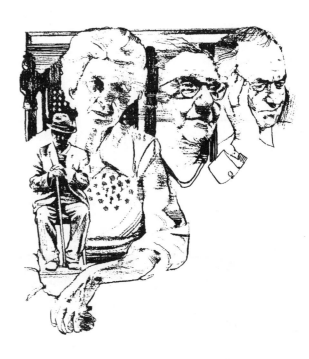

"Where's Johnny Today?"

Explaining the Death of a Classmate

Even though you might go through an entire teaching career without one of your students dying during the school term, it is certainly possible that a student might die from an illness or accident and you will be faced with an empty desk in your classroom. The easiest thing to do is to ignore the desk as though he (the deceased student will be called Johnny in this article) had moved to another school district.

But, is the denial of Johnny's death best for your students? We cannot protect the children or ourselves from the realities of death. To deny children the opportunity to discuss and learn about death and dying is to deny them a chance to understand death and learn to live with its eventuality.

The children's ability to cope with Johnny's death would have been easier if the teacher had introduced the topic before Johnny died. There are opportunities to teach about death as part of the health education and science curriculum; for example, death could be discussed as part of the life cycle of all living things. The death of a classroom animal used for health and science projects or the death of a student's pet can serve as a catalyst for starting discussions about death. However, before lessons about death are presented, teachers must prepare themselves for discussing the topic by coming to terms with personal feelings about death.

WILLIAM L. YARBER is assistant professor of health education, Purdue University, West Lafayette, Indiana 47907.

There is no one way to tell children about death. Within the past few years several books and materials have become available to assist the teacher and parent. From my resources I have made a list of do not's and do's for discussing death of a classmate with elementary children. Because of space limitations, the list does not address all possible issues or student questions concerning death, but it can provide a basis for developing your own style. Many of the suggested teacher statements were developed from the parent-child dialogue in Earl A. Grollman's book, *Talking About Death.*

Do Not's in Explaining Death

Do not deny the death of the student; acknowledge it

Our society is a death-denying society that attempts to avoid evidence of dying. Death and dying are no longer part of the family experience at home. Portrayals of death by the media and literature are often unrealistic and misleading, as a result, children have difficulty comprehending that death is a natural and inevitable end of life. The teacher might say: "Death is not like playing cops and robbers. Bang! I shot you dead. It is not like playing a game. Death is very real. Johnny is dead. He will never come back."

Do not tell the students what they will later discover to be false.

Teachers sometimes try to protect students from the realities of life by describing death with fictions and half-

truths. It may be less difficult to say that "Johnny has gone on a very long trip for a very long time," than to acknowledge Johnny's death. Describing death as a "long sleep" may cause fears and anxieties about going to sleep. Teachers should not give the illusion that someday the classmate will return. It is important to keep the students' trust by answering their questions honestly and sincerely.

Do not overexplain the topic.

Teachers sometimes go beyond what the pupils can handle. The questions asked are often the best clues as to what to discuss. Children usually do not ask for or need details. A complicated reply may confuse the child.

Do not focus on morbid details of death and dying.

Avoid describing the gory details of how death occurred and how the body is prepared for burial or entombment. For instance, if Johnny were killed in an automobile accident the teacher might say: "Johnny's head was badly hurt when the car slipped off the road."

Do's in Explaining Death

Do dispel guilt feelings

Children may feel guilty after the death of a classmate. In their experience, bad things happen to them because they were naughty. Earlier hostility toward Johnny might have included the wish that he were dead, and students might feel that they bear some responsibility for their classmate's death or might wish that they had done things differently. The teacher could say: "Are you worried you did something wrong and Johnny's death is a punishment to you? Of course not! You did nothing to make him die. But maybe you remember times when you were mean to him. You may have said terrible words or you may not have done the right thing. But all people are like that sometimes. You had nothing to do with his death."

Do help children understand what dead means.

Children may not know what happens when a person dies. They may ask what it is like to be dead. The teacher might say: "Remember when you saw a dog run over by a car. He was lying on the street still. He did not breathe or move, nor was his heart beating. The dog would never breathe or move again. He was dead. It is the same with people. The body does not move . . . it is still. The dead person does not breathe . . . the heart does not beat. The body is quiet and peaceful. There is no pain or hurt and there is no life."

Do present information in a nonmoralistic fashion.

Death education in the school should complement the information received in the home and church, but be basically nonmoral. Teachers should not project on their students their own personal beliefs about an afterlife. Stating that "Johnny was so good that God wanted him in heaven" or that Johnny's death was because of "God's will" may make children rebel against a god.

Children may want to discuss death in a religious context, in which case, teachers may choose to discuss various religious customs and beliefs about death. Children may ask if their classmate will go to heaven. The teacher might say: "Many people in the world believe in heaven or an afterlife of some type. Others do not. We cannot be sure. One thing is certain, the memory of the fun we had with Johnny will always remain with us."

Do keep the door open for discussions, doubt, questioning, and differences.

Do not convey the feeling to children that you have all the answers. In the end, children must struggle with defining the meaning of death for themselves. The discussion should not be rushed. Instead of being only concerned with saying the right things, be sure to be a good listener. Your smile and warmth will reassure them that you understand their feelings. The teacher might say: "I do not completely under-

Do allow the children to express sadness and grief.

Expressions of grief are normal and desirable; they provide a healthy way to minimize guilt feelings. Emotions should not be repressed. For both children and adults, tears are a normal expression of grief. Don't be afraid of causing tears. The teacher should not tell students to "be brave, don't cry, don't take it so hard." Tell the children that as time passes, so will our sadness. The teacher might say: "We miss Johnny so much that we might even cry. What is bad about that? Nothing. It is all right to cry. It is a way of showing how much we miss Johnny."

stand death. I, too, am trying to find some answers. Are you surprised that I don't know all the answers? Don't be. You can learn something from me and I can learn something from you. We can help each other. What is troubling you? Let's talk about it."

Some of us would shield children from the knowledge and experience of death. But, only after people have come to terms with death, can they learn to fully enjoy living. Discussions about death in the school will help children learn about the certainty of death and increase their joy of life. If a goal of education is the preparation of children for life, then death education should be a regular part of the health education and science curriculum of every elementary school.

Suggested Reading

Bensley. Loren B., *Death Education as a Learning Experience*. ERIC Clearinghouse on Teacher Education, Washington, D.C. 1975.

Berg, David W., and Daugherty, George G., *Understanding Death Series* (filmstrip/cassette tape program designed for intermediate and junior high grades). Education Perspectives Associates, DeKalb, Ill. 1972.

Green, Betty R., and Irish, Donald P., *Death Education: Preparation for Living*. General Learning Press, Morristown, N.J. 1971.

Grollman, Earl A., *Talking About Death*. Beacon Press, Boston, Mass. 1970.

Grollman, Earl A., (editor), *Explaining Death to Children*. Beacon Press, Boston, Mass. 1967.

Mills, Gretchen C., et al., *Discussing Death: A Guide to Death Education*. Educational Perspectives Associates, DeKalb, Ill. 1976.

Stein, Sara B., *About Dying*. Walker and Co., New York, N.Y. 1974.

A Unit on Death for Primary Grades

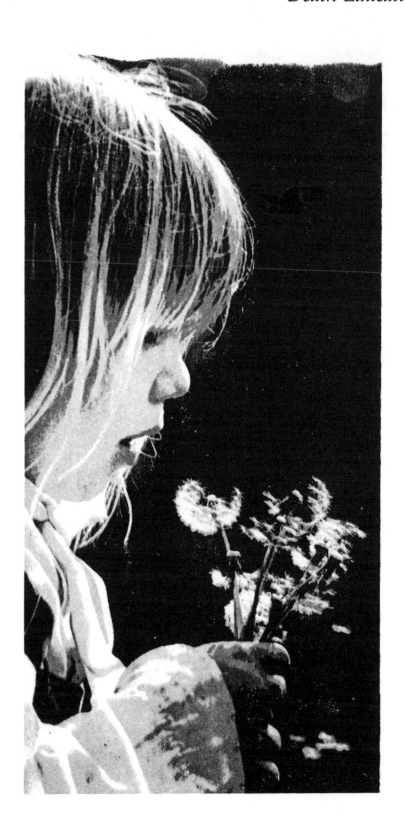

Teaching about death in grades 1 through 3 is a new idea, but many writers, experts in a variety of fields, think it is a good one. This unit is designed to answer some of the questions that children have about death. Ideally, children feel free to discuss their feelings and experiences, so it is likely that a responsive teacher might move into areas not included in the unit. The keys to good teaching in this unit are the same for good teaching anywhere: honesty, naturalness, sensitivity.

There are many ways to approach the subject of death. Poetry and music are excellent avenues. Field trips, speakers, and role-playing meet the needs of the older student. However, for young students, children's literature was chosen as a vehicle to open discussion. Lessons were kept short and the entire unit is only five days—taught in one school week or once a week for five weeks. It should be taught gently.

Activity 1—Basic concept: every living thing dies.

Objectives: The students will distinguish between living and nonliving things. The students will describe how a living thing is different after it dies.

Materials: A living flower planted in a pot, an identical flower which has been uprooted and is dry and faded.

TONI DAHLGREN and IRIS PRAGER-DECKER are both on the Capitol Campus of Pennsylvania State University, Middletown, Pennsylvania 17057.

Time: 15 minutes

Procedure: Ask students—What living things are in this room (plants, pet, students, teacher)? What things in this room are not living (desks, blackboard)? Is water living? Is the sky living? Is lightning alive? Is a teddy bear alive? or a doll? (We sometimes pretend they are, but they aren't really.) Is a rock alive?

What does a living flower look like? (Hold up the flower.) How is a dead flower different? (Hold up the dead flower.) What does a living bird look like? What does a dead bird look like?

Do you think that each living plant will someday die? Will each animal someday die? Will each person someday die? Every living thing must die. It is a natural part of life.

Evaluation: Some young children are confused about what is living and what is not living. Those who don't have this basic understanding will have special difficulty with the concept of death. Don't push children to understand more than they are ready to understand, but listen carefully to comments and questions so you will know their level of understanding.

Children may introduce comments about their own experiences which don't fit into the subject of this first lesson. Be flexible. Begin now to establish an atmosphere of honesty and a willingness to discuss what a child needs to discuss.

Activity 2—Basic concept: death is final and this makes it very sad.

Objectives: The students will listen to their teacher read *The Dead Bird*. The students will discuss the book and the "death" of cartoon characters and TV actors.

Materials: *The Dead Bird* by Margaret Wise Brown (Addison-Wesley, 1958).

Time: 20 minutes.

Procedure: Introduce the book—yesterday we said that every living thing must die. Sometimes we see animals which have died in the woods or in the roads or even in our yards. Have you ever found a dead animal? This is the story of a group of children who found a dead bird.
Read the book.
Ask the students: how did the children in the book know that the bird was dead? How do you think the bird may

have died? (It might have been very old; it might have been hurt; it might have had a serious disease.)
Why were the children so sad? (The bird would never fly again and the funeral was sad; they were saying goodbye to a bird which had been alive.)
Would the bird ever be alive again?
Discuss the way characters "die" in cartoons and the way actors die on TV. Do they really die? (Television deaths in stories and cartoons are just pretended. That's why they can come back again and again.)
Can any living thing which has died come back and be alive again? (No, death is final. That's why it is so sad. After you visit your grandmother it is sad to say goodbye, but you know you will see her again. If your grandmother dies and you know you will never see her in her house again, you are very much sadder.)
Did the children in this book really love the bird? (Not really. The bird was not a pet and not a part of their lives.) The book tells us that the children eventually forgot the bird. Is that alright? (Yes, since the children weren't deeply hurt by the death of the bird, their sadness went away quickly.)

Evaluation: Some children may tell you that "Jesus came back from the dead" or "I will see my grandmother in Heaven." There is no reason to contradict these statements in an effort to be scientific. Death is a mysterious and emotional subject—the teacher's main objective is to create a climate in which children can express themselves freely. The point may be made that when someone we love dies we will never see him or her on earth again.
Children often wonder what causes death. Discussing how the bird may have died can be generalized to all living things.

Activity 3—Basic concept: many feelings are experienced in grief.

Objectives: The students will discuss how Ben felt when his dog died. The students will discuss several feelings which might be part of grief.

Materials: *The Old Dog* by Sarah Abbott.

Time: 20 minutes

Procedure: Introduce the book—yesterday we read a story about a dead

bird and we said that the children who found it were sad, but not too sad. What if it were your dog who died? This story is about a little boy named Ben and about the death of his dog.
Read the book.
How did Ben feel when his dog died? What did he do? Was it alright for his mother to cry about the dog? Would it be alright for his father to cry? (Yes, sometimes crying helps to get the hurt out.)
Tell the students: when Ben's dog died, he felt grief. Grief is the hurt you feel when someone you love dies. Sometimes grief includes many different feelings. Ben might feel angry. Why? Who could he be angry at? What could he do if he were angry? He might be angry because his friend still had a dog or because it wasn't "fair" to lose his dog when he loved her so much and treated her so well. He might not know who to be angry at. He might feel like hitting his pillow very hard over and over. Would that be alright? He might feel like yelling at his mother. Would that be alright?
Ben might feel guilty. He might blame himself for his dog's death. He might think, "If only I had fed her more or petted her more, maybe she wouldn't have died." What could Ben do to get rid of his feelings of guilt? (He could talk to his parents; they would probably tell him that it wasn't his fault at all, his dog died because she was old and it was time for her to die.)
Ben might feel fear. He might be afraid to love another dog, because he wouldn't want to be hurt again. He might be afraid another dog would die too. Do you think it was a good idea for Ben to get a new puppy right away? (Ben probably needed time to get over his grief before he could really love another dog. Grief heals, but it takes time.)
This is concentrated material for children. Keep the pace as relaxed as possible with plenty of time for side trips and comments.

Activity 4—Basic concept: certain activities follow a death.

Objectives: The students will discuss what happens after death to the person and to the person's body. The students will compare the two funerals they have read about. The students will draw two pictures—one of death and one of what happens after death.

Materials: *The Tenth Good Thing About Barney* by Judith Viorst (Atheneum, 1975) and *The Dead Bird*. The dead flower. Paper and crayons for each child.

Time: 25 minutes.

Procedure: Introduce the book—yesterday we read about Ben and his dog. In this book Barney, a cat, dies and the two children in the book argue about where he is now.

Read the book.

Ask the students: Where did Annie think Barney was? Where did the little boy who owned Barney think he was? (In the ground.) What does that mean? How could he become part of the ground?

Take the dry flower and crush it between your fingers over a pot of dirt. Pass it around for the students to see.

Tell the students: no one knows for sure what happens after death; people have different ideas. Some people think we go to Heaven; some think that we live in the memories of people who love us; some think that we return to earth and are born again. We really don't know.

We do know what happens to the body after death. What do we do with the body of someone who has died? What did the boy in the story do with Barney's body? What did the children do with the body of the dead bird? How were the two funerals alike? (Show the books again.)

Why do you think we have funerals? (It gives us a chance to show how much we love the person or pet who died.) Have you ever been to a funeral? Have you ever held a funeral?

Ask the students to draw two pictures—one of death, one of what might happen after death.

Evaluation: The pictures should give the teacher some idea of how the children conceive of death. Young children often personify death and may draw it as a skeleton or scary person. Teachers are usually not well trained in psycho-logically interpreting children's art, so be cautious about reaching any conclusions. However, the teacher should be sensitive to what feelings the child is expressing through art and especially sensitive to what the child says about the picture. Don't be shy about asking a student, "What is this?"

Don't be afraid to tell children that you don't know what happens after death. Remember the goal is honesty with each other.

Activity 5—Basic concept: people often need help when someone close dies.

Objectives: The students will plan a funeral for a pet. The students will discuss how they would be able to help the children in the stories which have been read.

Materials: None needed.

Time: 20 minutes.

Procedure: Tell the students: We've been talking about death all this week. I wonder if we know a little more about how to deal with death now. Let's pretend that our class pet has died. Do you think we could plan a funeral for him?

Where would we bury him? What would we bury him in? What would we put on his grave? What would we say about him? What could we do to make his funeral special? How could we show how much we love him and would miss him?

How could we comfort each other? How could you comfort Ben when he was so sad about his dog's death? How could you comfort the boy who owned Barney?

What would you do if you came to class and found me crying because my friend had died? What would you say to me? Can a child comfort a grown-up? What would you want me to say to you if your friend had died?

Review: We have talked about death every day for a week. We said that every living thing must die. We said that death is sad because it is a final good-bye. We said that grief is the hurt that we feel when someone we love dies. We talked about what happens after death. What happens to the person and to his body? Today we talked about how we can deal with death. Are there any questions or is there anything more you would like to share with the class?

Evaluation: The students should be encouraged to realize that we can talk about death to someone who is grieving; we can listen sympathetically; we can hug him or hold his hand; we can do special, kind things for him; we can be patient with him and let him cry or be angry or withdrawn. We can plan or take part in a funeral for someone we love who has died. We can remember how special the person was and how much we love him. The goal of this final lesson is to show the children that we can deal with death in a positive and loving way.

Bibliography

Crase, D. R. and Crase, D. "Helping Children Understand Death," *Young Children*, 32 (November 1976) pp. 20–25.

Fredlund, D. J., "Children and Death from the School Setting Viewpoint," *Journal of School Health*, November 1977, pp. 533–77.

Grollman, E. A., "Explaining Death to Children," *Journal of School Health*, June 1977, pp. 336–39.

Hart, E. J., "Death Education and Mental Health," *Journal of School Health*, September 1976, pp. 407–12.

Koby, I. M., "And the Leaves that are Green Turn to . . .?" *English Journal*, October 1975, pp. 59–60.

"Learning About Death," *Language Arts*, September 1976, pp. 673–87.

LeShan, Eda, *Learning to Say Good-bye*, New York: Macmillan, 1976.

Wass, H. and Shaak, J. "Helping Children Understand Death Through Literature," *Childhood Education*, November 1976, pp. 80–85.

Yarber, W. L., "Death Education: A Living Issue," *Science Teacher*, October 1976, pp. 21–23.

Early Practice Essential for Dental Health

The need for dental health education is obvious when one considers the incidence of carious teeth among young people in America. By the time the average child reaches school age, he has three carious teeth; at age 12 or 13 the average child has five permanent teeth attacked by caries. One-fifth of six-year olds and three-fourths of 18 year olds have malocclusion. Dental health education is a vital step in an attempt to decrease dental problems and the younger the student is, the more significant the end result.

Professional services are necessary to care for diseased teeth or tissue, but only approximately

MARILYN McELLIOTT is assistant to the chairman, Department of Dental Hygiene, University of Maryland School of Dentistry, Baltimore, Maryland 21201.

1
Break off about 18 inches of floss and wind most of it around one of your middle fingers.

2
Wind the rest around the same finger of the opposite hand. This finger can "take up" the floss as it becomes soiled. (see figure 3)

3
Use your thumbs and forefingers with an inch of floss between them to guide the floss between your teeth. (see figure 4)

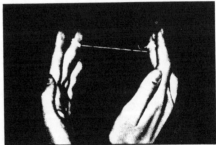

Figure 3

4
Holding the floss tightly (there should be no slack), use a gentle sawing motion to insert the floss between your teeth. Never "snap" the floss into the gums! When the floss reaches the gum line curve it into a C-shape against one tooth and **gently slide** it into the space between the gum and the tooth until you feel resistance. (see figure 5)

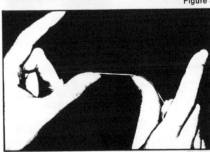

Figure 4

5
While holding the floss tightly against the tooth, move the floss away from the gum by scraping the floss up and down against the side of the tooth.

6
Repeat this method on the rest of your teeth.

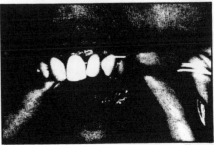

Figure 5

From *Cleaning Your Teeth and Gums,* American Dental Association, 211 East Chicago Avenue, Chicago, Illinois 60611

40-45% of the population obtains dental care. Perhaps through better dental understanding and appreciation for dental health the percentages can be favorably altered.

In its publication *A Dental Health Program for Schools,* the American Dental Association has outlined the following objectives for dental health education:

1. To help every school child appreciate the importance of a healthy mouth.
2. To help every school child appreciate the relationship of dental health to general health and appearance.
3. To encourage the observance of dental health practices, including personal care, professional care, proper diet and oral habits.
4. To enlist the aid of all groups and agencies interested in the promotion of school health.
5. To correlate dental health activities with the total school health program.

In designing programs for dental health education, it is important to be aware of the characteristic stages of children's emotional, physical, and mental development. Example of some characteristics and appropriate dental health education activities are shown in the chart below.

These are just a few ideas and a dentist or dental hygienist is a valuable resource person to gather additional information and approaches. It is essential that proper health habits are established early and encouraged through periodic reinforcement. The best place is the school health program.

CHARACTERISTICS	ACTIVITIES
Kindergarten	
—enjoy hearing stories	—tell animated stories about when to brush (immediately after eating)
—like dramatic pretending	—give a puppet show about non-carious causing foods.
First Grade	
—*why* is a favorite and often used word	—list the function of the teeth
—learn best from direct experience	—have a brush-in
Second Grade	
—losing primary teeth and getting permanent teeth	—demonstrate the pattern of eruption and the age for the total permanent dentition
—beginning to be safety conscious	—demonstrate the construction of a mouth guard and how it protects the oral cavity
Third Grade	
—have developed the ability to make decisions from known fact	—introduce nutritional data and the influence on optional dental health
—extensively use the word HOW	—review brushing methods and inform about the formation of plaque
Fourth Grade	
—enjoy competition	—develop a poster contest or essay contest for Children's Dental Health Week
—have acquired an interest and perspective of the community	—have a field trip to a dental office

Dental Floss

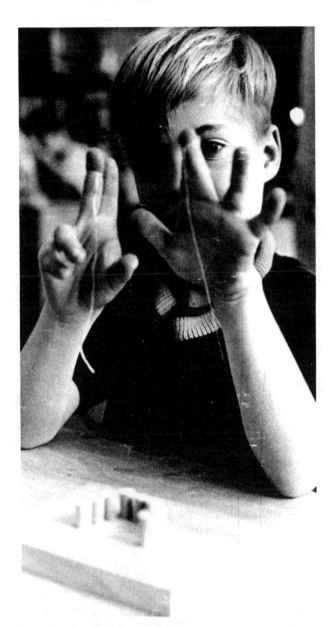

an oral hygiene tool for the elementary level

Dental health education has been inadequate in preparing our youngsters to care for their teeth. We have the knowledge to virtually wipe out dental disease, and yet 97 to 99% of Americans will probably contract some form of dental disease during their lifetime. The highest caries and gum disease rate today occurs in those individuals who do not practice beneficial oral hygiene techniques and/or in those who can't afford the luxuries of dental care. The low socio-economic neighborhood should be a prime objective of dental health education since today's effective oral hygiene devices are inexpensive and easily operated.

Dental floss and soft toothbrushes have been recommended by the American Dental Association and have been found effective in removing plaque or tooth debris along the gum line and on the surfaces of teeth. This article, however, specifically concerns the use of dental floss which has been proven to be beneficial in removing harmful debris from between teeth where toothbrushes, toothpicks, and water spray devices are not effective. It has been proven that teeth and gums will maintain their health as long as they are kept free of disease-causing bacteria. Dental floss prevents bacteria from accumulating and from causing disease by disrupting plaque's adhesive matrix that attaches to the teeth.

A limited number of investigations have been carried out to determine the effectiveness of a dental flossing program at the elementary-age level. A pilot study in San Antonio, Texas, described in the May-June 1972 issue of *School Health Review*, suggested that elementary students, K-6, can learn how to use dental floss effectively. Workshops were held to instruct teachers in dental disease prevention. Specifically, the program was directed towards the training of teachers to teach dental flossing and soft toothbrushing techniques which could eradicate the disease-causing plaque (a sticky matrix made up of bacteria, salivary products, food substances, and exfoliated cells from an individual's cheeks). Results of the two-year pilot study indicated that the most practical and effective classroom program involved two sessions of eight weeks each. Thirty

JAMES A. TERHUNE is an assistant professor of health education, San Francisco State University, San Francisco, California 94132.

to 60 minutes of instruction per day was required during the first two weeks of the program. The last six weeks required only 15 to 20 minute sessions twice a week.

Thirty-six teachers were involved in instructing more than 1,100 children in the above pilot program. Samples of groups within the total population demonstrated a marked improvement in gum tissue hygiene. The program seemed to be effective at all grade levels, but it was suggested that a modified approach to the instruction of dental flossing techniques, such as the use of manual flossing aids, might be appropriate for the K-2 levels.

Another investigation, carried out in two elementary schools in Lebanon, Oregon, proposed to determine how long it would take elementary students, aged eight, nine, ten, and eleven years, to learn an effective dental flossing technique.[1] Second and fourth grade youngsters from Santiam School and third and fifth grade youngsters from Queen Anne's Elementary School were separately presented a two hour general oral hygiene program. The children were divided into two groups of approximately 60 students each. The sessions concerned the causes and problems associated with dental disease, as well as the benefits derived from practicing positive oral hygiene techniques.

Fifteen students training to be dental assistants at Linn Benton Community College, a dentist, and a dental health instructor presented the dental disease education program. Students were shown slides and were directly involved with laboratory-type experiences, such as measuring the pH of various foods, determining the amounts of sugar left in their mouths after consuming a candy bar, and examining their oral cavities for dental plaque. A new and inexpensive instrument known as the Plak-Lite,[2] was used to enable the students to see the plaque on their own teeth. Two drops of sodium fluoroscein dye with the aid of a Plak-Lite provided the children an opportunity to discover exactly where they had failed to clean their teeth properly. The dye and Plak-Lite are excellent motivators, for they magically expose the hidden plaque, making it glow brilliantly. The dye is also quite adaptable for classroom use, since it is easily removed by a water rinse.

In the afternoon following the introductory dental hygiene program, individual classes of approximately 30 students each were given 50 minutes of group instruction on the flossing technique. Again, the 15 student dental assistants helped train the school children. The technique described for the students was proposed by O'Leary and Nabers.[3] They suggested that the floss be wrapped around the middle fingers, manipulated with the two index fingers between the lower teeth, and stretched between a thumb and index finger in order to clean the surfaces between the upper-maxillary teeth.

During each of the remaining ten days of the program, students were given up to 14 minutes of individualized instruction and 15 minutes of group instruction. Each day, for the final ten days of the program, five student dental assistants helped teach the children how to manipulate the dental floss.

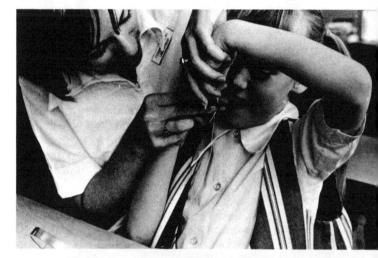

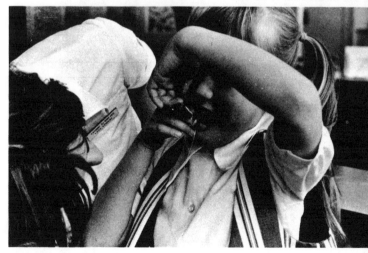

Every day the students were evaluated for their ability to pass two tests: the Direct Observation Evaluation (DOE) and the Flossing Performance Index (FPI). The DOE determined the number of days it took a student to learn how to manipulate the dental floss between each set of teeth. The FPI rated six teeth for the presence of plaque and indicated the number of days it took the school children to learn how to effectively clean between the teeth. The students passed the tests and were released from the investigation when they were able to manipulate the floss between all of their teeth and achieve a 50% reduction in plaque, within approximately eight minutes. Most children found that four of the six teeth evaluated in the FPI test were more difficult to floss than many of their other teeth. Thus, a 50% reduction in plaque would probably mean that the overall removal of plaque was substantially greater than 50%.

Analysis of the data on the 117 elementary children revealed that all of the eight, nine, ten, and eleven year olds were able to pass both flossing tests within ten, seven, six, and five days, respectively. This suggests that most elementary students have the manual dexterity to learn a dental flossing technique and that a dental flossing program can be taught to groups within our schools. It was also discovered that all children in the study could learn how to wrap and manipulate dental floss between at least two teeth by the end of one 50 minute program. This suggests that all students, aged eight years and older, would have the dexterity to begin to build a daily dental flossing habit after receiving 50 minutes of instruction.

In conclusion, both investigations used trained personnel to instruct the elementary children. The investigations also involved the students in an educational program that provided them with the motivation for developing an interest in and a positive attitude toward a dental flossing technique. The study in Lebanon, Oregon determined that all of the eight, nine, ten, and eleven year old children were able to learn how to clean their teeth with dental floss within a ten day time period. It was also discovered that all students could learn how to wrap as well as to manipulate floss between two teeth within a one 50 minute training session. The San Antonio pilot study found that all of the elementary students, K-6, could learn how to use dental floss. The pilot investigation also indicated that at least two years of reinforcement may be necessary for the formation of good flossing habits.

Implications for the Teacher

The two oral hygiene investigations suggest that school districts should begin training their teachers to deliver flossing education programs to elementary students. Workshops should be held to train teachers how to be effective in their presentations. Dental assistants, hygienists, and dentists should be invited to take part in the training program. High school students could be taught the procedures first and then used as aids to help practicing elementary teachers provide flossing instruction. Parents should be encouraged to cooperate and to take part in the flossing program. Bulletins should be sent home to keep the parents informed of the program's progress. Parents should also be invited to attend teacher's dental health workshops or asked to take part in setting up their own dental flossing training program. Local radio stations, newspapers, and shopping centers should be encouraged to advertise dental flossing programs as a public service.

Most importantly, once the program is initiated and students and parents begin to learn how to use dental floss, the education program must continue. Students should have five to ten minutes after lunch each day to floss their teeth and, of course, teachers should provide an example by taking the time to use dental floss in front of their students. Finally, since dental floss can be obtained inexpensively in large quantities, it should be provided upon request by each individual student. Providing floss for elementary children is an extremely important facet of the program, since successful habit formation can depend upon the availability of oral hygiene materials. Once children have the desire to maintain effective flossing habits, schools will no longer need to supply the material. If flossing education is started at the second grade level and reinforced continuously, most children will have a well-established habit by the time they enter junior high school.

[1] Terhune, James A., "The Effect of Age, Sex and Eye-Hand Coordination On the Ability To Predict the Readiness of Elementary Students To Learn An Effective Dental Flossing Technique." Doctoral thesis, Corvallis: Oregon State University, 1972.
[2] Plak-Lite Sales Department, International Pharmaceutical Corporation, Warrington, Pa. 18976.
[3] O'Leary, Timothy J. and Claude L. Nabers. "Instructions to Supplement Teaching Oral Hygiene," Journal of Periodontology 40: 27-32. 1969.

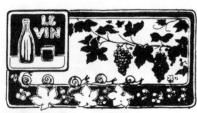

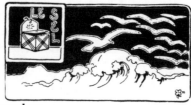

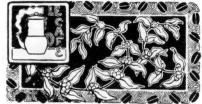

Empathizing With Addicts

PETER FINN is senior education and training analyst at ABT Associates, Inc., 55 Wheeler Street, Cambridge, Massachusetts 02138.

Most people who have never experienced a major addiction such as, alcoholism, drug dependence, compulsive eating, or cigarette smoking, have little understanding and often many misconceptions about what it feels like to have a persistent and irresistible craving for a substance or activity. An addiction is defined here as a craving for a substance or activity which a person cannot at the moment resist consistently or for a sustained period of time. In the following learning exercise, students gain insight into the nature of addictions by refraining for an agreed-upon period of time from an activity they have found extremely enjoyable for some time. As a result of this period of "abstinence," students may be better able to appreciate what an addicted person feels like and how they can best help relatives and friends who may have a dependency.

The exercise may also enable some students to realize that they have a strong and perhaps ungovernable urge for a substance or activity and to consider whether their compulsive behavior is healthy and what causes it. The exercise can foster insight into why everyone feels dependent on some activities and provide an inkling of how the students may feel if they are some day deprived of a substance or activity to which they have become accustomed or addicted.

This exercise has been used many times by me at the junior and senior high school level. However, it probably would be successful with elementary school students and adult groups, as well.

Procedure

Have students pick one or two activities which they would find very difficult—perhaps impossible—to stop doing. Then have each student agree in a written contract with the rest of the class to forego the activity for at least a week, but preferably for a month. It might be more enjoyable and educational for students to experiment with a friend or small group, with each person renouncing the same activity. Depending on their "passions," students might:

  use no salt or sugar in their food
  give up cigarettes
  stop seeing or talking with a close friend
  not kiss or touch their girlfriend, boyfriend, husband, or wife
  not make or answer any telephone calls
  get up at 4:00 a.m. every morning (not sleep late)
  stop watching television or listening to the radio
  give up Coke, coffee, or another favorite beverage
  give up a favorite sport or other form of recreation
  stop chewing gum

It may be helpful for the students to keep a diary of their behavior and feelings during the experiment to jog their memory when they relate their experiences to the class. Students can also talk into a tape recorder at the end of each day and play back excerpts to the class at the conclusion of the experiment.

Follow-up Discussion

After students have refrained from their activities for at least a week, have the class recount their experiences, then answer the following questions.

1. How many of you succeeded in refraining from your activities for the entire period of time stipulated in your contracts? How soon did those who failed give in? How do those of you who failed give in? How do those of you who failed feel about yourselves—disappointed? angry? indifferent? relieved? How do those of you who succeed feel—superior? sympathetic? resentful? neutral?

2. What did not doing the activity feel like? Did you miss it badly? Did you get angry? frightened? miserable? grouchy? bored? frustrated?

3. Did your relationships with other people change? For example, did you avoid certain people, or people in general, spend more time than usual with certain people, or with people in general, or relate to people differently such as, arguing more than normally?

4. Did talking or being with other students who were refraining from the same activity (or a different activity) help you resist the temptation to give in? Did you ask for, and get, help from other people in your attempts to forego the activity? How did they respond? How would you have liked them to respond?

5. Did other people change their behavior, attitudes, or feelings toward you as a result of your experiment? How did you feel about and react to that?

6. Did you start doing things that you don't usually do, such as forget things, become less observant, overeat, or develop physical symptoms such as headaches, stomach aches, tics, loss of appetite, insomnia, or unusual fatigue?

7. Did your other activities change at all? Did you compensate for the lack of your "forbidden" activity by participating more in some other pursuit? Did the substitute activity help take your mind off the thing you wanted to do? Did your efforts at compensation affect any of the people around you?

8. Were you confronted with an opportunity to "lapse," and did your willpower diminish in the presence of the forbidden activity or object? Were other people considerate in not mentioning the activity or substance, or helpful in suggesting a substitute?

9. Did you go out of your way to avoid the activity or substance, or things that might remind you of it? Did your avoidance behavior help reduce your craving?

10. Did you cheat at all? If so, did you try to engage in your activity just a little and find you couldn't resist resuming it completely? Did you bother to hide your lapses from other people? If so, did anyone catch you cheating? How did they react? How did you feel about being discovered?

11. When you finally did go back to the activity, how did it feel? Did you try to "make up for lost time"?

After the class has explored the issues related to these questions, students can discuss how their actions and feelings might be similar to those of an alcoholic, drug addict, cigarette smoker, compulsive eater, or other addicted person. The group should also consider how its experiences may have been different from those of truly addicted people. For example, the students knew they could resume their activity with impunity at the end of the test period, while an alcoholic, who has stopped drinking or an obese person who has begun dieting knows that to revert to their former behavior is to court disaster.

Students may also erroneously conclude, based on their own success, that addicted people should be able with relative ease to reject their self-destructive practices. The students' experience may have misled them because their own craving was a comparatively mild one and made even more bearable by the realization that it was only temporary.

Finally, focus specifically on how the students feel about addicted people. Do they feel the same way about alcoholics or drug addicts as they felt about themselves during their experiment? Should they? Did they gain any new insights into what it feels like to have an addiction and how addicted people can best be helped to shake off their dependency? Were the students able to identify any compulsive behaviors of their own and gain a better understanding of how to evaluate and cope with them?

One Way To Ascertain Drug Perceptions

PATRICK KIDD TOW is an assistant professor in the Department of Health and Physical Education at Old Dominion University, Norfolk, Virginia 23508.

Health educators occasionally run across students with misconceptions about various drugs and their effects. A good amount of drug information students retain seems to be from peer group sources. However, such sources are not always entirely accurate. Yet, students hold peer group opinions in relatively high esteem. This strategy is *not* intended to discredit the role of peers as information sources. On the contrary, peer influence on preventive health behaviors may be far more profound than that of health educators.

For this reason, all out attempts should be made to correct any misconceptions about substance use and abuse. Completion and scoring of the Drug Perception Scale (DPS) and the ensuing classroom discussions should help clarify some of the drug-related issues of concern. There are two prerequisites to administering this teaching tool to junior or senior high school students—health educators must become thoroughly familiar with the content of the scale and answers to students' questions must be based on factual information and not hearsay or personal opinion. Discrepencies between the drug information from teachers and student peer groups must be resolved as accurately as possible.

The teaching instrument to be used is depicted in a table below.

Examples of the process involved should be provided. For example, a student examines the relationship between beer and the likelihood of physical dependence. He may think it is seldom a possibility and assign a score of two. He

may perceive beer and psychological dependence as a more real and frequent danger and assigns a score of four. He may not perceive any possibility of overdose on beer and assign a score of one. The scores should be summed up in each row to represent the respective drug in the "total" column.

When everyone in class has completed the scale, the individual totals for each drug should be listed on the board. As the disparity or homogeneity among the given scores becomes apparent the class will begin commenting on the results of the scale. This teaching tool is beneficial for pre and post test analyses as well as a discussion stimulant. Respondents review their perceptions about the listed drugs while completing the scale and in the ensuing discussion period. Various viewpoints will surface and the health educator should facilitate any peer group interaction. The discussions about society, parent, and peer group disapproval may prove to be particularly interesting since the scoring in this portion is more subjective.

	Physical Dependence	Psychological Dependence	Overdose	Physical Damage	Society Disapproval	Parent Disapproval	Peer Group Disapproval	TOTAL
Beer								
Cigarettes								
Marijuana								
Cocaine								
LSD								
Amphetamines								
Barbiturates								
Coffee								
Heroin								
Whiskey								

The rows represent ten popular mood modifiers used by members of society. The columns represent predicaments which can occur. Students are directed to assign a score to each drug in every column to indicate the perceived likelihood of occurrence. The range of scores is: 5 = always; 4 = frequently; 3 = sometimes; 2 = seldom; 1 = never.

SODA: Models To Teach About Drugs and Self-Esteem

RICHARD M. BARRETT is the coordinator for Health, Secondary Physical Education, Henrico County School Board, Highland Springs, Virginia 23075.

The Henrico County, Virginia school system has been using high school students as role models for fifth and sixth graders for several years with great success. SODA, or Student Organization on Developing Attitudes, is a big brother and big sister approach to handling values education for younger students.

types of evaluations, a number of students are chosen each year to be a part of SODA. In the past it has been so popular among Henrico county students that as many as ten people have vied for one SODA vacancy.

Support from high school teachers and administrators has been strong. Despite

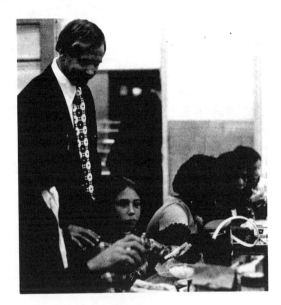

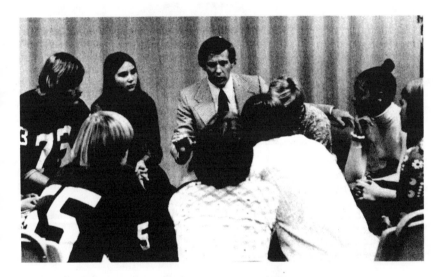

The program was initiated at first as a means of heading off drug curiosity before it becomes a drug problem in students. Through the years it has become a highly visible student-oriented contact program which instills positive values into twelve-year olds about drugs and themselves.

Carefully chosen teams of one boy and one girl are assigned to a fifth or sixth grade classroom for a year. During their visits, role models eat lunch with students, play with them, and talk with them. The high school people try to set an example for the impressionable pre-adolescents. They also discuss school problems and the difficulties of growing up. Often the high school teams show movies and lead group discussions which are designed to develop and reinforce positive values and attitudes.

The SODA students are chosen basically by the guideline that they must strive to be the kind of people they want their own children to be like. Through several

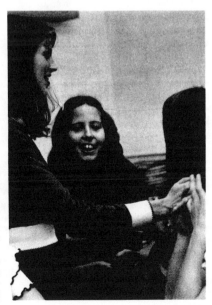

the fact that SODA members must periodically miss classes, teachers see SODA as a way to better classes in the future. They find the time to give SODA members a missed assignment or help them keep up with their academic work.

The Henrico County School Board provides funds for SODA, seeing it as an important humanizing aspect of the schools. Funds for the all-day training sessions of SODA members have been provided by the Board of Education and the Council on Drug Abuse Control.

SODA students are trained in understanding and communicating, not in teaching. This was one of the facts that had to be impressed on teachers and principals. The idea was to have the student role models act naturally, and hope the pre-adolescents will want to copy them.

Team members frequently give their fifth or sixth graders their home phone number and encourage the youngsters to call whenever they have a problem they want to talk about, whether it is about school, friends, or just chatting. It is these informal talks that are often the most productive and influential on the young students. They know they can get sound advice just by calling their older friends.

According to Barrett the SODA program is showing its impact in the higher grades "through better discipline, citizenship, and decreased drug usage."

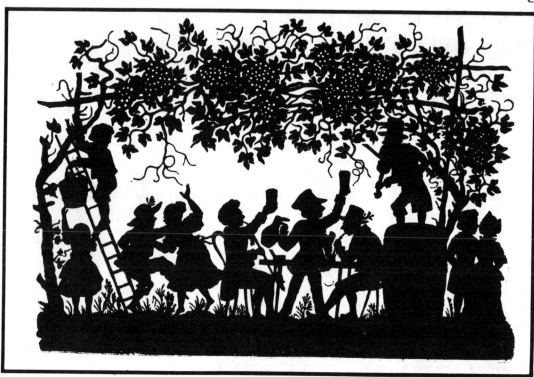

Drug Use Situations

BRUCE A. UHRICH is a former instructor in the Health Education Division at the University of North Carolina at Greensboro. He is currently a graduate student in the Department of Health Education at Temple University, Philadelphia, Pennsylvania 19122.

Under what conditions should the use of a drug be regarded as acceptable behavior in our society? To deal with this question I have developed, over the past two years, a series of statements which challenge student values and stimulate classroom discussion. I give students a handout with the following statements and these directions: "Read each statement carefully, then respond by rating each as an acceptable or unacceptable situation in which to use drugs. Be prepared to share each of your answers with the class, and to explain why you answered as you did."

Situation

1. Drinking an alcoholic beverage at a party.
2. Drinking an alcoholic beverage after work to relax at home.
3. Drinking an alcoholic beverage before driving several hundred miles.
4. Drinking an alcoholic beverage alone after an argument.
5. Drinking an alcoholic beverage at a football game.
6. Using a narcotic drug in a hospital for relief of pain following an operation.
7. Use of a narcotic drug by the head of a household in a lower socioeconomic area.
8. Use of a narcotic drug by a physician.
9. Use of a narcotic drug by students in an upper class high school.
10. Use of a narcotic drug as a cough suppressant.
11. Smoking tobacco in a high school restroom.
12. Smoking tobacco after dinner.
13. Smoking tobacco when meeting new people at a reception.
14. Smoking tobacco while riding in a car pool.
15. Smoking tobacco in class.
16. Using a sedative/tranquilizer to commit suicide.
17. Use of a sedative/tranquilizer to relax a neurotic personality.
18. Use of a sedative/tranquilizer to encourage sleep because of a loud roommate.
19. Use of a sedative/tranquilizer prescribed by a physician and then drinking heavily.
20. Use of a sedative/tranquilizer to relax before having to make a speech before a large group.
21. Utilizing marijuana at a dorm party.
22. Using marijuana after work to relax at home.
23. Refusing when handed a "joint" by your best friend.
24. Utilizing marijuana on a daily basis.
25. Using marijuana before an intramural softball game.
26. Starting each day with a cup of caffeine, before anything else.
27. Taking a "hit" of some stolen nitrous oxide.
28. Sniffing glue at a party.
29. Taking aspirin every time you feel any pain.
30. Receiving a painkilling drug from a paramedic for injuries at the scene of the accident.

Because the choices are limited to the extremes of acceptable or unacceptable, most students are highly motivated to verbally qualify their feelings. This situation allows the instructor to act as a true facilitator. For each statement, all students indicate by a show of hands which response they chose. Several students with acceptable and unacceptable ratings are then asked to explain their choice and supportive feelings. The result is class discussion, exposing all class members to a variety of opinions.

Who Me, Addicted?

Robert Stern is former director of community services, Greater Hartford Council on Alcoholism, and a former instructor of health education at Southern Connecticut State College and SUNY - Cortland. His address is 11 Regent Street, Hartford, Connecticut 06107.

Too often physical dependency is associated with the word addiction without enough consideration for its social and psychological components. Social dependency refers to individuals who consistently take a drug, not because they want it, but to be accepted by their peers or to be comfortable in a social setting. Phychological dependency occurs when people take a drug because they think they function better with the drug, for example people who smoke marijuana before a concert to enhance their enjoyment of the music.

Physical dependency is a state in which physiological symptoms occur when regular use of a drug has been stopped. These individuals no longer have the casual choice of the socially or psychologically dependent drug users. They must take the drug to avoid the pain of withdrawal.

While only a small percentage of drug users will ever become physically addicted to a substance, a large majority will become socially or psychologically dependent on their drug of choice. Therefore, in a drug education program, a discussion of addiction that is meaningful to the drug user's experience and complete in its consideration of all phases of drug dependency is essential. The Drug Dependency Inventory (DDI) was developed as one method of achieving this goal. It has been proven effective with high school and college students as well as teachers in in-service workshops. This strategy was designed to enhance classroom discussion and reinforce the following points.

1. What is drug addiction? Students share their definitions of addiction with their classmates. A discussion of addiction as a composite of social, psychological, and physical dependencies is held.

2. At what point is drug addiction considered destructive? These discussions center on the equality of life created by that individual's drug-taking behavior rather than the quantity of drug consumed.

3. Are you addicted to your drug of choice? After completing and analyzing the DDI, students assess their drug-taking behavior within the three areas of dependency as compared with their classmates.

4. How do you value your drug-taking behavior? Within the assessment, students place a value on the constructiveness/destructiveness of their drug-taking behavior.

Before administering DDI, participants should be aware that the results of the inventory are confidential and for their benefit alone. The effectiveness of the DDI depends on honest and accurate responses to each question.

Figure 1 is an example of a drug dependency inventory. Alcohol was selected as the drug, but with a few modifications, any drug can be substituted.

After the drug inventories are scored, they are anonymously collected and the class mean average is computed for each dependency index. This provides the students with an opportunity to assess their own drug dependencies and to compare their results with their peers. Based on the results of the scores received from students enrolled in a Drug Studies Workshop at the State University of New York at Cortland, the mean average score for the social dependency index was 10.2, the mean average for the psychological dependency index was 7.5 and a 4.4. was the indicated mean average for the physical dependency index. Of course, these averages will vary depending on the specific population being evaluated.

While the Drug Dependency Index has not yet been validated, this instrument has proven to be a relevant, safe, and effective mechanism for initiating valuable student dialogue in the areas of personal drug use, dependency, and addiction.

Figure 1. Drug Dependency Inventory

Here are some statements made by people to describe what they get out of drinking. How often do you feel this way about drinking? Circle one number for each statement. IMPORTANT: Answer every question.

I am the type of person who:	Always	Frequently	Occas.	Seldom	Never
A. Drinks to be socially accepted.	4	3	2	1	0
B. Drinks to be more myself.	4	3	2	1	0
C. Feels more comfortable in a party environment when drinking.	4	3	2	1	0
D. Downs (gulps) my alcoholic beverage.	4	3	2	1	0
E. Has experienced a loss of memory (blackout) during or after drinking.	4	3	2	1	0
F. Drinks when depressed, frustrated or angry.	4	3	2	1	0
G. Accepts a drink when pressured by friends.	4	3	2	1	0
H. Has gotten into fights or arguments when drinking.	4	3	2	1	0
I. Feels more superior when drinking.	4	3	2	1	0
J. Drinks when I am bored.	4	3	2	1	0
K. Feels more popular with friends or date after being relaxed with alcohol.	4	3	2	1	0
L. Likes to drink alone.	4	3	2	1	0

Scoring

Add up the numbers you have circled in items.
A × C × G × K = Social Dependency Index
B × F × I × J = Psychological
D × E × H × L = Physical Dependecy Index

Environmental Health

Health or Hazard? A Post-China Syndrome Game

Moon S. Chen, Jr.

Moon S. Chen, Jr. is an assistant professor of health education at Ohio State University, 215 Pomerene Hall, 1760 Niel Avenue, Columbus, Ohio 43210.

How important is it to teach about ionizing radiation or noise protection or industrial safety? For most students, these three topics seem remote and removed from the classroom. However, the movie, *The China Syndrome*, made the Three Mile Island incident and the hazards of radiation hauntingly realistic. Students and teachers in the Harrisonburg area were undoubtedly affected and students elsewhere certainly felt curiosity and a need to know more facts. What better place to bring together the topics of radiation and health hazards of the working environment than in an environmental health course or in a unit on environmental health? And how better to make learning more fun than with a game?

Fun and success with such a game, called "Health or Hazard?", are attributed to proper orientation and to student involvement and discovery. Orientation to the game consists of a cognitive introduction to the basic forms of radiation (e.g., ionizing—alpha, beta, gamma rays, and non-ionizing—microwaves) and how to use time, distance, and shielding for protection. A cognitive introduction to health hazards of the working environment should cover the detrimental effects on humans of noise, dust, gases, and toxic liquids. Protection measures would include environmental manipulation, medical surveillance, management decisions, and personal protection. Students should be taught to adapt such principles to specific hazards (that is where much of the learning occurs).

Following cognitive input, the teacher should divide the class into three equal-sized and intellectually-matched groups. One group will be student referees with responsibility for awarding points and making decisions regarding disagreements between sides. Their preparation will consist of correctly matching hazards with proper health protection methods.

The two other groups will be compet-

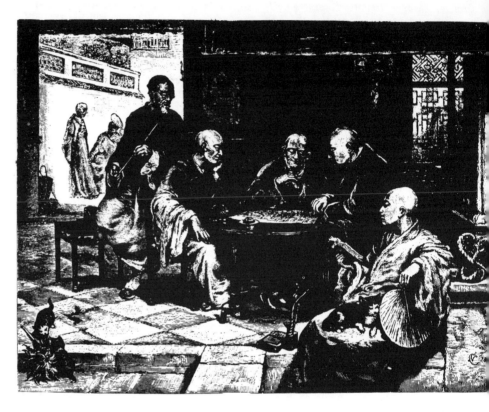

ing teams. Each team should prepare itself independently. Based on the cognitive information given in class, each team should prepare an array of "offensive" hazards and an arsenal of "defensive" health protection measures. Each hazard and each health protection measure should be written on a separate index card large enough so that it can be read across a classroom.

The spirit of competition between the two sides fosters a spirit of cooperation on each side. Team members naturally help each other in learning the associations between hazards and the proper health protection.

Competition begins after about fifteen minutes of preparation. Each side alternately chooses a player from the opposite team to "challenge." Each challenge is considered a "round." Each team alternately assumes an offensive and defensive position.

During the round the offensive player chooses a hazard with which to "attack" the defensive player. The hazard is hidden from view until the offensive and defensive players face each other in the front of the classroom. The defensive player brings his arsenal of methods. On a signal from the judge, the offensive player flashes his hazard. The defensive

player has fifteen seconds to respond by showing the card with the correct health protection measure against that hazard. If the correct health protection measure is not on one of the defensive player's cards, the defensive player has the same fifteen second time limit to write the proper health protection on a separate index card. No coaching from teammates is allowed.

A score results when either side wins a "round." Decisions regarding which side wins will be made by the student judge for that particular round. The student judge must decide whether the defensive player's response is correct and made within the fifteen-second limit. (The time should be kept by another judge.) If the defensive player displays the correct response within the time limit, the defensive side scores a point. If not, the offensive side wins a point. The first team to win a predetermined number of points wins.

For greater variety and excitement, more than one hazard can be introduced at one time, forcing the defensive players to respond more quickly. This game can be played at the pace of the students. It is fun, exciting, and a harmless way to learn health protection measures against radiation and hazards of the working environment.

The Paper Drive

We had made many important decisions for our class during our class meetings, but none of them affected us in such a profound way as our decision to have a paper drive.

At the end of our study of environmental conditions and after taking a close look at environmental health problems, my fifth grade class was determined to find a project which would make the community aware of some of the problems of ecology and would also benefit our community. When Chuck suggested that we collect newspapers, magazines, and other paper items for recycling, the class decided that this was the project they wanted to try.

During the subsequent class meetings, we set up committees to obtain permission from our principal for the school-wide drive and to locate the nearest recycling center and determine the amount paid for used paper. Finally, we set up the committees which would handle the details of the drive itself. Our principal approved of the drive, and we found that the nearby Apex Scrap Company gave 40¢ per hundred pounds of paper. It was decided that the drive would be held for six days—Wednesday, Thursday, and Friday of two consecutive weeks. To spur involvement and competition, a contest would be held among the classes. The class contributing the most paper—by weight—would win, and this class would decide how the school would spend the proceeds of the drive.

Posters advertising the drive were made and distributed. Letters explaining the purpose of the

Julie Crocker teaches fifth grade at the Magnolia Elementary School, Lanham, Maryland.

drive, the dates, and the procedure for bringing the paper to school were sent home to every family. Parents were asked to volunteer their station wagons and trucks to transport the paper to the recycling center. Everyone in our class was involved. Enthusiasm and excitement were high.

We thought we had planned well—but we had not anticipated the kind of community response which followed.

On the first day of the drive, our school driveway was jammed with cars and with people unloading paper. Children's wagons filled with papers and magazines were throughout the halls. Every student appeared to be carrying or pulling some kind of container filled with paper. Our original instructions had been that the paper must be bound and labeled by room number. It was to be stacked outside each room so that it could be weighed. Some of the paper arriving on our opening day was bound, but much of it was not. Few bundles were labeled. The halls were filling up with paper, and it was difficult to know which bundles belonged to which room. Parents continued to deliver paper throughout the day. Confusion reigned.

Slowly, the committees in charge began to reorganize the drive. Announcements were made by the students reminding them that the paper must be bound and labeled. One class volunteered to demonstrate how to correctly bundle papers. Delivery times for parents were set. The mounds of paper in the hallways were gradually brought under control. It had been a hectic beginning, and we were exhausted. But when the totals for the day were announced, cheers were heard throughout the building.

We had anticipated between 10 and 15 thousand pounds of paper for the entire drive. We reached 10,000 pounds the first day. Churches sent in old church bulletins, businesses cleaned their files, government offices contributed excess paper and old forms; few communities had cleaner attics and basements than ours. Even the evening paper had to be read quickly or else.

Our problems were far from over, however. More cars and trucks were needed to transport the backlog of papers which had developed. The paper had to be moved to an empty room until it could be taken to the center. This took time and muscle. Parents and students volunteered to help on Saturdays. Other classes wanted to help and did.

Each day the results of the drive were announced on the public address system and charted on a bar graph in the cafeteria. Everywhere students were discussing the drive. As the drive progressed, we became better organized. By the second week we were quite an efficient team.

When the final results were tabulated we had collected 22 tons of paper and had earned $126 for the school. We were tired, but elated. Mrs. Arnold's class had contributed eight thousand pounds and had won the contest. They decided to purchase a piece of playground equipment with the proceeds.

It is difficult to capture exactly the effect of the drive on each student and on the morale of our class and our school. How can you evaluate the effect of seeing your idea transformed into a successful venture? What value can you place on feeling so useful and important? How important is it to commit yourself to a project and work out each problem as it presents itself? How valuable is it to experience the benefits of cooperative efforts? These are some of the thoughts which occurred to me as I watched my class in action.

All that I can be sure of is that the drive became a turning point for the students in my class. Bill would be telling someone about a ball game and would mention "Oh that was the one before the paper drive," or Sally would be commenting on the date of her pajama party and would interject "it was about two weeks after the paper drive." Somehow "after the paper drive" we were different.

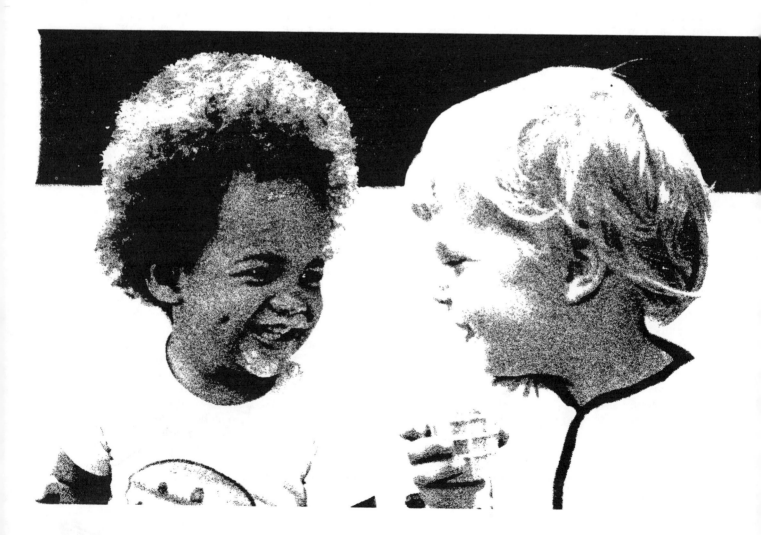

Environmental Health

Guidelines for a Recycling Project

George H. Brooks is assistant to the dean of the University of Northern Colorado Graduate School and chairman of the Greeley Committee on Environment.

Health educators and their students may become involved in local environmental action by helping to establish a community newspaper recycling program. One such program has been successfully operated since July 1971 by the Greeley (Colorado) Committee on Environment. The committee, appointed by the city council in 1969, originally consisted of about a dozen members—businessmen, housewives, teachers, and faculty members. Other members have been added, including a staff member of the local newspaper—a recent journalism graduate, keenly interested in the committee's work, whose added publicity efforts have greatly helped the success of the project.

The committee decided to undertake a newspaper recycling project after learning that 50% or more of the volume of municipal solid waste is made up of paper and paper products, and that about half of that volume consists of newspapers and magazines. They contacted a paper salvage company in Denver, which assured the committee that they would purchase the paper they collected.

A subcommittee was appointed to find a building to serve as a central collection center. In a long, unfruitful search they found building owners reluctant to permit storage of newspapers because of the potential fire hazard, or desiring to secure a long-term tenant. They investigated the possibility of securing a railroad car on a convenient siding, but learned that a car couldn't be spared. A local trucking firm, learning of the project, offered to spot a semi-trailer in a local shopping center parking lot on collection day, then haul the trailer to the paper salvage company in Denver. Permission was gotten to use the parking lot area —far enough away from the

main parking lot traffic pattern, yet permitting smooth in-and-out traffic flow along both sides of the trailer. Arrangements were made with the local police department for traffic control and with the city street department for portable barricades to channel traffic flow along both sides of the trailer.

The second Saturday of the month was selected and publicized as collection day. The Committee on Environment loaded the trailer that first Saturday, while a subcommittee sought volunteer groups to furnish labor for loading in subsequent months. The first day's collection yielded 27 tons. Seeing what the collection could amount to, the committee decided to share the monetary return from the sale of paper with the groups which offered to help —one-third to the committee, one-third to the morning volunteer group, and one-third to the afternoon group. The news media carried the story of the committee's plans for continuing the paper collection on the

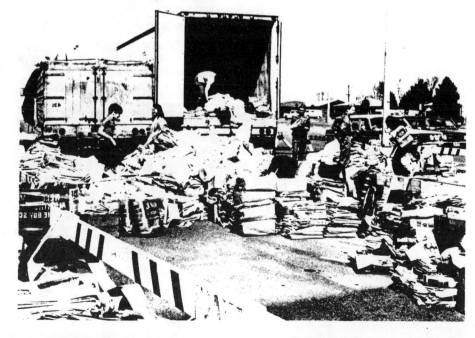

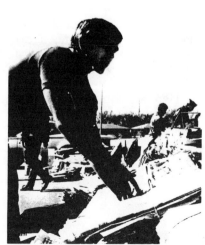

second Saturday of each month. Volunteer groups, wanting to earn money for their projects, were soon put on a waiting list as groups were assigned collection days several months in advance.

A telephone answering service agreed to receive calls from aged persons and others unable to bring their papers to the collection center. Trucks and station wagons, furnished by members of the groups working at the collection center, collected papers from callers. Most people who wanted pick-up service made their calls ahead of the 10 a.m. deadline on collection day. There was little cause for concern over abuse of the service.

The Committee·on Environment hopes that Greeley will soon combine its trash collection with recycling on a city-wide basis. However, though the technology is available for such an undertaking, the market for recycled materials needs to be expanded. Even paper collection alone is not yet feasible on a city-wide basis; the paper salvage company says it would be unable to handle all of Greeley's paper along with all the other paper delivered to its docks.

Greeley's Committee on Environment can boast of a great deal of first-hand experience with what has become a widely accepted but not always practiced dictum: man must live with his environment, not despoil it. People will cooperate, if properly informed and motivated with sound, well-planned projects.

Here are some suggestions for those who want to start their own recycling project.

A market for the materials to be recycled is a must. The company accepting secondary materials must be notified in advance of the start of your project.

Have adequate transportation available. Greeley's first Saturday collection filled a 40-foot van type semi-trailer. Every Saturday since, two trailers have been needed; in March 1972 a third truck was partially filled.

Advise city officials and the police department of your project.

Publicize each collection day, taking into account the different deadlines of daily and weekly newspapers and radio and television stations. Announce and adhere to opening and closing hours; remind people not to leave materials at any other time. Include phone numbers of key committee members and answering service, if any. Give clear instructions on how materials are to be tied, bundled, or boxed.

Liability insurance is a must.

Have adequate workers on hand —a minimum of 10 or 12— during all collection hours. At times even that may not be enough, though at other times it may be too many. Workers may need gloves for handling paper bundles. Lifting bundles by the heavy cord soon wears blisters on tender hands.

Someone should be responsible for receiving the checks by mail from the company purchasing the papers or other materials. A home address or Post Office box may be used. The same person should be authorized to write checks to the volunteer groups who furnish labor for your project, and should keep records of names and mailing addresses.

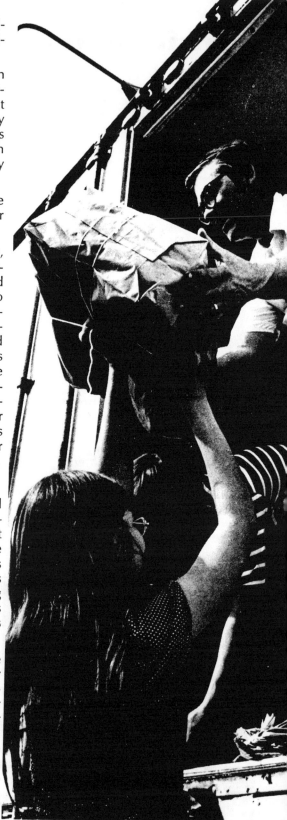

A Working Model for Simulation Techniques

GLEN G. GILBERT is instructor of health education, University of North Carolina at Greensboro, Greensboro, North Carolina 27412. Much of the material for this article is from the ongoing research by the author for his doctoral dissertation at Ohio State University.

Instructors of emergency care are faced with the challenge of educating personnel to deal with complex situations that require prompt and efficient treatment. The instructor, largely because of time limitations, is often forced to rely on "one shot" coverage of the individual skills involved. Commonly such coverage is followed by a paper and pencil test in an attempt to evaluate the students' ability to apply specific skills.

This article presents an alternative method of teaching and evaluating those skills dealt with in emergency health care classes. It promotes confidence in the students' ability to employ the newly acquired skills in real life situations, presenting a variety of situations that require the application of a multiplicity of first aid skills.

The use of simulated emergency care situations is not a new idea, but this article presents several new variations on simulation design and provides a working model for those persons unfamiliar with simulation techniques.

Simulated situations can be an asset to any emergency care program for the following reasons:

1. They provide examples of real life emergency care situations.

2. They provide practical applications of skills covered in the classroom.

3. They provide practice in the analysis and evaluation of emergency situations without possible injury resulting from judgment errors.

4. They provide an alternate teaching strategy for the instructor.

5. They provide a possible evaluation technique for instructors.

6. They provide students with practice in performing skills under stress and thereby should increase self-confidence.

Simulations can become an integral part of an emergency care instructional program from the onset. They can be used in a variety of ways, some of which are outlined below:

1. They can be used as a direct communication strategy by presenting the situation and the correct performance of first aid procedures by the instructor or the student.

2. They can serve as an instructor-student interaction strategy by presenting the situation and jointly (instructor and class) analyzing the proper course of action and reasoning.

3. They can be a group activity with several people working out a course of action and then undertaking it. This might be better in more complicated situations.

4. They can function as an independent student activity by setting up an area where students come in and perform skills in varied situations.

You may wish to devise your own simulation situations or ask your students to make them up for you, in which case each student should design one situation complete with symptoms and procedures. A file of such student situations can be collected and made available to students for review.

The Simulation Model: Scenario

The student selected to perform as a first aider selects a card, reads the number, and leaves the room.[1] While he is out of the room the situation numbered is set up. Other students are employed as victims with symptom tags, medical alert tags, or whatever is appropriate for the situation, placed on their person. These tags are put at the site of the simulated injury or symptom. The materials which are available to the first aider are placed in the area designated as the situation area.

The student re-enters the room upon notification and reads the card out loud to the class (he is allowed to keep it during the situation). He then examines the situation, makes a judgment based upon the symptom tags, and other information provided, and then performs the proper first aid procedures. The instructor rates the student's performance using a predesigned form.

The more realistic a situation, the better it is as a learning device. There are simulation kits available that include simulated injuries and simulated bleeding which can be used, but they require a much larger amount of time and the cost is often high. The major

---

[1]Selection of situation cards should be accomplished by shuffling and the taking of the top card each time or some other method at the discretion of the instructor. However, it is advised that a random device be employed so that students will not feel their situation was predetermined at the will of the instructor.

advantage of the system described here is that it is relatively fast and inexpensive while providing a good deal of realism.

You may wish to add certain realistic touches such as turning out the lights to simulate night time, adding more props, or even having victims chew cookies and simulate vomiting. The extent to which you carry this is limited only by your imagination.

Critique

Following the completion of situations it is recommended that a critique be held, explaining the proper procedures and clearing up any questions. This can be done after each situation, at the close of each session, or at the end of all the situations depending on the instructor's time schedule and wishes. Copies of the rating form may be distributed and used by fellow students during the performance, for comparison and to reinforce learning. They can also be collected by the instructor to aid him in his rating.

Another technique is to employ overhead projections (showing correct procedures) during the situation, but in such a manner that the participating first aider cannot see them. Flashing the projection immediately after completion of a situation is a technique which also saves class time that normally would be taken reviewing each different situation at a later time.

In the majority of situations several alternate first aid procedures are possible and appropriate. The design of evaluation forms should take this into consideration. Evaluation should be based only on the results of the first aid and not the appearance of any special bandage the instructor had in mind. The intention is to help save lives, not win a neatness contest. However, effective bandages are most often neatly applied.

Preparation for the Instructor

The instructor should develop and review the situations to be sure he understands the correct procedures and has all the proper materials necessary. Tags and other materials should be kept in separate envelopes and numbered for easy access. Masking tape can serve to hold tags in place. Assistants should be recruited and trained to ensure that the situations will be set up rapidly.

The instructor should review all instructions with participants and should present a sample situation.

The makeup of each class determines the situations. First aid for housewives should emphasize more household accidents and first aid for firemen should emphasize burns, smoke inhalation, and so on.

Careful selection of victims is necessary. Some situations require little acting ability (e.g. an unconscious victim), but others require a great deal of showmanship to be effective (e.g., drug freakout). Try to involve everyone at least once as a victim or bystander. You may wish to employ "professional" victims to ensure that the simulations will be well done.

SAMPLE EVALUATION FORM
TRANSFER-BREATHING-BLEEDING

Circle the appropriate number and total at the bottom. Values should be assigned according to the importance of each skill.

	YES Well Done	YES Adequate	NO
1. Was the victim examined quickly for all possible injuries?	3-2	1	0
2. Was the victim quickly removed from imminent danger by an appropriate method? *Note—lack of speed would be a deduction here.	6-5-4	3-2-1	0

3. Was victim given proper mouth-to-mouth artificial respiration until victim revives?
   A. Clear Obstructions (1)
   B. Proper head tilt (2)
   C. Timing (1)
   D. Dealing with difficulties (1)
*Note—in some cases mouth-to-nose, mouth-to-stoma or a manual method may be required.
	5-4	3-2-1	0

4. Was victim given proper care for mild bleeding?
   A. Direct pressure and elevation (1)
   B. Proper bandage (2)
	3-2	1	0

5. Was victim given verbal encouragement? *Note—just saying you will be OK isn't very good verbal encouragement.	2	1	0
6. Was victim treated for shock? *Note—remember shock treatment varies.	2	1	0
7. Was proper additional/professional aid called for?	2	1	0

Add ____+2____

Deductions _____

Total_____

Possible__25__

Comments:
—Additions can be used to equalize situations so they all have the same point values.
—Deductions include improper order such as treating a fracture before life threatening bleeding.

SAMPLE SITUATION

> **Situation:**
> Your brother is playing in the garage when you hear an explosion. There is smoke in the air and the roof appears in danger of collapsing.
> **Where:**
> Your home.
> **Miscellaneous Information:**
> No one else is home.

Above is the card that is given to the first aider. The information below is not seen by the first aider. It gives the directions for the conduct of the simulation.

Position of victim:
Face down.

Special Instructions for Victim:
Remain unconscious until signaled by instructor.

Special Instructions for bystanders:
No bystanders present.

Supplied Materials:
1. Home materials box (a box containing those first aid supplies generally found in the home.)

Tags:
1. No air going in or out (1) chest
2. Blue skin (1) face
3. Mild bleeding (1) right forearm

PARTICIPANTS INSTRUCTIONS

1. You must treat this *like a real life situation*. Nothing will be assumed—you must do all that you would in a real life situation. To receive credit for any procedure it must be accomplished completely. The only exception to this is procedures that cannot be done in the classroom such as making a phone call.

2. You may use only material *provided* in the testing area.
3. You may *not* use any notes or cards other than those provided.
4. For assistance you may use only those people provided and *you must give* explicit directions for any aid they administer. No undirected assistance or information is to be given by other students or victims.
5. *Time will be an important factor in life threatening situations.* A reasonable time will be allowed for less severe injuries, but do not waste time. (After having used a situation several times an instructor will have an idea of how long it should take to complete and may wish to set a time limit.)

SIMULATION TAGS

Simulation tags which have symptoms written on them are constructed for each situation and attached to victims by masking tape. They are coded by color—red for bleeding, blue for breathing difficulties and cold, green and yellow for miscellaneous symptoms.

Their size is appropriate for the symptom. This means that symptoms that would be obvious such as severe bleeding, have a large tag and clear fluid from the ear, are relatively small. No attempt is made to hide tags any more than in real situations. The objective is not to trick anyone, but rather to ensure a thorough examination.

Burns are listed by degrees for easy identification of proper first aid treatment. Bleeding tags are marked mild, moderate, or severe.

In appropriate situations medical alert tags and cards plus medications are supplied to further aid the first aider in diagnosis. Medications are given in several cases to ensure understanding of the Red Cross position on providing or giving medication. Names on medications and cards should be uni-sex (i.e., Pat) so that male or female victims fit into all situations.

Developing First Aid Skills

RICHARD K. WILSON is a graduate student in health education, Ohio State University, 1760 Neil Avenue, Columbus, Ohio 43210.

To successfully complete a course in first aid, a student must possess both the knowledge and skills necessary to administer first aid in a myriad of situations. For this reason, during my first aid classes, I placed a considerable amount of emphasis upon the skills or practical aspects of first aid.

To present situations which require application of first aid skills, I have developed a series of "practical situation cards." Each card describes an emergency and some pertinent information. It may include the location of the incident, the time of the incident, the number of people present, the environmental situation, and the materials available to the first aider.

By using the practical situation cards students practice skills as well as solve problems. Problem-solving could occur when the emergency requires more than one action by the first aider or when the instructor asks questions such as, what would you do first and why? Could you do anything differently? What would you do if *this* had occurred instead?

The following is an example of a practical situation card and how it could be used.

Situation: You and a friend are backpacking when suddenly your friend falls approximately 30 feet into a gorge.

Location: You are three miles from your camp site

Miscellaneous Information: The time of the accident was 11 a.m. and you are not expected back until dusk.

I prefer to use bound and numbered 3 × 5 cards. It is easy to flip through them to find the card relevant to that day's lecture.

I thought of many of the practical situations myself, but I have also had help from my students. During the quarter I permit those students who need bonus points to develop ten emergency situations. From the submitted situations, I select those which best meet class needs. I always have a wide variety of situations which are interesting and relevant.

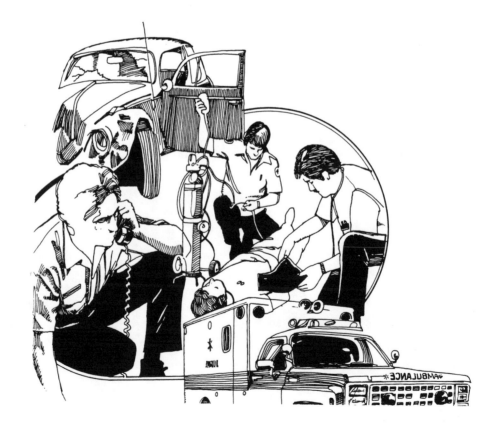

Health and Safety Education from the Trash Can

I. CLAY WILLIAMS is an associate professor of health education at Bowling Green State University, Bowling Green, Ohio 43402. JUDITH K. SCHEER is assistant professor of health education at the University of Toledo, Toledo, Ohio 43606.

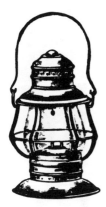

As educators, we constantly dream of ways to obtain effective visual aids to help us develop concepts; however, the difficulty of getting school monies appropriated for visual aids to enhance classroom presentations too often confronts us. I am going to share a secret of how to cope with, even *enjoy*, two problems of our everyday existence— teaching on a shoestring budget and taking out the trash! The trash can offers unlimited potential for collecting an abundance of effective teaching aids. My recent practice of accumulating discarded items provides a wealth of invaluable materials for the classroom that we can use effectively to develop important health and safety concepts.

In my collection is a necktie which is ripped and tattered. It makes me think back to early spring, several years ago. I was itching to get my boat in the water so, on returning home from church, I announced that anyone who wanted to go to the lake should be ready to leave in five minutes. My wife objected saying that I had promised to build some kitchen shelves for her and that I was not leaving the house until the job was done. Needless to say, I was in no mood to build kitchen shelves! Rushing like a madman, I started to cut a board with the circular saw and the next thing I knew, my tie was tangled in the saw blade which was rapidly approaching

my throat! Looking at the mutilated tie and thinking about the close call, I suddenly realized what a perfect visual aid this would make in teaching about hazard potential of various items of clothing. I saved the tie and it became the first of many items in my "trash can collection."

A plastic cup brings to mind a personal example of how an accidental poisoning might occur. I wanted to make a smoking machine out of a liquid detergent bottle so I went into our kitchen, grabbed the soap bottle, and poured its contents into a plastic cup, placed the plastic cup on the window sill and began making the smoking machine.

About a week later, Tom was making lemonade for the twins and found only one clean glass in the cupboard. Looking around, he spied the plastic cup on the window sill and filled it with lemonade for Robby. Robby took a big drink and started to cough and choke tearfully. His mother came running in and said, "What's the matter? Is your lemonade too sour?" She took the glass from him and sampled it herself to see what was wrong, and she's been blowing bubbles ever since! This is an excellent example of how poisonings occur in the home! We are fortunate that the glass didn't contain drain cleaner, automatic dishwasher detergent, or other

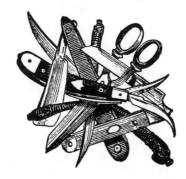

toxic substances which would have caused extensive tissue damage. By this example, we can learn quite a lesson about proper storage.

Other trash that can be used to teach about poisons is abundant. A paint can with a "lead-free" label is an appropriate visual aid when teaching about lead poisoning. A rusty, swollen or dented food can might be the focus of questions designed to stimulate an awareness of food poisoning.

Once your trash collection becomes well known, others will bring you items and stories to add.

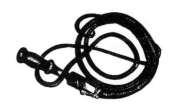

"I'd like to donate this to your trash collection," said one of my students as he handed me an old extension cord. The cord was peeling and cracked and dried out with wires exposed. He had used this under the carpet for several years. Instead of just telling students not to run extension cords under rugs, this cord can show how friction will break down the insulation. When students were asked to suggest ways that the cord might have become so abused, they told of pets which had chewed through extension cords and about times when heavy duty appliances were used on light duty extension cords causing the cord to deteriorate. One of the values of utilizing items from the trash can is that they act as discussion stimulators providing students with opportunities to share personal experiences.

One such experience involved a handmade sweater which our twins decided to use as a replacement for their lampshade when redecorating their room. The light bulb encrusted with charred wool and the tiny sweater with a hole the size of a grapefruit tell the rest of the story. Luckily, it was a wool sweater! Had it been made with synthetic yarn, it could have caused a fire instead of smoldering as it did. With the sweater and light bulb or other wearing apparel the concept of flammability in clothing could be explored.

The topic of home fires is rich with bizarre stories. This past summer, I heard a lot of commotion in the kitchen, so I came running in from the back yard and saw flames shooting out from behind the refrigerator. The coils on the back of the refrigerator had come into contact with the plug; over a period of time, vibrations had caused the coils to cut through the insulation. The melted plug is a good reminder that we should regularly check our electrical appliances.

In my trash collection I have a dish towel that touched the lower heating element in the oven. A section of it burned away when it was being used as a pot holder and the unsuspecting cook had a fire.

As a child, you probably enjoyed playing with tape measures. Jeff was no exception. While watching TV, he was reeling out a tape measure and watching it spring back. As he reeled it out, the end dropped between a chair and the far wall; Jeff flew out of his chair, eyes like saucers and hair standing on end. The metal tape had come into contact with the prong of a lamp plug which was not all the way into the receptacle. The other end hit the aluminum frame around the sliding glass patio door. At the contact points, the tape melted and charred. Jeff's tape clearly illustrates how seemingly harmless activities can be dangerous if the right conditions exist.

The average person can do little to prevent the unexpected; however, a safety conscious individual can take measures to guard against common hazards. When purchasing electrical

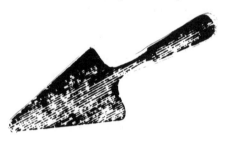

appliances how careful are you to look for the Underwriters Laboratory (U.L.) label? When I found a battery charger at an unbelievably low price I looked on the display card and found the U.L. label. It wasn't until sometime later that I realized the U.L. approval applied only to the cord and plug—not the battery charger. How often we have been led into a false sense of security by not reading the fine print!

Items like the extension cord, sweater, refrigerator plug, tape measure, and U.L. labels are discarded daily. Alert your friends and students to save these types of items for you. It has been our experience that students are much more willing to listen, share, and remember examples of home hazards than they are to memorize lecture notes of do's and don'ts.

Hundreds of suffocations occur in homes each year. Students become directly involved when I introduce the subject of suffocation by placing a plastic bag over my head. I demonstrate when plastic bags are and are not dangerous. A plastic bag, tied in knots, will illustrate the proper method for its disposal.

My mother-in-law receives shirts from the cleaners in plastic bags which

she uses for jobs around the house. When the twins were three, they discovered those bags in Grandmother's kitchen. They were just the right size to get over their heads. I happened to walk in just as Robyn pulled one down over her eyes and nose. Had she been more successful, she would have been in

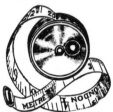

great danger of suffocation. A larger plastic bag in my collection was on a crib mattress at a hotel which could have tragic consequences if tired parents don't take time to check for such hazards.

Many other household helpers can be hazards. We all know that power tools should be handled with great respect, but often there is a tendency to abuse or be careless with "everyday" tools. You probably have a screwdriver with a blade that chipped because the tool was used as a chisel, a crowbar, or something else for which it wasn't designed. When there is finally an opportunity to tighten a screw, there's not enough blade. As you apply pressure, trying to turn the screw there is danger of per-

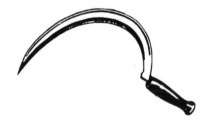

sonal injury as pressure causes the broken blade to slip from the screw head.

Another example is my 98¢ bargain hammer which was designed for light use such as driving tacks or small nails. When the kids decided to build a fort in the back yard, they used my hammer to drive spikes. Half the spikes went in crooked so they tried to pull them out. All of a sudden the claw broke, and there was a flying missile that might have put out an eye. These would-be-architects also damaged my hammer so that the head would no longer fit. To avoid upsetting me, they left it on the workbench just as they had found it, saying wrong. A week later, as I was working on a project the hammer head flew off and sailed

through the garage window onto the hood of my car. Are you saving your plastic bags, broken screwdrivers and hammers as aids in developing concepts relating to hand tools and home safety?

Annually, hundreds of youngsters are fatally injured as a result of home firearm accidents. Many of these accidents occur because youngsters don't understand the danger of firearms. It is not uncommon for children to consider .22 caliber guns as toys because of the small size of the cartridge. In an attempt to make students appreciate the destructive capabilities of a small bore gun, I showed them a soft drink can which was shot with a .22 hollow point.

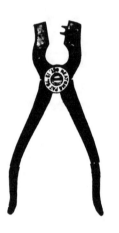

This mutilated metal creates a lasting impression when used to illustrate the damage a .22 caliber bullet could inflict on a human body. Gunshot wounds can also be explored with x-rays obtained from a radiologist. My x-ray of a skull that has been penetrated by BB clearly illustrates the importance of safe gun handling.

These items are examples of numerous objects that can be recycled from the trash to the classroom. As educators know, the more we can do to allow students to identify with our subject matter the more we can enhance the learning process. By using common items of junk as a focal point for discussing real life situations, teachers can help students develop important concepts concerning their own health and safety. Tight school budgets and rising inflation might be just the motivating factors to encourage rummaging through the trash for classroom stimulators.

52

TEACHING IDEAS

Health Services

Another Look at the Chiropractor

JOHN A. CONLEY is chairman of the Department of Health and Safety at University of Georgia, Athens, Georgia 30601.

The public has a vague notion that a doctor of chiropractic is a spinal specialist whose training differs from that of an M.D. but is not necessarily scientifically inferior. Is this an accurate picture of present day chiropractic?

Chiropractic originated in Davenport, Iowa by David Daniel Palmer. He was a "magnetic healer" who used manual adjustments of the vertebrae to "cure" deafness and heart trouble in 1895. From these cases he developed the theory that subluxated (partly dislocated) vertebrae emit heat, called "hot boxes," from pressure on the nerves.[1] These pressures caused almost all diseases. B. J. Palmer, the son of D. D., spread the philosophy to the rest of America and developed the B. J. Palmer Chiropractic Clinic as a model for all offices to follow.[2]

Today 15-17,000 active chiropractors are divided into two groups, the "straights" and the "mixers." The International Chiropractors Association represents the former, and follows the strict interpretation of Palmer's work, using only spinal adjustment in treatment. The American Chiropractic Association represents the latter, who added nutritional, physiotherapy, and acupuncture treatment to the traditional mode. Both groups discount all forms of medication, surgery, or vaccination.

The chiropractor's aim is to restore the patient's harmony with nature and to remove nerve blockages that interfere with that restoration.[3] He believes in a "force called Innate, a divine intelligence which directed its vital energy through the nervous system to all parts of the body." Chiropractic is a *science* that heals the sick, helps suffering, and keeps the well from disease. It is an *art* of sensitized touch that discovers and corrects the cause of disease. It is a philosophy and a religion that develops a way of life where man has a right to live fully in harmony with nature.[4] So say the advocates. Others are not so kind. The AMA maintains that it is a form of quackery and attacks practitioners on the basis of a lack of training and background to treat diseases. Others feel that any treatment methods that will not submit to science should be prohibited.

Following the lead of B. J. Palmer, hundreds of colleges of chiropractic sprang up all over the country, many offering correspondence courses to complete a degree. Others went to a school for a few months to get their degree. Soon, most states required that all who sought to practice healing had to first pass state examinations in anatomy, bacteriology, chemistry, and pathology.

By the 1970s, only 11 chiropractic colleges were still operating in the U.S. They offer a four-year course, often after a two-year precollege training period. In addition, there are many post-graduate workshops and courses attended by chiropractors on the professional and business aspects of practice. Some involve study in radiology and licensing procedures and many become certified x-ray technicians. Unfortunately, the qualifications of the faculty are poor. Only a few have even a B.A. degree. Also, many students are accepted without a high school diploma.[5]

Licensure has been a problem for the chiropractor since the beginning. By 1895, all states had passed the

Medical Practice Act prohibiting unlicensed persons from practicing medicine, so many early graduates of chiropractic schools were persecuted as quacks. All state legislatures have a form of licensure which requires passing more rigid tests than before. Practice in many states is a "limited medical" status for spinal adjustment only. To many prohibiting chiropractors from prescribing drugs or performing surgery is the most important part of licensing. However, according to the chiropractic doctrine, this is superfluous. Licensing requirements have been made uniform and more strict with review by a board with M.D. membership in the majority.

The Palmer College of Chiropractic was certified in 1974 by the Office of Education, HEW, as an institute of higher learning which made it eligible for federal funds. Perhaps this breakthrough will aid in the raising of standards of chiropractic education.

The heart of the chiropractic controversy is diagnosis and treatment. The conservative camp promotes the use of a thorough physical examination, x-rays, and neurocalometry to analyze potential problems. Some criticize the spinography technique of antero-posterior filming as having limited diagnostic value and give more support to small sectional x-ray techniques. Others criticize because nerves are not visible on x-rays and thus one cannot detect if they are being pinched by subluxations. Some medical journalists suggest that adjustments based on such methods actually cause breaks, pinches, and death. A 1968 HEW report recommended the exclusion of chiropractors from Medicare payment because they did not submit research for scientific validation.[6] Chiropractors do not diagnose specific diseases. They emphasize determining which vertebra(e) is misaligned. While the use of x-rays has given an aura of legitimacy, radiologists claim that such large (14" by 36") exposures are dangerous to the body.[7]

The chiropractor makes a superior merchandising effort, giving patients time for consultation and showing personal interest in their problems. Most are community oriented and involved in local medical needs and issues to a far greater extent than physicians.[8] Office visits are usually pleasant in surroundings with little or no waiting, and inexpensive when compared to medical practices.

Presently a scientific research attempt to validate claims is being done by C. H. Sue and others at the University of Colorado at Boulder. This, and other spinal research, has shown that muscle spasms and tight ligaments can cause pain and decreased joint movement from an adverse influence on nerve function. The emphasis on physical examinations, long a source of controversy for physicians, has prompted at least one major life insurance company to authorize chiropractors to do insurance physicals.[9] Chiropractors have always had many followers who readily give testimonials to the success of various treatments. These are a mixed blessing since some are easily attacked, but others have proven to be quite valid.

As with the field of acupuncture, chiropractic has a wide range of successes and failures. The most common areas of successful treatment have been with backaches and muscle spasms. Support is also widespread for physiotherapy type treatments, of joint injury. Headaches and lower back pains have wide, but lesser claims of success. The greatest questions are raised when treatment is attempted of asthma, bronchitis, allergies, visual problems, digestive trouble, diabetes, heart ailments, diarrhea, hives, dermatitis, ulcers, pneumonia, appendicitis, multiple sclerosis, nutrition, emotional disorders, tuberculosis, diseases of the reproductive organs, liver, kidneys, etc. Many feel that chiropractors are not trained to diagnose such severe conditions, and that the treatment of spinal adjustments may only serve to delay "proper" medical care.

Should chiropractic be restricted to treatment by manipulation? Should these therapeutic techniques be controlled and regulated? abandoned? unrestrained? The role of the chiropractor for most of our society is still not defined, yet the consumer of medical treatment for a wide variety of pains and ills is faced with making a decision where helpful factual information is scarce or not available at all.

---

[1] Ralph Lee Smith, *At Your Own Risk*, (New York: Trident Press, 1969), p. 62.

[2] A. Aug. Dye, *The Evolution of Chiropractic, Its Discovery and Development*, (Philadelphia, Pa.: By the author, 1939).

[3] Marcus Bach, *The Chiropractic Story*, (Los Angeles, California: De Vorss and Co., Inc., 1958), p. 26.

[4] Ibid., pp. 57, 64, 189.

[5] Ibid., p. 103-08, 153.

[6] Albert Q. Marsel, "Should Chiropractors Be Paid with Your Tax Dollars," *Readers Digest*, July 1971, p. 4 of reprint.

[7] Ralph Lee Smith, *At Your Own Risk*, (New York: Trident Press, 1969), p. 160.

[8] *International Review of Chiropractic* 27, no. 7, November 1974.

[9] *The Digest of Chiropractic Economics* 17, no. 3, November/December 1974.

53

TEACHING IDEAS

Using Para-Professionals in the Arkansas Health Education Programs

EMOGENE L. FOX *is an extension health education specialist, Cooperative Extension Service, University of Arkansas, Little Rock, Arkansas 72203.* JANE WEWER LAMMERS *is an instructor, Department of Health Education, University of Central Arkansas, Conway, Arkansas 72032 (former extension health education specialist).* RUNYAN E. DEERE *is state leader — health education, Cooperative Extension Service, University of Arkansas, Little Rock, Arkansas 72203.*

Numerous approaches are being taken to reach and positively influence individuals and families to increase their concern for, improve and maintain their personal health. A new approach was taken in Arkansas by the Cooperative Extension Service, University of Arkansas. Indigenous homemakers were employed as community health education aides in Cross and Drew Counties in one of six special projects funded by the Bureau of Health Education, Center for Disease Control, Public Health Service, Department of HEW.

Health aides are certainly not new, but aides who provide only educational service to the people in their community have been less widely used. Usually, various types of health aides provide one or more health related services in addition to education. For example, aides employed to work in migrant health projects under the 1962 Migrant Health Act are trained not only in basic human skills but in technical skills of nursing, health education and sanitation.[1]

The Extension health education aides grew out of the aide concept which the Alabama Extension Service piloted five years before the national program of the Expanded Food and Nutrition Education Program of early 1969. EFNEP is directed entirely toward low-income families. The health education program is made available to all families regardless of economic level. This program seeks to upgrade the diets of low-income families through education. Feaster[2] describes the program as follows.

> Food and nutrition education has always been a major activity of the Extension Service, but the EFNEP represents a substantial change in magnitude, orientation, and approach from past efforts. Changes include a broadened scope of food and nutrition education with special focus on hard-to-reach families in poverty, many of which are minority groups living in urban areas. Also, the Extension Service is now using paid nonprofessionals to extend the efforts of professional home economists in helping families improve their food knowledge and food consumption practices . . . . Additionally, families are provided information on resources and Government programs in the community that may provide assistance in improving their dietary practices and living standards.

In 1975, the Arkansas Cooperative Extension Service created six half-time health education aide positions in both Cross and Drew Counties. The counties were chosen on the basis of population, geographic location, and abilities of the county Extension staffs. Although the aide concept was not new with the Cooperative Extension Services, the concept of health education aides as teachers was the first to be undertaken by the organization nationwide.

Objectives

The overall goal of the health education aide program is to demonstrate the effectiveness of health education aides in working one to one or in small groups with target audiences to increase their health knowledge, promote desirable health attitudes, and positively influence their health behavior. The paraprofessionals were instructed to teach the program families: (1) how daily living habits influence their health; (2) to use preventive health practices; (3) when and how to use self-care and when to seek medical care; (4) how a clean, pleasant home and surroundings contribute to positive health; and (5) to understand the local health care services. As the paraprofessionals work with families, they refer them to the available health care resources in their county and after referral, follow-up to encourage better use of the local health care delivery system.

Audiences and Materials

Families were selected through referrals and direct contacts. Target audiences included economically deprived families but were not limited to them; several middle income families were also enrolled. In order of priority, the aide chose families from among new parents, economically deprived families with children or grandchildren, middle-aged families, and elderly people living at home.

Two state extension health education specialists and the state leader for health education utilized the EFNEP model to develop the materials and guidelines. All the subject matter materials for the program are prepared in the form of mini-lessons, written by the health education specialists and reviewed by the faculty at the University of Arkansas for Medical Sciences. When the aides visit their program families, they teach one mini-lesson to the homemaker and leave a summary of the material for the homemaker to study and refer to if necessary. Supportive materials left with the homemaker are prepared simply and creatively so that the homemaker can easily understand them.

Training

The health education aides were involved in an initial intensive three week—120 hours training program, including an overview in selected subject areas of health education. An underlying theme or philosophy was adopted—each individual should assume the responsibility for maintaining his or her own health, rather than expect health professionals to assume this responsibility. Both aide training and their teaching is designed to promote this philosophy.

This training also included specific information on such things as: recognized risk factors involved in coronary heart diseases; cancer education emphasizing importance of early detection; diet and weight control; diabetes; venereal disease; basic first aid for life-saving; mental health; health quackery; pre-post natal care; dental health; basic home sanitation.

Health education aides have a minimum of high school education. They are assigned to work in their local communities and because of similarities of age, education, and socioeconomic levels, they can more easily relate to women with whom they work on both a one-to-one and small group basis. To further enhance these relationships, skill-building activities in values clarification, decision making, inter and intra personal skills were also included in the training.

In order that the health education aides better understand their local health delivery system to more effec-

tively make referrals, local health agency representatives explained facilities and services through public health departments, mental health centers, other state agencies, and other volunteer and service agencies. This was a vital part of the training program.

Assessment

Assessment of each program family's progress is being done through a Family Review Form. This is first administered when the family is enrolled and assessments are made at six month intervals. The review form contains clusters of questions relating to health practices, health knowledge, knowledge of facilities and services available.

After a six month period of individualized instruction with 121 of the enrolled families, the following changes took place.

The percentage of homemakers who could name the risk factors involved in coronary heart disease increased 193.9%.

Identification of seven warning signals of cancer increased by 205%.

The percentage of women who practice regular monthly breast self-examination increased by 67%.

Percentage of women who had a blood pressure reading during the six month period increased by 30%.

Recognition of local health facilities and services increased by 45%.

Number of homemakers who go to the dentist regularly rather than with a dental crisis increased only 1%.

No appreciable change in weight of individual homemakers. (It was found that those people who need to lose only 10–20 pounds have more success in weight reduction than those who are 60–70 pounds overweight.

[1]Hoff, Wilbur, *The Use of Health Aides in Migrant Health Projects*, U.S. Department of Health, Education and Welfare, Public Health Service, Health Services and Mental Health Administration Division Health Care Services, U.S. Government Printing Office: 1971 0–408–207, p. 3.

[2]Feaster, J. Gerald, *Impact of the Expanded Food and Nutrition Education Program on Low-Income Families: An In-depth Analysis*, U.S. Department of Agriculture, Economic Research Service, Agricultural Economic Report No. 220, U.S. Government Printing Office, February 1972, p.1

Health education aides participated in an initial intensive training program. The underlying theme was that each person, not the health professional, is responsible for his or her own health. Training also included information on specific diseases, basic first aid, dental health, and basic home sanitation.

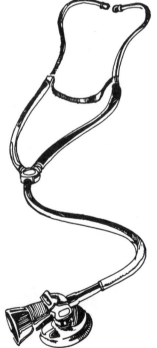

A Physical Examination for Sixth Graders

In May 1973 a school nurse from one of the six elementary schools located in the area served by the Community University Health Care Center, a comprehensive children and youth health care project, asked the Center's community health educator for suggestions on how she could motivate 6th grade students to receive a physical examination prior to their entry into 7th grade. The staff from the Health Care Center, the school nurse, and the 6th grade teachers met several times to discuss ways students could become involved in a program to learn about basic components of a physical examination and why it is important to have one before entering 7th grade. As a result of these discussions, a three-part physical examination education program was developed.

The primary purpose of the educational program was to help each student understand what a physician looks, feels, and tests for, as well as listens to, during a normal physical examination. The program was designed so that each student would become actively involved in each segment of the program—seeing and handling the instruments used by a physician during a normal physical examination, and also doing several of the accompanying lab tests.

Year 1—May 1973

A three part program was developed for the 6th graders. During part 1, a multidisciplinary team from the Health Center consisting of health educator, a medical student, a pediatric nurse practitioner, a physician, and a school nurse met with each 6th grade class to discuss

DAVIS B. MILLS is an instructor and field placement supervisor in the Program in Health Education. K. KAY DeROOS is an instructor in the Program in Health Education and director of health education at Community University Health Care Center. BARBARA SCHULTE is a pediatrician in the Community University Health Care Center. All are at the University of Minnesota, Minneapolis, Minnesota 55455. This article is taken from a presentation given at the American Public Health Association, 104th annual meeting, Miami Beach, October 1976.

why it is important to have a physical examination; what is done during the examination and; how the students can make it a true learning experience. The students were given ample opportunity to ask questions and express their concern about any aspect of a physical examination.

Following this discussion, the students were divided into three small groups and each group was assigned a set of body systems to study. One group worked with the nervous and sensory systems; another with the heart, respiratory, and gastro-intestinal systems; and the third group with the genital-urinary and circulatory systems. Each group of students was asked to prepare a list of questions about their assigned body systems. The students were to obtain answers in the second part of the program.

During part 2, each class took a field trip to the Community University Health Care Center. The medical and nursing staff at the Center were divided into three groups corresponding to the students' groups. Each student group was given the opportunity to handle the instruments used during a physical examination of the body systems assigned to that group. For example, one group used an otoscope and an ophthalmoscope, a tuning fork, a tonometer, and an eye chart. Another group used a stethoscope, a blood pressure cuff, and viewed x-rays of the heart, lungs, and G.I. tract. The third group performed some basic lab work, such as hematocrits and urinalysis, viewed slides of blood cells through a microscope, and observed positive and negative strep throat cultures.

During part 3 the staff from the Health Center returned to the classroom and each group of students gave a report to the class on what they experienced during the field trip. The reports were followed by general discussions on the importance of receiving a physical examination before entering 7th grade. Students were then given the school health examination forms to take home to their parents and were encouraged to get a physical examination as soon as possible.

Year 2—May 1974

More input from the students and teachers was obtained this year and the program better reflected the needs and interests of each class. Teacher and student questionnaires were developed by the school nurse and the community health educator. The teachers were asked to describe what they had taught about physical examinations. Students were asked: (1) what would they like to know about a physical examination; (2) what questions would they like answered when they go to see the doctor; (3) what worries them the most about going to the doctor; (4) what would they like to know about what happens to them when they visit the doctor. These responses were used by the Health Center staff to revise the program.

Due to increased health service demands, the medical staff at the Health Center recruited two second year medical students to work with the program. The length of the program was changed from three to two sessions which meant a reduction of information presented during each session. This year the students did not visit the Health Center; instead the health care team went to the school.

The basic content of the program remained the same, only this time students rotated through each of the three groups of body systems. Some new material was developed to help the students summarize what took place in each group. Torso, eye, and ear models were also used to explain what happens during specific parts of a physical examination.

During the first session, the team from the Health Care Center led a ten-minute discussion about the basic components of a good physical examination. The students then broke up into three groups to explore each set of body systems for approximately 30 minutes. After all students had gone through the three sets of body systems, they met again as a class and the school examination form was given to them to take home to their parents. Each class was asked to reflect on what they had experienced and to prepare questions for the next session.

A week later the second session was led by the community health educator and one of the medical students. The pupil health history form was used as a discussion guide and its importance as part of a normal physical examination was stressed. Students were encouraged to take an active part in their physical examinations by asking the physician to answer questions and explain the results of the examination.

A simple evaluation was done with the students. Before breaking up into groups, students were asked to describe what happened to them the last time they went to the doctor, especially if that visit was for a physical examination. After participating in the program, each student was asked to list three things a physician looks, feels, and tests for, and listens to during a physical examination. The answers from this exercise were compared to the answers from the first question. The students were able to describe more procedures after participating in the educational program.

Year 3—May 1975

The program presented the third year was similar to that of the previous two years. Two sessions were held for three different 6th grade classrooms. The second session was conducted by the school nurse alone.

Year 4—February-April 1976

Due to the positive student-teacher response the previous three years, the program was expanded to all six area elementary schools during the fourth year. Because of the expansion, only one two-hour session was held for each classroom. The students rotated through four groups spending 20 minutes in each. A short discussion was held before and immediately after rotation.

The 1976 program was expanded from a "physical examination" to a "health assessment" educational activity. The role of the entire health care team was emphasized, not just the physician's. A fourth section, dental health/nutrition, was added. In this section students identified and tasted foods conducive to good dental health habits and some which were not.

Students in each classroom evaluated the educational activity subjectively. They were asked which sections they liked best and least, what they learned, and whether or not they enjoyed the activity. Table 1 summarizes the results of this evaluation.

Each of the four years the program changed somewhat in order to accommodate health resources and time available for implementation. Teacher, student, and health care team evaluations accounted for the changes in program format and material over the years. The program has been able to demonstrate several things:

(1) A multidisciplinary team from a community health care center can work cooperatively with a school nurse and 6th grade teacher to develop and carry out an experiential health education program for sixth grade students.

(2) Students liked the idea of being able to see and handle the instruments used by a physician or nurse during a physical examination.

(3) Students do respond to programs which they have helped to develop.

(4) The members of the health care team were able to work cooperatively and provide a valuable role model and learning experience for medical, nursing, and community health education students who helped with the project.

(5) The school nurse and the Health Center staff were able to expand the program from one school to all six schools in the Health Center's service area. Health personnel involved in the 1976 program included medical student, pediatric nurse associate, registered nurse, dental assistant, nutritionist, community health educator and student, well child worker, school nurse, and nursing student.

There were several problems that plagued the project each year of its operation. Initially, the health education team wanted to followup children who participated in the program to determine: whether or not they did complete a physical examination prior to entering seventh grade; their comfort during the examination; and whether they learned something. The extreme mobility of the children in this project area (over 60% turnover in some of the schools each

Table 1. Tell Us What You Think (Student Evaluations) Year 4—1976

Program Area	Liked Best		Liked Least	
	Number	Percent	Number	Percent
Heart/lungs	101	37.8%	23	8.6%
Nervous/sensory	41	15.3%	48	17.9%
Lab	21	7.8%	64	23.9%
Dental/nutrition	96	35.9%	40	14.9%
None of above	10	3.7%	68	25.4%
No answer	2	0.7%	31	11.6%

Learned	Number	Percent
Many new things	136	50.9%
Few new things	81	30.3%
Nothing new	8	2.9%
No answer	42	15.7%

Program was	Number	Percent
Fun	74	27.7%
Fun and interesting	23	8.6%
Interesting	139	52.0%
Boring	10	3.7%
Waste of time	3	1.2%
OK	2	0.7%
No answer	6	2.2%

(N = 267)

year) prevented the education team from accomplishing these tasks. Furthermore, due to lack of money and personnel, the transfer of medical information on physical examinations could not be coordinated among the parents, schools, physicians, and health education team. Because of these problems a relatively subjective evaluation of the program and its usefulness to the teacher, students, and Health Care Center staff had to be relied upon.

During year 4 over 80% of the children learned something new from the educational program. A total of 88% of the students considered the program "fun" and/or "interesting." Thus, on a very subjective level the program has been a success. The teachers also expressed similar views about the program and all of them felt it was a positive addition to their health education units.

Conclusions

The major conclusion drawn from this project is that it is feasible for a community health care center to work cooperatively with a school nurse, 6th grade teachers, and 6th grade students in developing a participative educational program about physical examinations. The students, teachers, school nurse, and educational health care team from the Health Care Center were satisfied with the interaction and personal involvement in each session. But most of all, the staff participating in the program were pleased with the interest and excitement students showed.

In the future, we hope to expand the program into the junior high school and perhaps set up some type of followup procedure to determine whether or not the 6th graders received a physical examination and their reactions to it. On a very limited basis, we might try to work cooperatively with several of the local physicians and nurses to determine their reactions to the way the 6th graders behaved during their physical examinations. The potential for future research in this area is great. One thing remains certain, we must continue to provide positive health education experience to children throughout elementary and junior high school for them to be informed, participating members of our health care system.

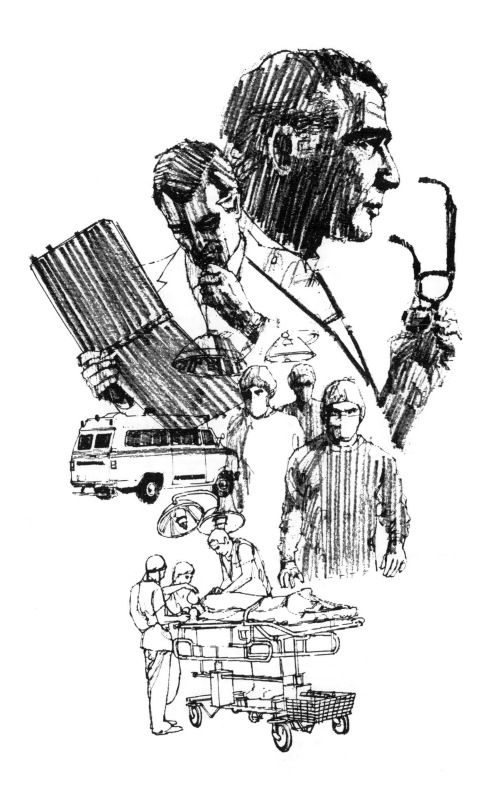

Making Screening Testing Educational for Elementary Pupils:
A Pre-Professional Exercise

Robert J. McDermott is in the Department of Curriculum and Instruction at the University of Wisconsin-Madison, Teacher Education Bldg., 225 North Mills Street, Madison, Wisconsin 53706.

Phillip J. Marty is in the Department of Health, Physical Education and Recreation at the University of Minnesota-Duluth, Duluth, Minn. 55812.

The authors are indebted to Warren H. Southworth, Professor of Health Education and Preventive Medicine, University of Wisconsin-Madison, for his input in developing this exercise with undergraduate students in health classes.

The professional educator faces the challenge of influencing the understanding, attitudes, and behavior of children and youth, so that pupils know not only the facts, but also the correct application of this information to healthful daily living. Probably nowhere is this task more arduous than in the realm of motivating personal health care.

The Joint Committee on Health Problems in Education of the National Education Association and American Medical Association[1] pointed out more than a decade ago that school health services can enhance pupil knowledge and understanding of health and problems related to health. It also stated that health services have an excellent educational base from which attitudes toward health personnel could be positively influenced. Furthermore, Mayshark and Foster[2] stated:

Health services in the school setting have an educational base that we must endorse and encourage. When students learn the important elements of personal health care through actual participation as well as abstract discussion, the promise that they will exercise positive action in the same areas as adults is enhanced.

The educational potential of school health services may be even greater than indicated in the above quotation. With careful planning, school health services can promote an immediate participation in the health care system. Cronin and Young document that in some communities children and youth are often excluded from the health care system. As the adult-parental models are often passive about matters of personal health, this finding is not surprising. From a cognitive-developmental perspective, however, the exclusion of young people from the health care system need not happen. Palmer and Lewis[4] point out that children as young as eight years of age are capable of determining their need for outside health service. Dennison[5] advocates "activated health education"—an approach that is aimed at getting the consumer involved in his own health assessment, and avoids the role of passive recipient. It is therefore reasonable to expect that participation in health services provided by schools (such as screening procedures) can be meaningful from both a cognitive and a behavioral perspective.

The educational "side effects" derived from pupil involvement in school health services are well-documented in the literature. Mills, DeRoos, and Schulte[6] demonstrate the appeal of involving sixth graders in their own physical examinations and the feasibility of a community health care center working with the school nurse, teachers, and pupils to develop a participative educational program about physical examinations. Guskin and Taylor[7] show that TB testing of sixth graders, when combined with information about TB, increases a person's beliefs about their own susceptibility to TB. Susceptibility beliefs are indicated by Becker and others[8] to contribute significantly to personal decisions about health behavior.

In spite of the seeming preponderance of literature advocating the marriage of health services and instruction, Eisner and Callan[9] report:

Our observations of various health care programs show that workers rarely plan for an educational effect or manage to implement the potential for making health services a learning experience.

The divorce of the two health components is explained by Mayshark and Foster[10] as a consequence of the gradual decline in the overall emphasis placed on school health services in the past three decades. The service component of the comprehensive school health triad continues to be passed over as a means of increasing health awareness.

Health awareness needs to be made more relevant for young people. As Parcel[11] explains:

The concept of health is a difficult abstraction for children to understand and is often made more difficult by health education programs that have little relationship to the real-life experiences of children. There is a need to identify a few basic health skills that can be learned by young children and then develop learning activities that will enable the children to practice these skills in real-life situations. For young children, experimental learning activities should be the major emphasis of health education. Learning by doing is most likely to lead to the development of health skills.

The Simulation Technique, a teaching strategy aimed at maximizing the educational aspects of school health services (cited by Eisner and Callan[12] as advanced by Schindler/Rainman and Lippitt), is easily adapted to the type of screening procedures readily used in the schools and performed by school nurses, teachers, or volunteers. The strategy utilizes a three-step approach: rehearsal and preparation before the procedure is performed; the actual testing; and follow-up exercises that enhance knowledge and reinforce the usefulness and desirability of the screening procedure and others like it.

The Simulation Technique was used by students enrolled in a course entitled "Health Information for Teachers," at the University of Wisconsin-Madison. The students participated in a two-hour exercise giving and taking three types of screening examinations, including: a test of visual acuity, utilizing the Snellen Eye Chart, the Massachusetts Test of Visual Acuity, and the Titmus Vision Tester; an examination of hearing acuity, conducting an audiometric sweep test with a puretone audiometer; and a measurement of physical growth, with a beam-type platform scale.

After having practiced the three screening procedures, students were asked to develop strategies that would enhance the educational potential of the tests when given to children and youth. The following examples were developed from their suggestions.

Visual Acuity

Preparation Activities for Teacher and Pupils

- Explore the structure and function of the eye, using diagrams.
- Discuss the effects of light intensity on vision.
- Explain the rationale for early detection of vision problems.
- Ask pupils to speculate on how good vision is important in many aspects of daily living (learning, communicating, driving, appreciating one's surroundings, etc.)
- Differentiate between various terms which apply to the eyes, such as retina, pupil, and lens.
- Discuss appearances, behaviors, and complaints of children which might indicate a disorder of the eye or of vision.
- Indicate the importance of nutrition, physical health, and heredity in regard to vision.
- Explain the need to protect one's eyes from illness and injury.
- Discuss the importance of cooperation among pupils during the actual screening procedure.
- Demonstrate the equipment to be used in the screening and emphasize that the procedure is not painful.

Activities During Screening

- Allow pupils who have completed the testing to participate as proctors or as recorders of data on facsimiles of their permanent health records.
- Permit pupils to observe, disassemble, and reassemble a plastic model of an eye.
- Have pupils view a variety of glass lenses which distort vision and illustrate different types of visual defects.
- Have pupils build and observe a peephole box (where images are superimposed upside down as occurs in the eye) to show how images are actually focused on the retina.

Follow-Up Activities

- Discuss what is meant by 20/20 vision, 20/30 vision, and others.
- Explain how various defects are corrected with glass lenses.
- Discuss corneal transplant, cataract surgery, treatment of glaucoma, eye donations and eye banks.
- Blindfold one or more pupils and have others become "their eyes" under careful teacher supervision.
- Discuss the roles of the health professionals such as opticians, optometrists, and ophthalmologists.
- Secure animal eyes from a local abattoir or bioscience supply company for pupil or teacher dissection and observation.
- Invite a blind person to the class to demonstrate braille and other forms of "touch" communication with pupils.
- Design sensitivity exercises such as touching, feeling, or hearing, which will help children to increase their sensory awareness.
- Visit an ophthalmologist's or optometrist's office or a hospital where eye surgery is performed to show pupils the medical advances available to treat the more serious eye disorders.
- Review vision screening procedures and their purpose, and discuss when future testing will be conducted.

Hearing Acuity

Preparation Activities for Teacher and Pupils

- Obtain or draw a picture of the ear and discuss its function, structure, and care.
- Discuss the hazards of loud noise to hearing.
- Introduce the relationship of infection and injury to balance, equilibrium and hearing.
- List various childhood diseases which can temporarily or permanently affect hearing acuity.
- Explore types of hearing impairment (sensorineural vs. conductive) and describe how they might be prevented.
- Have pupils speculate on the relationship between periodic health examinations, nutrition, safety and good hearing.
- Have pupils try to identify various sounds with their eyes closed (whistle, train, bell, drum, etc.)
- Have pupils discuss factors which influence one's ability to hear, such as distance, intensity, frequency, and background noise.
- Explain the importance of remaining silent during the hearing screening procedure.
- Provide instructions and demonstrate the screening equipment, deemphasizing the "testing" nature of this procedure.

Activities During Screening

- Allow pupils to observe a model of a human ear (obtainable from a medical clinic or bioscience supply house.)
- Have pupils draw the major anatomical parts of the outer, middle and inner ear.
- Allow students to use an inexpensive stethoscope to illustrate how such a device can aid a physician in his ability to hear normal and abnormal sounds made by the body's organs.
- Secure and place earplugs in pupils ears to demonstrate how a person with defective hearing perceives sound.
- Ask pupils who complete their hearing test to record their own screening result on a facsimile of their permanent health record.
- Under supervision, permit pupils to use the equipment on each other.

Follow-Up Activities

- Visit an audiologist or other hearing specialist for a demonstration of the types of hearing-aid devices that are available.
- Plan a field trip to a school for the hearing-impaired and have one of the teaching specialists demonstrate sign language.
- Develop silent skits which pupils can perform in mime to develop an appreciation for non-verbal communication.
- Have pupils design, plan, and build a model of a human ear or a "superperson" ear, using readily available materials.
- Have pupils speculate on why people do not have the very keen sense of hearing which some animals have that helps them to survive.
- Demonstrate how people in other countries have languages different from our own.
- Visit a foundry to evaluate methods industry uses to reduce the effects of noise on employees.
- Review the hearing screening procedure and its purpose, and explain when future testing will be conducted.

Physical Growth

Preparation Activities for Teacher and Pupils

- Discuss the importance of overall health to physical growth and development.
- Describe various types of health problems which can affect height and weight.
- List and explain the important elements of a nutritious diet, describing the effects that hypernutrition and malnutrition have on the body.
- Compare body structures of people from different countries and cultures.
- Discuss the effect of heredity on growth and development. Have pupils try to outline their "family tree."
- Formulate an experiment (encouraging pupil input) using juvenile white laboratory rats, give one group a nutritious diet and the other group a deficient

diet and compare growth after two weeks.

- Help pupils develop a healthy body image and positive self-concept by explaining that a wide range of individual differences in height and weight occur.
- Have pupils find the names and biographies of historical characters who were very tall or very short.
- Describe and demonstrate procedures and the equipment to be used in physical growth screening.

Activities During Screening

- Ask pupils to record results of the height and weight screening on a facsimile of their physical growth or health record.
- Place a chart of standardized norms for height and weight on the wall and let pupils assess their present level of physical growth.
- Have pupils convert their height and weight measurements into the metric equivalents.
- Allow pupils to use other height and weight measuring devices such as a yardstick and a bathroom scale to determine if some differences occur.
- With teacher supervision, allow pupils to operate the scale (beam-type platform) and take some measurements.

Follow-Up Activities

- Arrange a class visitation from someone who has recently had a cast removed from his arm or leg. Have pupils measure the affected and unaffected limb to illustrate the effect of immobility on muscle mass and development.
- Have pupils conduct mathematical problems on the accumulated data like

the lists of possible activities are lengthy, they are far from being complete. Classroom teachers can add to each list or generate new ones. The only limitations are those of the teacher's imagination and creativity and his or her ability to plan ahead. The activities are general ones and specific adaptation is left to the teacher depending on the needs of each class.

Doing this exercise with teachers-to-be is important for several reasons. It demonstrates: 1) how the Simulation Technique can be used as an educational device for the introduction of methodology in pre-professional settings; 2) the ease with which supplementary activities can be developed which go beyond traditional textbook approaches; 3) that teachers can make personal health more interesting to young people; 4) that teachers can help young people the sums of heights and weights, averages, gains, and losses, etc.

- Have pupils do a caloric count of all foods eaten over a 24-hour period.
- Discuss the role of regular exercise and fitness in promoting optimal physical growth and development.
- Have pupils collect food labels and create a collage of the collected materials indicating certain nutritional themes.
- Compare different types of foods by analyzing ingredients on the label.
- Have pupils keep track of the foods they eat over a seven-day period, and have them develop a profile of their personal eating habits.
- Review physical growth screening procedures, and indicate when future testing will be conducted.

The activities shown above represent the combined brainstorming efforts of forty future elementary teachers. While

develop positive attitudes about personal health, and take an active role in their own health assessment; and, 5) that there is a close relationship between instruction and services in a comprehensive school health program. The suggested educational activities clearly delineate the natural blend of instruction and service components.

[1]Wilson, C. C., (Ed.). *School health services* (2nd ed.). Washington, D.C.: National Education Association and American Medical Association, 1964.

[2]Mayshark, C. and Foster, R. A., *Health education in the secondary schools: integrating the critical incident approach*, 3rd Ed. St. Louis: C. V. Mosby Co., 1972, p. 72.

[3]Cronin, G. E., and Young, W. M. *400 navels: the future of school health in America.* Bloomington, Indiana: Phi Delta Kappa, 1979.

[4]Palmer, B. B., and Lewis, C. E. Development of health attitudes and behaviors. *The Journal of School Health*, September 1976, *46* (7), 401–402.

[5]Dennison, D. Activated health education. *Health Education*, May–June 1977.

[6]Mills, D. B., DeRoos, K., & Schulte, B. A physical examination for sixth graders. *Health Education*, July–August 1977.

[7]Guskin, S. L., and Taylor, R. M., Educational effects of a school tuberculin testing program. *The Journal of School Health*, April 1968, *38* (4), 219–226.

[8]Becker, M. H., (Ed.). The health belief model and personal health behavior. *Health Education Monographs*, Winter 1974, *2* (4): 324–508.

[9]Eisner, V., & Callan, L. B. *Dimensions of school health.* Springfield, Illinois: Charles C. Thomas Publisher, 1974, 82.

[10]Mayshark & Foster, op. cit.

[11]Parcel, G. S., Tiernan, K., Nader, P. R., & Gottlob, D. Health education for kindergarten children, *The Journal of School Health*, March 1979, *49* (3): 129–131.

[12]Eisner & Callan, op. cit.

TEACHING IDEAS

A Hospital Visit for First Graders

A visit to the hospital for first graders? Why frighten them with such an experience before it is necessary? The visit, in fact, does just the opposite.

The director of public relations at the Rochester Methodist Hospital, Rochester, Minnesota discussed with the Public School Health Curriculum Committee chairman the possibility of helping children learn firsthand about hospital procedures. Most children of this age have never had the experience of even visiting a patient in the hospital because of hospital rules. The director knew that the Rochester Public Schools were revising their *Health Course of Study* and proposed that a visit to the hospital be included as part of the curriculum.

The purposes of the visit are fourfold; it is designed to help children:
1. To learn about regular hospital routines
2. To know what to expect if they were hospitalized
3. To see what doctors, nurses, and other hospital personnel do
4. To understand that hosiptals are places where people are helped to become well.

Each first grade class in Rochester is scheduled to visit the Rochester Methodist Hospital sometime during the school year. It is suggested as a culminating activity of the one week unit on the subject of hospitals, doctors, and nurses.

The concepts outlined in the *Course of Study* are these:
1. Hospitals are places where one gets special care which cannot be received at home.
2. Doctors and nurses take care of us in the hospital.

WARREN W. ZIMMERMAN is elementary principal, Jefferson School, and chairman of the Health Curriculum Committee for the Rochester Public Schools, Rochester, Minnesota 65901.

Teachers may use a variety of methods to teach these concepts. One suggested method is to read stories such as *Curious George Goes to the Hospital, Johnny Goes to the Hospital,* or *How Hospitals Help Us.* In discussing these stories, teachers can discover what fears, anxieties, or misconceptions children may have about hospitals. In this way they can talk about taking temperatures, checking the heart and lungs, getting shots, the need for staying in bed, and other related information. The visit to the hospital not only confirms some of the ideas presented by the teacher but also adds many others.

Two nurses were selected by the hospital staff to work with the children. Their friendly, easy manner helps children realize that most things that happen to them when they are patients do not hurt. Children are selected to play different roles such as the patient, his mother and father, the doctor and nurse. The "patient" actually gets into a hospital bed so that all can see how it can be elevated at the head or foot, why they put side rails up for very sick people, and how one is made comfortable.

A child is selected to play the role of the doctor. He is dressed in a complete surgical outfit and the reasons for the dress are explained.

The use of a bedpan and urinal are discussed and the reasons for testing the urine are explained simply. The nurses take temperatures, listen to the heart, take blood pressures, and each time ask the patient, "Does this hurt?" The children, of course, reply, "No." Each time this helps build on the concept that there are many, many things that happen to a person in the hospital which do not hurt.

The nurses discuss very frankly things that might hurt, such as a "shot." They show the children the syringe and needle and explain what a child can do to help make the "shot" less painful, that is, "By relaxing the muscles in the buttocks the penicillin goes into the tissues more easily."

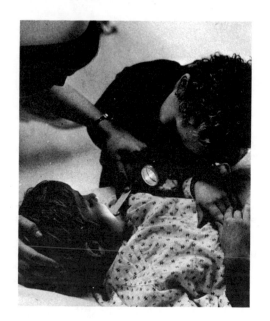

The nurses are skillful in noting when children become restless. They have built-in plans for getting everyone "into the act." At such a point, they might explain how an x-ray of the chest is made. Each child stands up with hands behind hips, takes a deep breath, holds it, and then relaxes. Then the nurse asks if this would hurt, again reinforcing the idea of many painless things taking place. Another time that the children are able to empathize with the "patient" is when the "patient" is anesthetized. Each child does the countdown, taking good deep breaths, and then "going to sleep" on "0."

As the children leave the hospital they are given a small bag containing things like a cotton ball, band-aid, tongue depressor, a surgical cap, a cardboard nurses cap, or a reflector band.

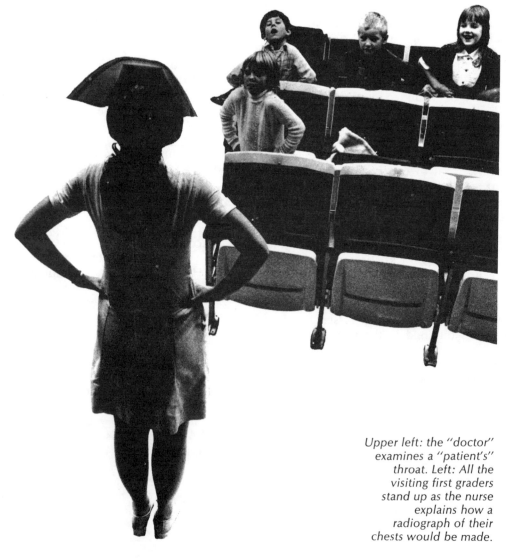

Upper left: the "doctor" examines a "patient's" throat. Left: All the visiting first graders stand up as the nurse explains how a radiograph of their chests would be made.

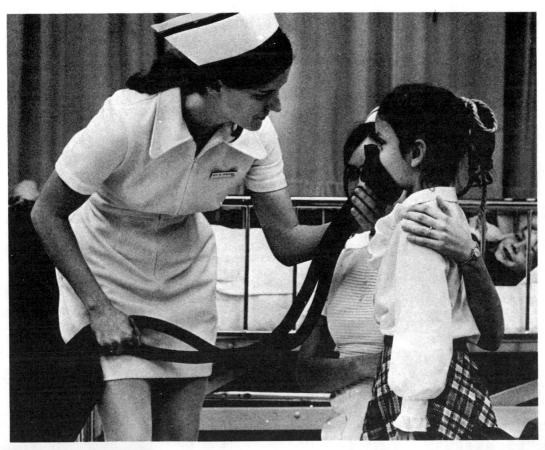

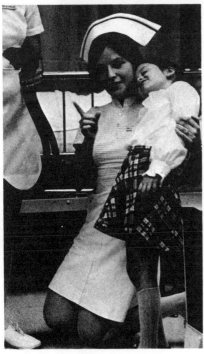

A youngster learns how it feels to have the mask over her face, and after the nurse explains anesthesia the "patient" goes to sleep.

The enthusiasm displayed by children upon returning to the classroom indicates that they have a *good* feeling about hospitals, which is a positive reason for providing this experience.

The creative drawings done by the children as a follow-up activity indicate that they understand the concepts taught. For several days after the visit the children made comments like:

—"Some things hurt but not for long . . . like shots."
—"We learned about going to the bathroom in the hospital."
—"We can take some toy with us if we stay over night."
—"The doctor and nurse kits were cool."
—"It was fun to know how we get put to sleep for operations."
—"I didn't know beds could go up."

Our evaluations of the program to date indicate that this is of more value to children than we had thought it would be. It seems to prove our thesis that children want and need to know about everyday happenings.

57

ROBERT GUINN is an assistant professor of health education at Pan American University, Edinburg, Texas 78539.

Promoting Mental Health in the Bicultural Classroom

Renaissance in ethnic pride in America has resulted in resistance to assimilative pressures by minorities and educators alike. This trend reflects the growing realization that diversity among people is to be valued and has survival value in a rapidly changing society. It also seems inevitable.[1]

Multicultural curriculums have never been more critically needed than in mental health education programs involving the Mexican-American student. Of the estimated 9,200,000 people of Hispanic origin in the United States, approximately 5,100,000 are Mexican-American.[2] Successful promotion of mental health among Mexican-American children depends upon an awareness of the many forces involved in assessing their mental health needs.

Caplan[3] defines mental health as the ability to solve problems in a reality-based way within the framework of the person's traditions and culture. The state of mental health among Mexican-Americans has been one of controversy largely due to their failure to conform to established norms of the majority Anglo-American culture. In reporting on the irrelevancy of traditional mental health services for urban Mexican-Americans, Torrey[4] points out that whenever therapists from one culture diagnose and prescribe treatment for patients of another culture, there is an inherent probability of professional misjudgment.

This concept of intrinsic culture conflict underscores the fact that mental health needs of the Mexican-American must be consonant with his values and culture. Mental health education in the school must also be structured considering the dominant cultural values of the Mexican-American learner to be effective.

La Raza

Throughout the United States, Mexican-Americans consider themselves members of *La Raza* which can be literally translated as "the race," but carries the broader meaning of a group of people united by common values and customs. In Mexico, the term *La Raza* carries strong connotations of the spiritual strength of the Mexican people. In the United States, Mexican-Americans use the term to characterize themselves as a minority group within the Anglo-American culture and to distinguish themselves from the Anglo members of their particular community.[5] Performance of religious duties, good manners, and high moral standards are focal values in this concept. The instructor working with Mexican-American students should foster this spirit of brotherhood and work within its framework as a means of strengthening self-esteem and personal pride.

La Familia

As a Mexican-American social institution, the concept of *La Familia* has a profound and positive influence on their thinking and lifestyle. After marriage the Mexican-American family does not fragment as does the Anglo family, but develops into an extended family system, including spouse and children, parents, grandparents, uncles, aunts, and cousins. To be a member of a *familia* is to have that all-important feeling of belonging, psychologically secure in the knowledge that members of the extended family are equally concerned with one's physical and emotional well-being.

Jaco[6] after finding Mexican-Americans under-represented in residential care facilities for the mentally ill, argues that the extended family system provides warmth and support during periods of high emotional stress. He concludes that familial support is one reason for a reduced rate of mental breakdowns among Mexican-Americans. Komaroff[7] found that Mexican-Americans rate death of a spouse or close family member and major personal injury or illness as less stressful than do Anglos or blacks. His interpretation is that the tradition of the extended family offers solace which Anglos and blacks cannot rely upon.

Teachers must be aware and encouraging of these strong family ties. Seeking support from the extended family should not be associated with dependence, passivity, or immaturity. It should be viewed positively as adaptive, anxiety-reducing, and problem solving due to the great emotional sustenance derived from it.

Health and Illness

In the traditional culture of Mexico, illness is related to an individual's life, relationships, community, and religion. Illness is not considered a chance event as it is in Anglo American culture.[8] This fatalistic concept is reportedly widespread among Mexican-Americans, particularly in the Southwest. Mexican-American folk medicine diagnoses illness on the basis of natural or supernatural causes. Folk diseases such as *susto* (fright), *embrujado* (bewitchment), and *mal ojo* (evil eye) stem either from physical causes or from psychological conflicts. In areas where such beliefs are upheld, the *curandero* or folk healer[9] is relied on.

Curandesimo is a traditional, cultural form of psychology which shares many striking similarities with contemporary psychology. It is successful in Mexican-American society because it offers security through adherence to traditional values, reduction of anxiety through confession, and active involvement in the therapy. This is accomplished through maintenance of close relations with both the patient and his family. The folk healer patiently explains the cause and nature of the affliction and the reasons behind each step of the treatment. These explanations are meaningful to the Mexican-American culture and much interest is taken in them. The *curandero* often uses great skill in manipulating interpersonal relations within the family to relieve pressures that produce stress and anxiety in the patient. Madsen[10] reports of *curandesimo* being successful where established psychotherapeutic techniques have failed.

Using folk practitioners in the Mexican American community as mental health allies is an alternative solution for the types of emotional problems for which most Anglos would seek more commonplace psychiatric treatment.[11] The teacher should avoid attacks on *curanderos* whenever possible. Cooperation among the school, medical profession, and the folk healer could be particularly valuable in cases of mental illness which respond to treatment better in a home environment than in an institution. This would increase the number of cases referred to physicians by the *curandero* if their curing techniques fail.

Sex Roles

There is no "typical" Mexican-American family, however, there is agreement that masculine and feminine roles are more clearly delineated than in Anglo culture. A review of the literature describes males in terms of ideal attributes: proud, dignified, reliable, vengeful when dishonored, and controlled. Women seem submissive, cultivating the quiet quality of womanliness which makes a man feel virile.[12]

Staples[13] emphasizes that during adolescence, Mexican-American boys have much greater freedom than girls. He points out that this is consistent with the cultural assumption that men are superior to women and that women should lead more sheltered lives than men. In the home the wife depends upon the husband to maintain discipline.

Foremost among the traits essential to male prestige is the quality of *machismo*. Aramoni[14] defines *machismo* as an attitude toward existence. It reflects the way a special type of man responds to conditions of life. Physical courage is stressed; a man must not weep if injured. An affront from another man requires restitution of honor, often through retaliation.

The Mexican-American child coming from a father dominated home into a female dominated classroom is confronted with an experience very much at odds with his cultural upbringing. Much empathy is required of the teacher in order for the child to overcome this difference and at the same time preserve his ethnic identity.

Awareness of Mexican-American cultural values is the first step, but what competencies should teachers in the bicultural classroom possess? Generally, prospective teachers should have undergraduate specialization in cross-cultural education, language skills, application of educational psychology to the bilingual learner, and directed teaching in the bicultural classroom.

The Mexican-American culture has a rich and proud heritage and deserves understanding and respect. In this era of high divorce rates, mental breakdowns, drug abuse, and suicides, we have much to learn from our Mexican-American citizens about family solidarity, child rearing, respect, and religious values.

[1]Elam, Stanley. "The Prime Goals of Desegregation/Integration Are Social Justice and Domestic Tranquility," *Phi Delta Kappan*, 56(8): 514, April 1975.

[2]"Census of Population: 1970," in *Characteristics of the Population*, Series PC (1)-B, Washington, DC: U.S. Dept. of Commerce, 1973.

[3]Caplan, Gerald and Ruth. "Development of Community Psychiatry Concepts in the United States," in *Comprehensive Textbook of Psychiatry*, Alfred Freedman and Harold Kaplan, Baltimore: Williams and Wilkins, 1967.

[4]Torrey, Fuller E. "The Irrelevancy of Traditional Mental Health Services for Urban Mexican-Americans," paper presented at the meeting of the American Orthopsychiatric Association, 1970.

[5]Madsen, William. *Society and Health in the Lower Rio Grande Valley*, Austin, Texas: the Hogg Foundation, 1968.

[6]Jaco, E. Gartley. *The Social Epidemiology of Mental Disorders: A Psychiatric Survey of Texas*, New York: Russell Sage Foundation, 1960.

[7]Komaroff, Anthony; Masuda, Minoru; and Holmes, Thomas. "The Social Readjustment Rating Scale: A Comparative Study of Negro, Mexican, and White Americans," *Journal of Psychosomatic Research*, 12(2): 121-28, 1968.

[8]Kiev, Ari. *Curandesimo: Mexican-American Folk Psychiatry*, New York: Free Press, 1968.

[9]Creson, D.L.; McKinely, Cameron; and Evins, Richard. "Folk Medicine in Mexican-American Subculture," *Diseases of the Nervous System*, 30(4): 264-66, 1969.

[10]Madsen, William. "Value Conflicts and Folk Psychiatry in South Texas," in *Magic, Faith, and Healing*, Ari Kiev, ed. New York: Free Press, 1964.

[11]Kline, Lawrence. "Some Factors in the Psychiatric Treatment of Spanish-Americans," *American Journal of Psychiatry*, 125(12): 1674-81, 1969.

[12]Geismar, Ludwig and Gerhart, Ursula. "Social Class, Ethnicity, and Family Functioning: Exploring Some Issues Raised by the Moynihan Report," *Journal of Marriage and the Family*, 30(3): 480-87, 1968. Penalosa, Fernando. "Mexican Family Roles," *Journal of Marriage and the Family*, 30(4): 680-89, 1968.

[13]Staples, Robert. "The Mexican-American Family: Its Modification Over Time and Space," *Phylon*, 32(2): 179-92, 1971.

[14]Aramoni, Aniceto. "Machismo," *Psychology Today*, 5(8): 69-72, 1972.

Mental Health

THE MIRROR GAME[1]

ROSA SULLIVAN is a health education teacher at Herbert Hoover Junior High, Lackawanna, New York 14218.

It is so extremely important for individuals to be able to look back on themselves in order to be evaluative of their personality traits. Many times people cannot detect their negative faults or, in contrast, tend only to find negative traits. A mentally healthy individual should be able to search on both sides and progress to working out "bad" traits. The following activity is one way to work toward this.

Objectives

1. To have a better understanding of who you are as you see yourself.
2. To have a better understanding of how others see you.
3. To recognize and understand that others always do not see you as you see yourself.
4. To appreciate the fact that you have negative points and evaluate how to change them if you wish to.
5. To evaluate how others see you and decide if that is your true image.

The Game

Duplicate a list of 20-30 personality traits suitable to the students' age group. (The group I used this game with was 14 years of age and enrolled at a junior high school.) Set them up in columns with room for graduated ratings of self and partner. (See example.)

Procedure

1. Have each student pick a partner with whom they are familiar.
2. After passing out the list, stress that they are not to talk while they are evaluating themselves or their partner.
3. The groups have 10-15 minutes to make their judgments.

4. They then compare what they marked about themselves and each other. This should reveal a number of differences between their self-impressions and how they are perceived by others. This may take as long as 15-20 minutes.
5. During the last 5 minutes in class and continued as a home assignment, students should write on the back of their papers three things they learned

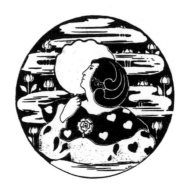

about themselves that they did not know before. They should also explain what these three things mean to them.

Follow up

(15-20 minutes of another class or as a home assignment)

1. With your class go over the list and mark each word as either positive or negative (example: if you marked always or sometimes for sensitive then it is positive; if you marked seldom or never for sensitive then it is negative).
2. A sheet containing the following questions is then passed out and the teacher requests the student to be as truthful as possible in responding since no one will see their answers without their expressed permission.

What image did you project to your partner?

What are some of the traits you feel you possess but others do not feel you possess?

Why do your perceptions differ from others' perceptions?

Do you have a strong self-image? (Do you like yourself or if you weren't you, would you like you?)

Do you have more negative or **positive traits? Why?**

Everyone has traits they do not like. Think about two of your negative ones and explain how you can go about changing them.

[1] Adapted from *Go To Health* (New York: Dell Publishing Co., Inc., 1972), p. 98.

TRAITS		SELF				PARTNER			
		Never	Seldom	Sometimes	Always	Never	Seldom	Sometimes	Always
1. Sensitive	+								
2. Arrogant	−								
3. Silly	−								
4. Trusting	+								
5. Tender	+								
6. Two-faced	−								

Perceptions of Me

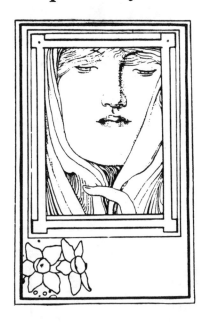

JERROLD S. GREENBERG is coordinator of health education, State University of New York at Buffalo, Buffalo, New York 14214. He serves as contributing editor for this SHR department, which is designed to be of particular usefulness to the classroom teacher at all levels.

Though realizing the degree of immodesty of which I can be accused, let me risk stating that the most interesting topic to me is me. Further, the most interesting topic to you is probably you. That's nothing startling. We all are interested in ourselves. Realizing this phenomenon, educators recommend that learnings in school be related to the life experiences of the learner. It then seems to follow that with the learner himself the topic of study, the efficiency and effectiveness of the learning process would be maximized.

The question of the appropriateness of oneself as a topic for study within a school setting, however, remains. Since one behaves on how one perceives reality rather than upon reality itself, one's perceptions of oneself will determine many health related behaviors. For example, one

possessing a positive self-concept might be expected to walk tall (upright) while one with a negative self-concept might walk slumped over to physically indicate "lowliness"; or one with a positive sense of sexual self-esteem might be outgoing and pleasant, whereas one with a negative feeling about oneself sexually might behave in a shy, withdrawn manner.

Based upon the importance of perceptions of oneself, and, in addition, how others perceive one (since they will behave toward others based upon their perceptions of them) activities should be developed and conducted with students to help them to:

1. More realistically perceive themselves and others.
2. Explore the relationship between their perceptions and how they act.
3. Make whatever adjustments they deem necessary to become what they want to be. Presented in this article are examples of such learning activities.

Sentence Completions

Unfinished sentences which require the student to react by completing them, allow for self-inquiry of a kind to which people are not accustomed. Examples of such questions indicate the breadth of possibilities and range of topics which can be explored with this instructional strategy.

1. I often _____
2. I seldom _____
3. I'm bored when _____
4. I love to _____
5. Other children _____
6. I will _____
7. I must _____
8. I am very _____
9. I wish I could _____
10. My friends are _____
11. My parents _____
12. I wish _____
13. I feel _____
14. I'm happy when _____
15. My body _____

Whereas the completion of these sentences requires the student to think about himself, processing the responses in small groups allows

students to explore other childrens' perceptions of themselves. It is hoped that surprises about certain responses will help children be more accepting of others and better understand themselves. If the class trusts the teacher sufficiently, the reading of the responses by the teacher might also aid the teacher to better plan instruction which pertains to the needs of the students.

Discussion Questions

Using questions to stimulate group discussions is not a recent educational innovation, but the types of questions suggested for use here differ from those employed elsewhere.

1. What is the one thing that scares you the most?
2. When are you most hurt?
3. What is the very first thing that you remember?
4. What is the saddest thing that has ever happened to you?
5. What is the best thing that has ever happened to you?
6. What do you dislike most about school?
7. What don't you like about yourself?
8. What do you like most about yourself?
9. What would you rather have: wealth, intelligence, or physical attractiveness?
10. Who is the most influential person in your life?
11. What do you wish?
12. How can you be happy?
13. What do you love to do the most?
14. What was the strongest feeling you had last week (anger, joy, grief, etc. . . .) and what caused that feeling?
15. What is something you can tell us now that you wouldn't have felt comfortable telling us before?

Each group should be reminded that there are no right or wrong answers to such questions and, therefore, they should expect each person to respond differently. The group members' role should be to ask questions of the respondent which will help the group to better understand the response, rather than to attempt to get the group to agree on what would be the "best" answer. As a result of this exercise, it is anticipated that each student will have a more accurate picture of both himself and his classmates than prior to the exercise.

Question Sociogram

An activity which can be used to aid students to see themselves as others see them is the Question Sociogram. Unlike a regular sociogram which asks children to list a number of people they would like to attend a movie with, etc., the Question Sociogram asks children to place the name of the person in the class *most likely* to fit the description implicit in the question. Examples of questions which can be used will help to clarify this technique:

_____ 1) Who most likely is afraid of mice?

_____ 2) Who most likely cannot resist eating a donut?

_____ 3) Who wakes up often with nightmares?

_____ 4) Who loves cowboy movies?

_____ 5) Who loves romantic movies?

_____ 6) Who most wants a lot of money?

_____ 7) Who watches a lot of television?

_____ 8) Who most likely will be a scientist?

_____ 9) Who will be a politician?

_____10) Who will make the best mother or father?

_____11) Who will never get married?

_____12) Who will never use drugs?

_____13) Who is most likely to cheat on an exam?

_____14) Who will be the most thoughtful lover?

_____15) Who will be a talking liberal who won't do anything?

_____16) Who will insist on a small wedding?

_____17) Who would be the best teacher?

_____18) Who is apt to do anonymous favors for people?

_____19) Who will always be physically attractive?

_____20) Who would make the best friend?

To the left of each number, students are required to place the name of one student in their group or class. Only one name can be written on the blank line and each blank line *must* have a name on it. After the responses have been made each child can ask each other child which descriptions he most fits, thereby acquiring others' perceptions of himself. To better know oneself is the first step in improving oneself.

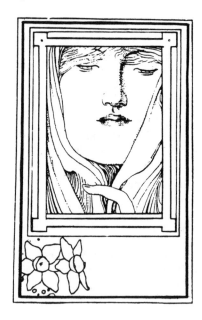

Intimacy Questions

Once trust has been developed in a class or group of children, questions of a more intimate nature can be explored. Best discussed in pairs to provide a close relationship, some of the following questions can be employed by a teacher willing to take risks to provide meaningful educational experiences:

1. What do you feel most ashamed of in your past?
2. What have you deliberately lied about? Why?
3. When do you hurt people?
4. What turns you on the most?
5. Do you have any health problems? What are they?
6. What are your least attractive features?
7. Do you believe in God? Organized religion?
8. Are your parents happily married? Why? Why not?
9. How do you feel when you love?
10. What makes you swear?
11. What do you think about homosexuals?
12. Do you like yourself? Why? Why not?
13. What was your greatest failure? Greatest success?

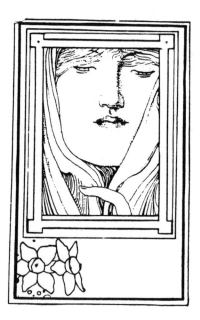

14. Who would you be if you could be anyone else that you wanted?

These questions develop greater closeness between two people who are honest and trusting to begin with, and likewise can develop greater distance between two people who feel threatened by such openness. It is important, therefore, to employ this activity only with a group that has matured and can take advantage of such an opportunity to mature further.

The Neglected 'R'—Responsibility

What is it really saying? The red line on the wall chart rises gradually and then suddenly leaps and then leaps and leaps again. Underneath in perfectly printed lettering is the identifying "Incidence of Gonorrhea." What does it really say? Perhaps more accurate subtitles would read "Incidence of Irresponsible Behavior" or "Incidence of Selfishness." Isn't that what one is really talking about when one talks about the spread of venereal diseases?

Riddle: Which of the following practices is more likely to have far-reaching results: (a) teaching students where they can get treatment for veneral disease, or (b) helping students realize the need for responsible behavior? Teaching facts about venereal disease can be likened to treating cancer. We must, at the same time that we treat the current cases, identify the causes and seek means of prevention. This charge to educators will finally result in *total* education about venereal disease.

Three principles should guide a total program of venereal disease education. First, *begin early!* Kindergarten is not too early to begin stressing principles of responsible behavior, concern for the welfare of others, and identifying one's own needs for love and security. Each succeeding year should continue to build on these and other principles of self-awareness and interpersonal relationships. Then, when students learn what sexual intercourse is, whether it is in fifth, sixth or seventh grade, they should be aware that diseases can be spread in this man-

BETTY KAY STEIN is health coordinator at Minnetonka West Junior High School, Excelsior, Minnesota. Her article is reprinted from Minnesota's Health, *published by the Minnesota Department of Health.*

ner. It may not be necessary to go into any more detail, but the awareness should help accentuate the need for responsible behavior.

Secondly, venereal disease education, as well as all health education, must be person-centered rather than fact-centered. Activities which *involve students* in thinking about themselves and their relationships with others should be a major portion of the curriculum. Planning for such activities requires time and creativity, rather than vast amounts of expensive materials and elaborate scheduling of people and things.

Finally, the basic objective should be to discover and deal with the primary causes of the spread of venereal disease. Notice the typical chart which demonstrates the "chain of infection" of venereal disease. Those sterile black duplicated figures on white paper show little emotion and require even less from the onlooker. Ask the students to select one such figure and write a biographical sketch about him or her. What happens? Now the figure becomes a person, with feelings and emotions, with needs and desires, relating to others effectively or ineffectively. Upon further evaluation, students should be able to discern what the real causes of the figure's behavior are. Behavior is what accounts for the spread of venereal disease.

What concepts should be included in a people-centered curriculum? Listed below are a few I think are important, along with at least one activity which might be used to clarify each concept. These are only samples, and the list is far from all-inclusive.

Concept: Each individual must accept responsibility for his actions.

Activity: On a sheet of paper, each student lists new freedoms he has acquired within the past year. Opposite each one, he lists the added responsibilities he has acquired

along with the freedom. Then discuss: From whom did you get these freedoms? To whom do you have responsibilities? What will result if you do not accept the responsibility? Whom will it affect? How will you feel about yourself if you fulfill the responsibility? if you do not?

Activity: Have a small group of (volunteer) students role-play any or all of the following situations and the resulting consequences:

a. student decides not to do his homework.

b. man speeds on the highway because he is late.

c. boy convinces his girlfriend to drink on a date.

d. girl receives a birthday gift.

e. boy is elected captain of the wrestling team.

Afterwards, discuss: Did the person accept the responsibility involved? What do you think were his reasons for accepting or rejecting the responsibility? What other results would have occurred if he had acted differently? How would he have felt about himself? How might this affect his future actions?

Concept: Communicating one's feelings to another aids in maintaining a relationship of trust.

Activity: For one day, students observe and record (on paper) accounts of people communicating with others. Note the presence or lack of honesty in what they reveal about their own feelings. Discuss: Give examples of people who did and did not express their true feelings to others. (Identify only by role, etc., not by name.) What were the results? Which person would you be most apt to believe? In which case is a lack of understanding most apt to result? Which person would *you* most prefer to talk to? What does this tell you about yourself? Think of some people to whom you feel you can speak honestly. (Do not name names.) Why is it possible for you to speak honestly with them?

Concept: Everyone has a basic need for love and security.

Activity: Assignment for students: Write a detailed obituary for yourself as you would someday like it to appear. Afterwards, consider these questions: What does this reveal about your goals in life? What feelings would you have about your accomplishments? Which feats will produce feelings of love and/or security? Will these satisfy those needs?

Activity: Divide students into groups for music, movies, TV programs, books and poetry. Have each group analyze the currently popular items in its medium, e.g., music group analyzes current hits, etc. In analysis, answer these questions: What proportion of items analyzed dealt directly with human needs for love and security? What percent did not deal with it at all? What solutions, if any, were offered for solving those needs? Do you think these solutions are realistic? Would they really satisfy the need?

Concept: One person responds to another in proportion to the power he gives that person over him.

Activity: Students are asked to respond to several lists of people-roles, e.g., (a) best friend, father, teacher, sister; (b) next-door neighbor, clergyman, policeman, doctor; (c) little brother, grandparent, mother, self. In each case, he lists the four in order from the person who has the most power over him, to the person who has the least. Discuss: Are you able to identify the people who have power over you in your life? What reasons can you think of for giving them that power? Are there some people who have more power than you really want them to have? What reasons might a person have for giving another power over himself?

Discussions in all of the above-suggested topics should be voluntary. Some students may not feel confident enough yet of their feelings to share them with others.

Teachers must respect the rights of the individuals for privacy. However, all students should be encouraged to consider the questions posed, and to ponder them in relation to their own lives.

These concepts, which deal with understanding self and others, should lay a good foundation for venereal disease education. Obviously, as the age of the students involved increases, a teacher can link these understandings more directly to discussions about venereal disease. It should become apparent to older students, for instance, that promiscuous behavior can be linked to a need for love and security. The final challenge to the teacher is to enable each student to evaluate his own behavior, and to assist him in assuming responsibility for it. And somehow, the home, school, and society must provide youth with experiences in which they can enjoy the positive feelings which result from demonstrating responsible behavior.

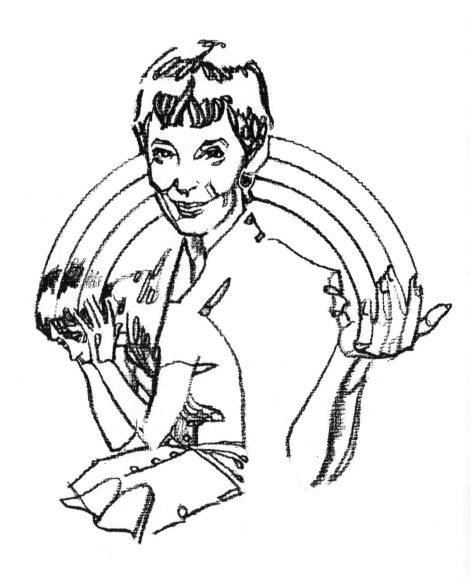

ME POWER

JACK POESKE, GARY COTE, and LEON-
ARD ANDERSON team teach the sixth
grade at Panther Lake School in Kent,
Washington 98031.

What do you do when the district curriculum says that health is a required subject to be taught and the district is in the
process of getting a new book to replace
those good old 1959, dull health texts you
hated when you were in school? We
found ourselves in this predicament with
three choices: (1) use the old text; (2) bag
teaching health; (3) make up our own
program, which is what we did.

We shared ideas picked up from different workshops and magazines and decided to try them out in our rooms. Most
were great, but a few turned out to be bad
in our particular situations. This article is
intended to try to help teachers who may
be caught in the same bind.

Teachers are always catching kids
doing things wrong and kids do the same
thing. We decided to try the opposite—
recognize the good things kids did. In
each class we described a positive act and
explained that we'd like to hear about
good things kids do. We took a big section of butcher paper and drew a cartoon
character on it under which we wrote "I
caught someone doing good." We taped
the paper on the door and told the kids to
write down the name of anyone they saw
doing something good and what it was.
Teachers should contribute, too. For
example, "Jimmy opened the door for
Mary" or "Kurt put Eddie's chair up for
him." The idea is to fill the paper with
good things.

Stars and Valentines

This idea worked so well that we tried a
similar idea called blue star, gold star.
This again used butcher paper taped to a
wall or door with the name of each class
member written on it and blank spaces
beside each name.

We talked about good actions (positive) and bad actions (negative). The kids
were told that each time they saw something good to put a gold star by that person's name when they came into the
room. If they saw someone doing something bad, then they were to put a blue
star by that person's name. This idea did
not work. They concentrated on looking
for negative things in others and it soon
degenerated into a contest to see who
could get the most blue stars.

For Valentine's Day we tried a combination of projects to make a gigantic Valentine's card. We passed around a complete
class roster to each kid in our class with
the instructions to write one *personal*,
positive thing about each person in the
class on the space next to each person's

name. The only restriction was that what
they wrote was not general like "Jim is
nice," or "is cool."

After everyone turned in their positive
comments, each student's remark was
clipped and given back. Then each student had 30 positive things about himself
from his classmates. Next the students
paired up and drew silhouettes of each
other. Students filled in the silhouettes
with the things that the other kids had
said about them, or made a collage of
their self-image.

Then we used a three foot by three foot
section of colored butcher paper or a
large sheet of construction paper folded
in half to form a card. On the front of the
card, the kids made anything having to do
with Valentine's Day, on the inside card
the words "What My Classmates Think of
Me," were printed and the silhouette
pasted in. If the kids made a collage on
their silhouette, they either wrote in or
pasted in the other kids' remarks.

On the other inside page titled "What I
Think of You," the kids drew or wrote
good things about their parents. This is
what they give to their parents for Valentine's Day.

Experiments and Questions

After spending some time building up a
students' self image, we moved into more
concrete areas. The first unit was smoking. We decided not to preach, but present facts about the possible hazards of
smoking, and let the kids make their own
decisions. We started out by telling the
kids to make up a cigarette commercial
and we were surprised to find out they
came up with every gimmick the tobacco
companies use.

During the tobacco unit, a cancerous
lung in a jar on display is always an attention getter. It makes the cancer statistics
of smokers compared to non-smokers
mean a little more. The local Cancer Society probably will loan one to you.

We ran a couple of experiments dealing
with smoking and its effects on the nervous system. For example, we asked students to take and record the pulse of a
smoker before he lit a cigarette. After
smoking a cigarette, the kids took the
smoker's pulse right away then every five
minutes till the pulse got down to normal.

By this time we had the kids' attention
concentrated on some measurable effects of smoking. We showed some films
and filmstrips that dealt with smoking and
effects on the heart and lungs and then
brought in a man from the lung association to talk about emphysema. He
brought in four slides of lung tissue that

ranged from a healthy lung to the last
stage of emphysema.

The last thing we did was to make up a
questionnaire to ask a smoker: (1) Why did
you start smoking? (2) When did you start
smoking? (3) What do you get out of
smoking? (4) Has anyone asked you to
quit? (Who?) (5) Have you tried to quit
before? (6) Why did you start again? (7)
Have you noticed any physical problems
you can attribute to smoking? (8) How did
you feel after you quit smoking? (9) If you
knew then what you know now about
cigarettes, would you have started smoking? (10) Do you want your children to
smoke? Why?

Talks with Addicts

We covered alcohol and various drugs
by showing films and filmstrips that dealt
with each group. The children could do a
report on a particular drug, make up a
chart of the slang names of drugs, or draw
the parts of the brain affected by drugs
and alcohol, all as background for the last
part of the project—two young drug addicts from a halfway house came to talk to
the kids about an addict's life. The last
thing we did on drugs was to take the
class and their parents into the halfway
house to talk to the addicts who are desperately trying to stay off drugs.

These last two activities really impress
the kids, and the speakers have been impressed by the good questions our kids
have asked them, which we attribute to
the preparation work.

The nutrition unit can come either first
or last. We study the four food groups
(your state dairy council is a goldmine of
free and interesting teaching aids) and
how they help the body to grow. Films
and filmstrips supplement what we have.
A good activity to do after going through
the four food groups is to have kids bring
empty food boxes, cans, and cartons
from home. Set them up as groceries on a
table divided into five sections, one for
each food group and the fifth for "nutritional garbage." Nutritional garbage is
food that contains "empty calories" (food
with no nutritional value, just calories).
After doing this, see how fast kids can
group the groceries. Usually they'll be
surprised to see how many foods fall into
the garbage class.

A "Me" Book

We found an interesting way to keep all
the information we had been studying in
health. We called it a "Me" book, because all the information in the book pertains directly or indirectly to the student.
We made our "Me" books out of tag
board in notebook form. The students

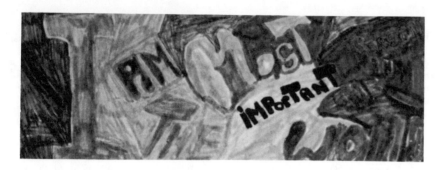

fore we start the actual physical part of health, we talk to the kids about the body as if it were a machine with a lifetime guarantee. After discussing just what a guarantee is, we pass out a retroactive guarantee to be filled out by the student, signed by the parent, and pasted on the inside cover of the "Me" book. Then we start the physical health sections.

In the section "Things I Need to Maintain a Healthy Body" (proper diet, rest, recreation) all nutritional information is recorded.

The section entitled "Things That Hurt My Body (shorten lifetime guarantee)" contains all drug and tobacco information.

The Most Important Person

The last thing we do with the kids is to ask them two questions: 1) Who is the most important person in the world?; 2) What is love and are there different kinds of love?

The answers will vary to question one, but the answer we seek is "I am the most important person in the world."

The definition of love will be up to the teacher, but we feel that if a person loves himself, he will act kindly (treat others with love) towards others. The last project is to make a sign out of the tag board. On one side the theme is "I am the most important person in the world" and on the other side the theme is "Love Yourself." The signs should be colorful and contain drawings or designs. The exact words don't have to be used, just so that the thought comes across. One of our students summed up the whole project with his sign that read "ME POWER."

could design their cover around the theme of "Me." For example: "The Wonderful World of Me," "All About Me." For the first few pages, we asked the students to bring in pictures of themselves growing up, preferably one picture that shows them at each year to present grade. The kids can actually see the changes that have been going on as they grew. It is a natural motivator. You can have kids write captions under each picture, and the kids with no pictures can write an autobiography to date.

The next section is entitled "Things I Want to Be." Here they list everything they want to be. Next is "Things I Can Be." These are things that the child can actually be. They'll have to think about them.

"Things I Like in Others" is next. List all traits they like and admire in others.

"Things I Like About Myself." Everything kids like about themselves is listed. Kids have a hard time with this.

The next section "Things I Don't Like About Myself" is tricky. We tell the kids that we won't look at this page when checking over the notebook.

The section "Things I Can't Change About Myself" gives kids a chance to list the things that they are stuck with in themselves. After they have done this, they must pick out two of these things and write out a plan as to how they can live with these things.

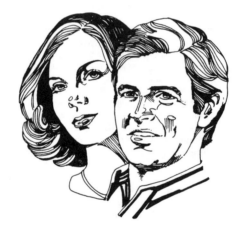

In "Things I Can Change About Myself" the kids list things they can change, pick two of them and write out a plan to follow to actually change those two things.

These first sections are discussed while working on positive image building. Be-

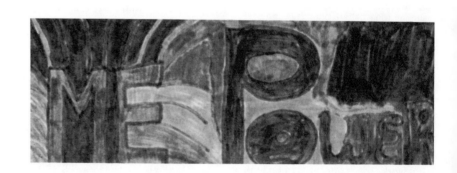

Mental Health

Exploring Emotions with Young Children

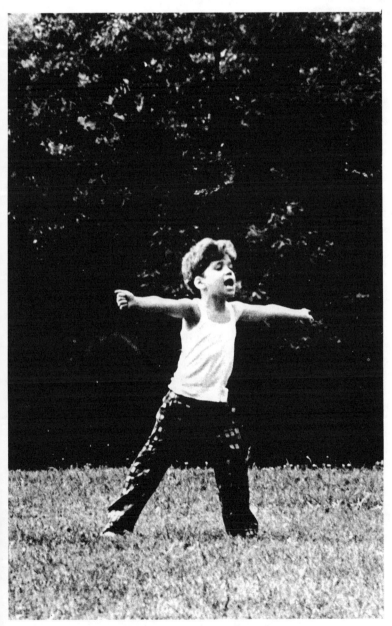

Happiness is winning.

Is mental health a viable content area for inclusion in the school curriculum? Yes; possibly no aspect of education is more important than the promotion of a healthy personality within each student. Much lip service is given to the ability of teachers working with emotional development, but little is being tried systematically. How well are we accepting this responsibility? And when? Most are aware of the inclusion of personality, psychology, etc. at the secondary and college levels, but the idea of dealing with mental health at the elementary school level on a cognitive basis is probably foreign to most people. In essence, the mental health responsibility of the elementary school lies in the provision of services, a warm and accepting environment, and instruction concerned with the development of a self-concept which the individual can accept and understand. Are we doing all that we can and should in each of these areas?

Our project illustrates one way of dealing with the teaching of mental health at the elementary school level—the understanding of emotion. Read and Greene [1] suggest some concepts to be dealt with in the elementary schools. The one we have chosen to implement is "Emotions are expressed in many different ways" and arise from a variety of life situations.

Emotion here is defined as a response of the entire human being to a stimulus, not necessarily to be confused with a basic drive—the reaction that follows the satisfaction and/or frustration of a basic need. All emotions involve both physiological and psychological adjustment. Usually, but not always, these adjustments are temporary. An important distinguishing factor is the intensity of the emotion. All these ideas can be explored and expanded upon with elementary school children. The study of emotion is a study in synthesis. One must concentrate on the study of single emotions

HERB JONES is professor of health science at Ball State University, Muncie, Indiana 47906.

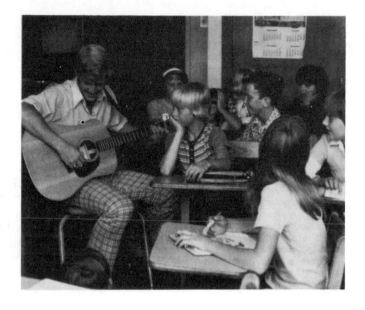

Happiness is being together.

in order to make observations about the emotional behavior of children.

To reach a better understanding of how children deal with emotions, we decided to work directly with the children. To do this, we attempted to capture emotions through photography. The study is only a beginning but has produced much useful information. Children at the elementary and preschool levels were photographed in a variety of situations. They were then asked to comment on the emotions being expressed in the photographs. Essentially we dealt with happiness, love, sorrow, fear and anxiety, anger, and loneliness. What follows are the children's responses. The reader will be able to see the myriad of activities which might follow some of the exploratory sessions with children about their emotions.

The first series of pictures dealt with happiness. This universal emotion really needs no introduction since most have experienced the results of having a basic drive fulfilled. When asked to complete the statement, "Happiness to me means . . . ," this is how the children responded:

Second graders
    A day off from school.
    To never work.
    To sleep with my cousins.
    A trip to Florida.

---

[1] Read, Donald and Greene, Walter. *Creative Teaching In Health*. New York: Macmillan, 1971.

Fifth graders
    When I make one of my friends happy.
    No school.
    Getting a 100 on a test.
    Winning something.
    Sleeping.

Sixth graders
    Being captain of patrols.
    Winning.
    Kissing your mother (a male response).
    Freedom.
    Being together.
    Having a *Playboy* magazine.

When the child is very young he loves no one except in a most self-centered sense. He lives in a world dedicated to himself and his needs. As time goes on, however, his experiences change his character so that he develops an ability to feel for others, to express sympathy for them, and to enjoy contributing to their happiness and well-being. But what causes a child to manifest love in his myriad of ways? What does love mean to elementary school children? Despite the influence of the mass media, fifth grade children failed to speak in terms of romantic love. They, instead, expressed love as:

When I love my mother.
Love is a family.
When I kiss my mother.

On the other hand, changes seemed to take place and a more sexual connotation was attached to love:

A sexy girl.
Kissing and hugging.
Laurie and Peter.
Having a girl friend.
Kissing your girl friend.
Finding that the prettiest girl in the class likes you.

Yet, perhaps the most meaningful definition of love came from a second grader who said, when asked the difference between liking and loving something or someone, "Liking something is for a very short time. Loving is forever." Sometimes children see the truth more clearly than do adults.

At the other end of the emotional spectrum, students were asked to respond to pictures which depicted sorrow. Interestingly enough, sorrow for many of the children meant death of some kind, of either a relative or a pet. Death is one of those dark mysterious forces that have always stood somewhere just outside man's consciousness. This "fear" is not only a fear of actual physical death, but often of spiritual regressive death as well. It is only recently that the subject of death has become academically respectable, and then usually at advanced levels. Should we explore this concept with children? With sympathetic understanding can we give a child something to hang on to? Can we instill an acceptance of life and death in children so that they can better manage their fears? Here is how the children responded to the emotion of sorrow:

Second grade
Sorrow is feeling sad (almost everyone expressed this).

Fifth grade
Sorrow is death.
When I feel I've hurt somebody that didn't deserve it.
When I do something wrong.
Crying, feeling down.

Sixth grade
When someone dies.
Nixon—four more years.
The agony of defeat.
Having your *Playboy* taken away.
Losing a friend.

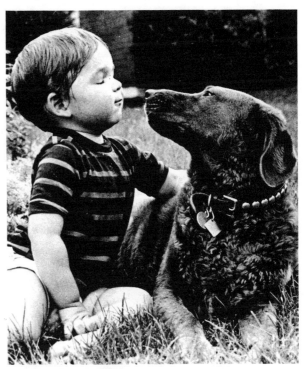

Love is Duke.

Sorrow is crying.

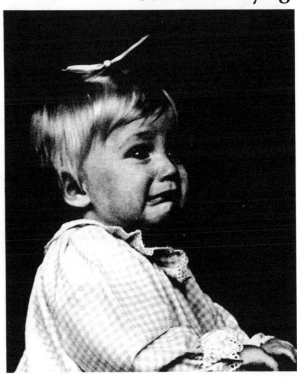

We all usually think of fear as a reaction to a situation of physical danger to ourselves. These types of fears we understand because they deal with our concepts of survival and self-preservation. But there are other fears which we possess that are not so clear to us. Fortunately, when we discuss our fears with others, we often discover that they were imagined rather than real. Examples of such fears might include fear of sex, fear of sexual knowledge, fear of sin, and fear of elemental emotions such as rage and jealousy. We do not always try to cope with these fears and tend to make efforts to separate ourselves from them. For young children as well as older people, fear of the dark, of being alone, and of imaginary creatures are common. But how do elementary school children respond when approached with the concept of fear in a structured educational setting?

Second grade
   Fear is a bad dream.
   When the lights are all off.
   A high wire act with no net.
   Jumping off a cliff.
   Being on a high bridge.

Fifth grade
   When it is pitch dark in my room and I hear noises.
   Knowing someone is going to beat you up.
   Being alone at night.
   Not having your homework done.

Sixth grade
   Being lost in a cave.
   Being afraid to speak up.
   Being alone, and unhappy.

Anger is undoubtedly one of the most studied of all the emotions. A baby becomes angry if he is not fed when hungry, not changed when wet, or if inhibited in movement. Small children become angry when someone takes a toy away or when they must share or stop an activity which they are enjoying. When we asked elementary school youngsters about anger, they almost always responded with social situations.

Second grade
   Anger is when I have to set the table.
   When someone hits me.

Fifth grade
   My brother messing up my room.
   Living with boys.

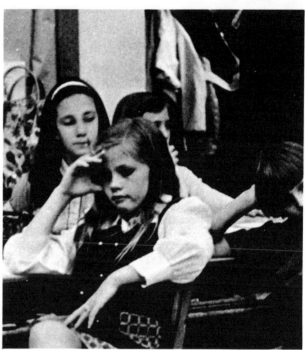

Fear is not having your homework done.

Anger is living with boys.

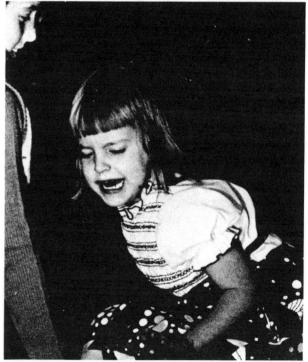

Getting in trouble for something someone else did.

When someone pulls your hair.

Sixth grade
Getting in a fight.

Interestingly enough, it was extremely difficult to photograph angry children.

Frustration and loneliness are two emotions which we would not consider to be problems for young school-age children, at least on the surface. Knowing the social nature of young children, we would guess that they are seldom lonely. Read

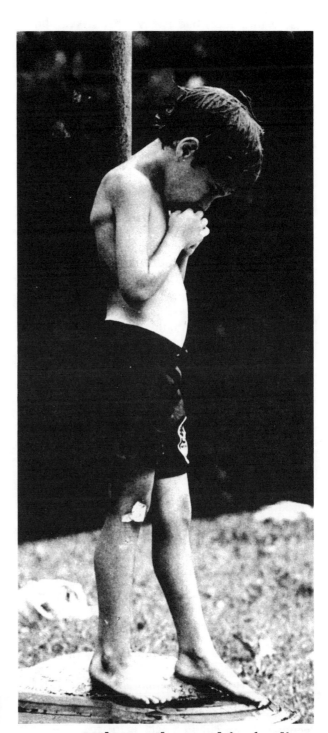

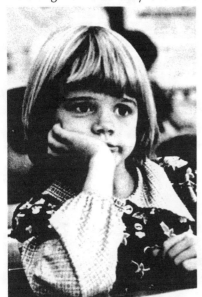

Frustration is trying to solve a problem.

Frustration is when nothing works.

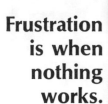

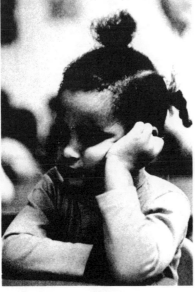

When I have this feeling of loneliness, I go somewhere and see if anyone misses me.

what sixth graders had to say when asked about frustration and loneliness. Frustration is:

Trying to draw a person.
Trying to solve a problem.
Giving up.
When nothing works and you get mad.

Loneliness is:
Having no boyfriend.
When I'm lost.
Being left behind.
Fear and anxiety.

One youngster responded, "When I have this feeling of loneliness I go somewhere to be by myself and see if anyone misses me."

Finally, we captured one child on film whose pose we felt had something to offer, though it defied classification as an emotion. For want of a better term, we call it daydreaming. It is a situation that we all find ourselves in, sometimes to withdraw from a frustrating situation, but often only harmless fun. When viewing a picture of a child daydreaming, this is what the children had to say:

She was thinking of things far away.
She was thinking of her school work.

The important point to consider here is the extreme difference in the two responses.

Judging from these examples, it seems that the study of emotions is not enough by itself to classify and understand behavior. How to utilize emotions in the classroom is left to the ingenuity of the classroom teacher. We have only tried to illustrate one way in which such study is possible. Emotions and mood are not necessarily the same. Emotions can be expressed in a variety of ways, yet with a lot of similarities. Some suggest that emotions are either attack- or withdrawal-oriented, that there is no other basis for emotion. Since emotions tend to characterize a society's values, the study of emotional behavior of man, including children, will continue to be of interest and is a fruitful area for consideration in each classroom. Hopefully all children will have a solid background to work from as they tackle the social and academic challenges of school and of life in general. Most children will learn to cope with these challenges without our help and without long-lasting emotional scars. It is our thesis that we can help them handle emotions by making them a legitimate part of the curriculum in health education.

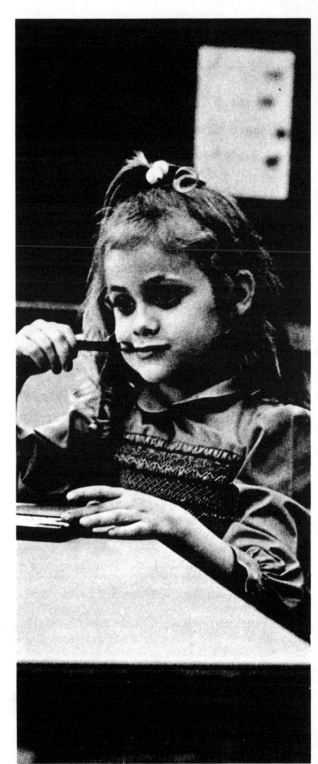

She was thinking of things far away.

Catch Somebody Doing Something Good

"This is really a happy classroom. You feel it when you walk in." Rodney Larson, principal of Ruston School of the Tacoma District in Washington State, made this comment to Carolyn Patterson, the teacher, as the children left for recess.

It wasn't always so. Earlier in the year the children in this third and fourth grade class tattled a great deal, argued, and verbally tore each other to shreds. Little work was being done. Crying, complaining, and fighting filled their days. Mrs. Patterson had tried several things with the class but nothing seemed to work.

She discussed the situation with Lou Fine, the school social worker. He had been reading stories to the class and seeing some of the children individually. They decided to talk with the children themselves to see how they felt about what was happening.

The class didn't like the way things were going but didn't know what to do about it. All of their methods were bringing negative rather than positive results. Mr. Fine suggested, "Instead of catching somebody doing something bad, let's *catch somebody doing something good* and let's write it down and keep track for a week."

One skeptical child said, "Aw, we'll never do it!" Mr. Fine replied, "Well, maybe so . . . I'll tell you what, little buddy. I'll betcha a bag of peanuts that the kids do it and if they don't, I'll give *you* two bags of peanuts. And for the rest of the class, for each one of you who catches somebody doing something good and can honestly say it, there's a bag of peanuts too."

The children quickly became enthusiastic and put up a chart. They also decided to keep a tally sheet next to the door for marking down the times they felt like tattling but didn't. They made posters for the hall outside their room showing the good things they might catch somebody doing.

When the group met again at the end of the

CAROLYN PATTERSON is a teacher at Ruston School, and LOU FINE is in pupil personnel for the Tacoma Public Schools, Tacoma, Washington 99201.

first week, most felt that things had gone better. Fifty-two items of "something good" had been tallied from the chart. "Somebody helped me up when I fell on my skates." "Someone thru a pace of papper in the garbich." "I got in a fight with a frend and I said I was sorry."

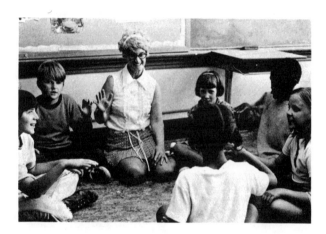

Each item was discussed, circled, and numbered. The children were given verbal reinforcement and recognition for their positive behaviors and 27 bags of peanuts went into their tummies!

Mrs. Patterson and Mr. Fine realized that the project would not work solely in isolation and it would have to be a part of everything the children did. Mrs. Patterson involved the children individually and in small groups, in discussions of feelings—of helping children find the good in another child—of finding ways of expressing the good to others.

The children made a *Catch Somebody Being a Good Sport* chart. Somebody caught somebody who "Threw a ball over the fence and the other girl went to get it so they were friends." Someone else saw somebody "Forget to go down to her friend's classroom but when she saw the person again the person wasn't mad."

They had fun with a *Happy Chart*—things they enjoyed—using pictures from magazines or drawings of their own. On this chart, Mrs. Patterson and Mr. Fine found: "Happyness is tiing your bother's shoes." One child wrote, "Happyness is reading lots of books" to which another added: "And enjoying them to."

They learned to make various kinds of graphs, charting how the tattling was going down. And as one fourth grader remarked at the end of the third week, "We needed a big tattle paper at first, but now we don't need any at all!"

And they sang. Mrs. Patterson and the class found songs that were fun to sing and that made them feel happy. When there were rough times—and there *were* rough times—often someone would say, "Let's sing—I feel better when we have troubles and we sing."

By the end of the fifth week the teacher and social worker found that the theme was catching on. The children were moving outside themselves, trying to help each other and willing to say "I'm sorry" when the inevitable slips happened. Quarreling had lessened; work was up; smiles and laughing were much more in evidence. Other staff members made comments that problems on the playground no longer involved the children from this room.

Lou Fine said, "I think we should have the parents in one evening and fill them in on what's been happening—see if they've noticed any differences at home and figure where we go from here."

A letter was mailed to each parent, followed by phone calls by the children. Out of a class of 27 children, 17 parents attended an evening meeting held in the classroom.

Some parents had noticed differences, and others hadn't been aware that the project was even going on. Those who hadn't known were pleasantly surprised and *all* were anxious that it should continue. As one father put it, "We've always let our kids know when they do wrong but how often do we, as parents, make an effort to say 'That was a good try or a nice thing to do for your sister.' "

The group decided to have the program extend to their homes, to *catch their own children doing something good*. They also decided to call the absent parents and tell *them* what had been happening. And they wanted to meet again—to discuss how things were going and to exchange ideas.

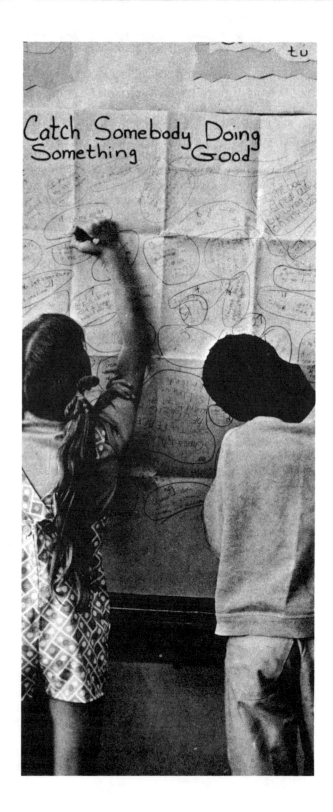

Freedom To Think in Elementary School

CHILDREN FACE many problems in day to day living, and the decisions they make are based on what they believe, on what they feel are important values. How can we help them and guide them toward decision making?

For many years, we have done this through modeling or attempting to impose our values and life styles, hoping to thereby set examples of meaning to children. For many reasons, this method is no longer effective (if it ever was). As teachers, we do hope to directly influence our children, but more than that, the goal is to aid them to make their own decisions in such a way that rational thinking processes are involved and their values and beliefs are recognized also.

Schools today are different and exciting. There are many new ways to learn, as well as traditionally effective ways. Learning is no longer just cognitive. We are attempting to teach in all the domains, and the affective and psychomotor domains are utilized in day to day learning—and the children are enjoying it.

BONNIE BRACEY is a teacher at the Long Branch Elementary School, 33 North Fillmore St., Arlington, Virginia 22201.

There are many new programs and a multitude of professional reference texts to help the teacher make a start. The use of interviews, quizzes, group dynamics, charting, and process approaches is recommended. Sometimes just the reading of the philosophical theories provides enough insight to get started, if it is possible to sort out "affective," "humanistic," and all the other new designations for programs of this sort. It is difficult sometimes to keep from getting entangled in something that is only slightly related to the information you are seeking.

There are classroom kits with records and filmstrips on values, with valuing as the basis of group activity.

There are particularly good creative writing booklets that provide a teacher with some limited and interesting insights into what children think of themselves as they compare themselves to a flower, a fruit, a number, a color, or an animal. A skillful, nonjudgmental teacher can find out a lot about the individual child, through his mind-stretching activities.

Unfortunately, though, after using most of the new programs and relying on old favorites, there is still a void. We teachers still end up making the decisions, selecting our values, without really giving the children freedom to think.

Inside-Out Brings Success

I have used a program, however, that *can* do the job. I have many examples of its success. It is called "INSIDE-OUT," a series of approximately 30 programs, developed by National Instructional Television to deal with the day-to-day problems and emotions of children from their point of view. There are programs on all the characters found in a typical classroom (whatever that is). The children meet the bully and the practical joker. They deal with such crisis situations as competition between the children in a family, when to ask for help, developing responsibility. Programs present some topics we have generally avoided that need to be examined and presented to children in other than real life examples. Television news, or secret discussions, such as a death in a family, strong feeling, child abuse, and divorce. NIT says the series of programs takes into account the vital elements that form the wholeness of self, both inside and out. My enthusiastic children say that the program brings the feelings inside, out to discuss, think about, and use. They say that they can make decisions with the help

"I Dare You" Best Program

1st

Inside-Out is an educational T.V. program.
Inside-Out is a good, funny program.
Inside-Out is a show on which kids can show their feelings.
Inside-Out is a good program because if you were in that situation you would know what to do.

Poem Inside-out is about children's problems when they spout but if they don't know you see they'll never learn His-tor-y but if they don't know History they'll never learn to see and if they didn't see inside out they couldn't say me!

of these programs.

In our utilization of the programs, many of the children's problems were exposed, but we treated all of these problems as universal problems, which indeed they are. No children were singled out and specifically addressed, ever.

Let's review some of the programs, and let me tell you what I observed as a result of individual problems.

Several of my little girls had a "Divorce Club," they were all in families that were separating, or in the process of divorcing, and the girls were at first very secretive about what they were talking about. They did not talk to other children who were not knowledgeable about what was going on and they were so involved in not facing reality that one girl stopped almost all of her work, was apprehensive all of the time in school, would not eat very much, and took to sulking. The club was going to help her get her father back. They pooled all their collective experiences and ideas and set out to help each other. They liked me as a teacher and a single person, and clung to me for affection and attention, but they would not share their discussions, decisions, with me or any other adult. I was told about the club only if I promised not to break it up. What could I do? The children did not want the school personnel to help, they rejected any advances made by the child development consultant. Thankfully, the "Inside-Out" series began, and the format of the programs, nonjudgmental, open-ended, allowed the children to form their own opinions. When the program "Breakup" was viewed, these girls for the most part sat silently and entered into the discussion only a little. The mother and father in the film defined divorce, and the children had many of their questions answered. The discussion identified children who had gone through this problem and who described things that had happened following the divorce or separation and talked about their feelings. Several weeks after the program, the girls disbanded their club. Some of them talked to their mothers for the first time without

accusation. Some went to the school's child development counselor and talked rather openly about their fears. The important thing was that Katie's smile returned and she started to do her work with the same zest. They all began to play during recess instead of huddling together and planning to run away.

In one drama, "I Dare You," a new girl in the neighborhood is asked to take an unsafe dare to be accepted if she wishes to keep her friends (who, incidentally, also performed dares before being accepted but of different danger levels). The purpose of the program is to help children to decide questions involving a choice between risk and personal safety with group pressure, and to help them feel comfortable with the feelings that accompany such a crisis.

We viewed the program and during the follow-up activity discussed ways to solve Clarissa's dilemma. The children shared openly and rather excitedly their opinions, and gave examples of their participation in daring activities or lack of such. (The people who say that children should not be exposed to programs that give them ideas, such as daring, should have heard the actual things children shared that were *performed* dares!) The children focused on why you take a dare, when you should take a dare, and if you should ever even discuss such a thing. We went on rather spiritedly for some time and a small voice piped up in the back. "That's why I don't have any friends, because I don't like to be bullied and I don't think taking a dare means anything. I would just as soon not have any friends. I don't see what those children were trying to prove anyway, just like the children in my block. Don't they play any real games, or read, or have plays?"

A little boy who liked this child very much, who happened to be a daring child, said, "Well, sometimes I think the children can't really mean to go that far, and you can be friends with them anyway. Probably tomorrow, they will forget about it or maybe they will remember, when they get

Inside-Out is a program on television about peoples feelings and insidents in childrens lives what kids do when they are in a rut. Inside-Out probaly teaches teaches about kids feelings.
Inside-Out is funny plus it teaches you something

Insideout

I. I like your shows
N. Nothing like them
S. Serious people
I. Interesting
D. Dare program
E. Even better then tv.

O. Original
U. Under over

= insideout

T. Tempting !!

hurt, that you were wise enough not to take the dare." The discussion was a long one, and we did not even have time for the suggested follow-up activity. But, I can report that the children started volunteering reasons for not doing things other children wanted them to do and began to freely discuss minor problems.

This year (at a new school, with a new group of children), my class repeated much of the same discussion. Several weeks after the program, a child brought in an article about three boys who were playing, taking dares on a railroad track, and one of them was killed. She deplored the fact that, since they were older and could not talk things out, or had not seen "the program" the boy had died. "His teacher could have saved a life you know," she ended.

Last year a gerbil died in my room, in its owner's hand. Surely, this is not the only time this has happened, and surely it can be assumed that children who have animals become acquainted with death. As I was on my way to the child wondering what to say, a bevy of children surrounded him and gently began to ask what had happened. Here was the class whirlwind, the know-it-all, reduced to real tears. Here was the little guy who had answers for everything. "I had him for 3 years and he is my only true friend that knows me. Poor Herman," he cried. His heart-rending sobs stopped all activity in the class room. I thought he might be ridiculed by the other boys. But what happened? One of the little girls, who had a parent recently die, put her arm around him and said "You should not feel so bad, I felt worse, it was my mother, but I do know how you feel." One boy began to question him about the animal. "You could write a story about him to preserve his memory, and we will help you to bury it in a safe place." "No!" said another boy, "If you really love him, bury it when you get home, and you can go and think quiet thoughts about it, when you miss him." "I had a dog once that was killed. I tried to be a big shot. I said that I didn't care about it at all, but I cried

lots of times when I thought no one would know it," said another. Thus comforted, the children resumed their work.

We saw the program "In My Memory," and later when a child lost his father, it was handled even better. The programs seem to teach children to care, and to be tolerant of others also.

I have never attended the utilization workshops, or viewed the teacher workshop kits, but they are available through NIT, with games, photographs, films, slides and transparencies. I gained my experience with the series by use of the teacher's guide and the format in which they are presented by our local channel. I view the program on any day during the week, in the half-hour immediately after school. I think about the program, about my feelings, then I sort out children, who might react unfavorably in some way. If necessary, I consult with some supportive health personnel regarding the subject. If I really feel unprepared or sensitive, I ask for help in planning follow-up activities. I was particularly sensitive about the program "But Names Will Never Hurt." Being black, I assumed that the race problem might come up, so I viewed the program with some apprehension. The setting was far removed, and though there were strong parallels, we were discussing a universal problem. I did not have to put on my protective armor. What a wonderful way to present the problem. You must see this program, to really appreciate it.

One great thing about the series—the children are not picked, one black, one white, one the minority, in the phony way that children deride. Some of the programs show all black children, some all white, some are mixed. There are various real settings and situations, and the actors are believable. My children say they do the same; that is their life, those are their problems.

If you see several of these programs and study a teacher's guide, you will understand my enthusiasm and the enthusiasm of the supportive personnel who have to help solve the problems that are a little deeper.

Natural Food

"Naturally grown prunes" read the homespun looking tag attached to the plain plastic bag of dried fruit and, in smaller print, "potassium sorbate added as conservative." This was in the regular produce section of a supermarket, not in a health food store, and the brand was a large "establishment" one.

Natural is "in," and preservatives are "out"—even if it means skirting honesty with a synonym.

Are "natural" and "organic" foods better? Are our foods poisoned with synthetic chemical additives? Are they processed so that they are no longer nutritious? Frequently, the answers given are, on the one hand, an unremitting series of horror stories, or on the other, the assurance that everything is virtually perfect.

Let's have a closer look at these questions. "Natural" is used to connote the opposite of processed, synthetic, chemical. It implies the "real thing," wholesomeness, and the way things are *supposed* to be. However, what is natural is not always good; there are natural poisons in mushrooms and shellfish, natural toxic factors in legumes, tubers, and other foods.

It is true that processing frequently reduces nutritive value. Milling of wheat and rice does remove much of the vitamin, mineral, and protein content. Heat processing (cooking, canning, etc.) does destroy a certain amount of vitamins. On the plus side, however, heat processing increases storability, palatability, digestibility, and sometimes even nutritive value; e.g., the cooking of soybeans destroys several toxic factors and increases the nutritive value of the protein. In the canning of orange and grapefruit juice there is some loss of vitamin C, but this is minimized by the processing time and temperature employed. This vitamin is also lost from the oranges and grapefruit stored in your refrigerator. The important consideration is whether sufficient nutrients to nourish us well remain in the food we consume.

SIGMUND GELLER is a lipid chemist in the Department of Clinical Sciences at Colorado State University, Fort Collins, Colorado.

How about natural versus synthetic or chemical? Synthetic has connotations of being fake or inferior and chemical, of being harmful, if not poisonous. A fundamental fact of chemistry is that a compound has a definite composition no matter what its source. Water distilled from sweat-soaked gym socks is identical to that obtained from fresh mountain dew. Likewise, synthetic vitamin C is identical to the vitamin C isolated from foods.

"Organic" is a curious word. It is currently used to mean "organically grown," i.e., grown without synthetic fertilizers or pesticides and in soil fertilized with humus and manure (organic matter, i.e., derived from living things). However, organic has a more established and precise meaning: an organic compound is a compound containing the element carbon. It is this meaning that the hucksters of shampoos and soaps trade on in their advertising.

The "organic" advocates claim that their food is more nutritious than that grown with synthetic fertilizers. There is no evidence for this claim. The plant utilizes synthetic, inorganic nitrate and ammonia, for example, just as well as nitrate and ammonia derived from animal waste. And, in general, the composition of the soil has a relatively small effect on the nutrients in the plants; the effect is mainly on the yield of the crop. "Organic" food has no legal definition. It may or may not have been grown as advertised. Although organic foods are generally more expensive, there is no evidence for their claimed superiority in safety, taste, or nutritive value.

Are chemical additives in food toxic? This may appear to be a simple question, but isn't—for two reasons. First, there are many different kinds of additives; for example, salt, vitamins, anti-oxidants, emulsifiers, flavors, colors, etc.—thousands of them. (Some, but not all of these, e.g., propionate and citric acid, occur naturally in foods and in the metabolism of the body.) Second, whether something is toxic or not is, unfortunately, not a yes or no matter. *Amount* is of crucial importance. A little salt or a little vitamin D is not harmful. In fact, they are essential for life. But a lot can be harmful, even fatal.

When additives are tested for safety, huge doses are given to experimental animals. Often the results are not clear cut. A button does not light up indicating "safe" or "toxic." A judgment must be made. Additives cannot really be *proven* to be absolutely safe. Subsequent investigations may demonstrate harmful effects not previously found. Therefore, a conservative approach in allowing additives is desirable.

Why then are additives used? For flavoring, preservation, nutrition, or eye appeal (can be read as "deception" if one is so inclined). Also, to make possible the production of the simple-to-prepare convenience foods that are so popular.

How safe and wholesome is our food supply? Answer: Pretty safe and pretty wholesome. Sure, there is room for improvement, but a nutritious diet is available from any number of combinations of choices from the supermarket—and none needs to be chosen from the "health food" section.

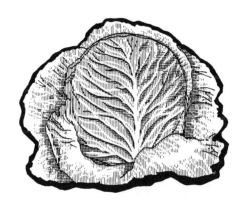

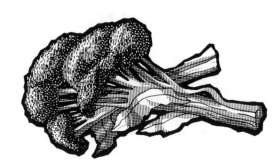

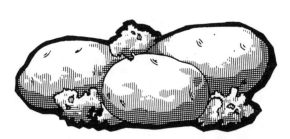

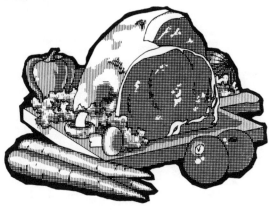

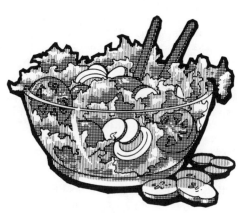

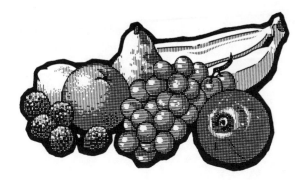

Decision Making and Fad Diets

RICHARD ST. PIERRE and KENNETH S. CLARKE are at Pennsylvania State University, University Park, Pennsylvania 16802.

The American public spends an estimated $10 billion a year on a variety of foods, devices, pills, and services designed to shed excess pounds.[1] The Hollywood image of a slender, alluring, or virile figure as a prerequisite for success and popularity has caused millions of Americans to seek easy, rapid methods to lose weight. Health problems related to being overweight compound the cosmetic concern. The problem, from a consumer standpoint, is that the realm of weight reduction is beset with influences that cloud the decision-making process. Not all fad diets are bad. If an individual uses a fad diet knowingly for a short period of time just to get off to a good start on a weight reduction program, this could provide the necessary motivation for more permanent long term weight control regimen.

Weight Reduction in Perspective

Wise consumerism evolves through a sequential decision-making process.[2] First, is weight reduction justified? The high school wrestler who must lose ten pounds to reach a specified weight level or the teenager who desires to lose ten pounds so that spring clothes fit better must make this decision. In many cases this basic issue is clouded by particular factors which will be identified later in this paper. The consumer who rationally considers his present condition, however, often will not find that his weight represents a physical or an emotional concern, rather his desire to lose weight is a result of a goal based on outside influences. The first step is to identify the goal and the values associated with it.

In the next step the wise consumer should seek a nutritionist's or physician's advice and learn about the dynamics and implications of weight control. As a secondary source, reliable books on dieting are available.[3]

The third step is to explore the available alternatives. Certain foods are more accessible or desirable to an individual. That, coupled with the convenience of physical outlets may mean the difference of faithful compliance with a planned program or not. Armed with facts about weight control the consumer can better evaluate the efficacy of various approaches to both dieting and physical activity. After the alternatives have been considered, the consumer evaluates the potential benefits and hazards associated with each, including likelihood of noncompliance as well as false promise. In other words, the risks involved in various approaches are considered in light of the known facts and the individual's own personal value system.

The fifth step is to decide on the alternative with the greatest potential benefit and the most desirable consequence. A decision constitutes an action, a demonstrated selection of a course of action. The final aspect of the decision-making process involves the consumer's rational evaluation of the actual consequences and the related costs (in all respects) of the action taken.

The alert reader should be able to see where the following five factors enter into the rational approach to weight control and often lead to irrational decisions. Hopefully, the health educated consumer will be capable of selecting actions having more health producing than health limiting potential by developing skill in the pursuit, analysis, and application of meaningful information.

The Nature of Obesity

Most individuals faced with a weight problem have difficulty accepting a basic tenet of obesity: most excess weight is due to too much eating and too little exercise. The rationalization that a given weight problem is due to heredity, faulty metabolic condition, hypothyroidism, or physiologic dysfunction is much easier to accept. By calling it overweight instead of obesity, the sting (and the commitment) is reduced.

Failure to understand or accept the basic cause of their weight problem places most consumers at a serious disadvantage when attempting a weight reduction program. To put this dilemma in perspective, for every 3,500 excess calories ingested, one pound of body fat is gained. If an individual's activity level remained constant and the only change in his food intake was an extra piece of candy (50 calories) each day for one year he would gain five pounds during that year or 50 pounds over a ten year span. Impatience interferes with reversing this process. An equivalent negative caloric balance takes an equivalent amount of time to take off pounds. Thus the idea of creeping obesity, gradual weight gain over a period of years, must be applied oppositely, creeping weight loss over a period of years.

Overeating is a learned behavior maintained by a variety of reinforcements. A person does not become obese overnight or without a reason. The factors that encourage overeating are developed over time leading to deeply ingrained behavior patterns that are not responsive to short term dietary alterations. In many cases these behavior patterns require a change in total lifestyle, a commitment far greater than called for in most fad diets.

Hunger indicates a physiological reaction to food needs. Most overweight individuals never experience true hunger, instead, their eating is controlled by their appetite. Unlike hunger, appetite is responsive to environmental conditions, the sight and smell of food, advertisements, and social situations conducive to eating all influence appetite. Unfortunately, most self-prescribed diets are designed to reduce hunger and have little influence on the true cause of obesity, appetite.

The ratio of muscle mass to fat tissue also plays an important role in obesity.[4] As muscle mass decreases, less energy is required by the body because fat tissue does not use nearly as many calories as muscle tissue at rest. Many people become overweight because they use less calories while doing nothing than they used when they had more muscle tissue.

Societal Conditions

We live in a society that both glamorizes and chastises excessive weight. Many people believe that being overweight is a simple character weakness and anyone who does not desire to be obese could easily do something about it. As a result, many people are forced to seek quick solutions to their weight problem. The same society that equates plumpness in infants as a sign of good health, talks about the jolly fat man, and idolizes Santa Claus, is quick to ridicule the obese adolescent or adult.

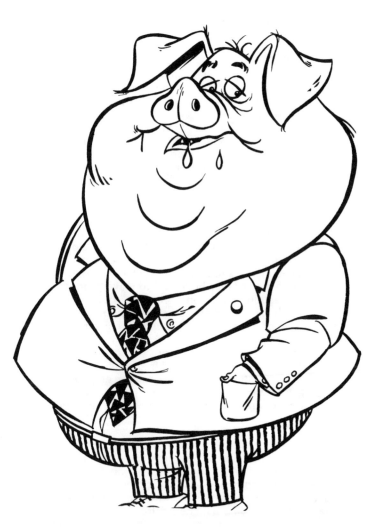

In a health conscious country such as ours the harmful effects of excess weight are well publicized. Most overweight individuals are aware of the relationship between obesity and heart disease, diabetes, kidney disorders, and other maladies. This emphasis on the physical effects of obesity can interfere with rational decision-making. Edward Hart[5] has demonstrated the role of anxiety or fear arousal in accepting or rejecting health information and concludes that the greater the anxiety level the less effective will be approaches to change behavior positively. The implications for health education are that too much anxiety could lead to impulsive behavior (i.e. selecting the first diet product available) or that not enough anxiety could lead to apathy. Health educators must deal with the delicate balance needed.

Peer Pressure

The importance placed on attractiveness compounds society's influence on the obese person. The overweight individual is almost forced to believe that success, popularity, and happiness can result only at a desired weight level. Adolescent girls in particular are faced with peer pressures demanding adherence to codes of dress, style, etc. Since this is a period when peer acceptance reaches its utmost importance, fad diets flourish. The motivations to diet can be group initiated. For example, three girls might go on a diet in mid-November to lose weight by Christmas, thus allowing them to overeat at the holiday.

Adolescents in particular feel the severe pressure of peer conformity. Group norms on body size, clothing styles, and food fads often force the obese teenager to seek questionable alternatives to dietary change. The youthful consumer may be forced to make product or service selections based on secondary sources. Continually relying on others for decisions or rebelling against others' decisions is not intelligent consumerism. Unfortunately, peer pressure often results in such a situation. The adolescent who skips the school lunch in favor of a bag of potato chips and friends illustrates this point. Society's stress on slimness and the emphasis on the negative effects of excess pounds is a strong barrier to a rational, long-term approach to weight reduction.

Advertising

One of the greatest barriers to a rational decision by the prospective dieter is consumer products and services advertising which is usually accompanied by an incessant and impressive advertising campaign. The typical advertisement involves an attractive model, an emphasis on fast results, statements stressing that you can eat all you want, and testimonials from people who experienced tremendous success with the diet. This barrage of information simply confounds an already complex situation. When one considers the difficulty inherent in long-term dietary rearrangement which leads to successful weight loss, the appeal of fad diets becomes even more apparent.

The diets that supplement their advertisements with testimonials from consumers and "authorities" avowing to the effectiveness of the product further complicate the consumer's rational decision-making process.

The wise consumer should consider the following points when contemplating the selection of a diet based on the appeal of the advertisement:

1. Fast weight loss is only possible under two conditions: dehydration or amputation.
2. Effective weight loss is accomplished only from long term dietary changes.
3. A diet that stresses rapid weight loss affects water balance and should be avoided.
4. You cannot increase caloric expenditure passively.
5. Avoid emphasis on carbohydrate foods; they do not satisfy hunger and thus encourage snacking.
6. Weight loss is due to the ingestion of fewer calories than your body expends.
7. The body can take an unbalanced diet for a short time, but then must have its needs met even if at a low calorie level.

Magnitude of Products and Services

The complexity of decision-making is compounded when the alternatives are increased. Adequate comprehension of all the products and services is impossible. They range from diet books that rank among the nations' leading sellers and machines designed to roll away fat to macrobiotic diets and candies to diminish hunger. The consumer is faced with a bombardment of products in the dietary field that, in itself, prevents rational decision-making.

Summary

Fad diets represent a major investment of time and money by today's consumers. By being informed about the various factors which influence the decision-making process in this area, educators can structure learning activities designed to reflect this sensitivity. All health behavior requires some level of decision-making and students should be encouraged to examine the motivational factors involved. The brevity of a satisfaction one finds when evaluating the consequence of a decision process works well in tandem with the task clarification that begins the decision process.

[1]D. A. Schanche, "Diet Books That Poison Your Mind . . . And Harm Your Body," *Today's Health,* April 1974, pp. 56-61.
[2]Kenneth S. Clarke, "Accident Prevention Research in Sports: An Exploration of Reform," *Journal of Health, Physical Education, and Recreation,* Vol. 40, p. 45, February 1969.
[3]J. Mayer, *Overweight, Causes, Cost, and Control,* (Englewood Cliffs, N. J.: Prentice-Hall, Inc., 1968), and N. Solomon, *The Truth About Weight Control,* (New York: Dell Publishing Co., 1971).
[4]"Weight Training for Energy and Weight Control," *The Health Letter,* Vol. 5:4, February 28, 1975.

Sensible Dieting

MARILYN MUDGETT is associated with the Health Education Department, Group Health Cooperative. DOROTHY CULJAT is presently evaluating the weight control program of Group Health Cooperative, 200 15th Avenue East, Seattle, Washington 98112.

Dieting is an obsession for many Americans. Money readily spent on fad diets, exercise devices, over-the-counter weight loss aids, miracle foods, and national self-help organizations all add up to a billion dollar weight reduction industry. Physical activity has been taken out of the realm of the natural and is under the domain of big business—health spas, athletic clubs.

The search to be thin can be confusing and costly to the consumer. Students need accurate, unbiased information to make decisions about weight control and learn how to protect their pocketbooks at the same time. The following assignments are methods of educating the potential consumer.

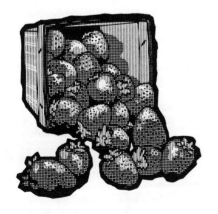

1. Investigate commercial health spas and community recreational facilities. Compare cost, services offered, equipment available, and reputation. Investigate commercial diet clinics comparing type and length of "treatment," promises made, food plan, consideration for changing food habits, and success rate.

2. Make a study of doctors who specialize in weight control. Examine professional qualifications, length of treatment, types of treatment (pre-packaged foods, pills, shots, hypnosis, etc.), success rate, and possible health dangers.

3. Visit the local drugstore and make a list of the over-the-counter reducing aids available or visit a library or bookstore and note the number and titles of books on dieting.

4. Compile magazine and newspaper advertisements on diets, diet aids, and slimming devices. Evaluate the reliability of these advertisements analyzing the use of objective facts, pseudo-scientific words such as "cellulite" and "diuretic," or claims to do something for nothing such as, "lose ugly fat while you eat the foods you love."

5. Write to adolescent summer weight camps and adult "fat farms" for brochures. Figuring length of stay and desired weight to be lost, determine how much each pound of weight loss would cost.

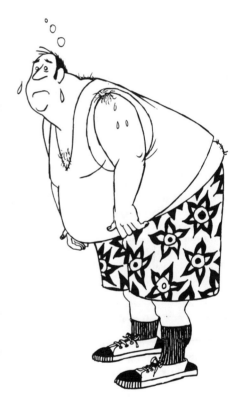

6. Make a survey of family and friends to determine if they ever dieted; types of diets; aids, products and/or facilities used; success rate, and cost.

Two excellent resources for consumer education and weight control are *Thin From Within* by Jack Osman and *A Diet for Living* by Jean Mayer.

EGG BABIES: A SIMULATION ON PARENTING

Linda Burhans Stipanov is an associate professor and Kathy Koser is an assistant professor in the Health Science Department at California State University, Long Beach, 1250 Bellflower Blvd., Long Beach, CA 90804.

The current teenage pregnancy rate is epidemic. Births among unwed teenage mothers have more than doubled since 1960, and the rate of births to girls under 15 years of age has increased 33% in 10 years.[1] Over 50% of the unwed mothers in the nation today are teenagers.[2] According to the Department of Health and Human Services, one-fourth of the teen-age girls in the United States have had at least one pregnancy by the time they are 19 years of age.[3] Approximately one million girls under 19 become pregnant each year; and of the total, about 300,000 are under 15 years old.[4] One in five U.S. births today is to a teenager.[5]

Teenage pregnancy causes serious economic, social and physiological problems for both the teenager and her child. Pregnancy is the major cause of school dropouts among teenaged girls in the U.S.[6] Approximately 70% of the pregnant teenagers do not finish high school.[7] For those pregnant teenagers under 15 years of age, approximately 90% drop out of school.[8] The divorce rate is three to four times higher for those married in their teens than for other age groups.[9] Another social consequence of teenager pregnancies is the need of the girl to depend upon public welfare. The cumulative social welfare cost for one illegitimate child is about $100,000 over a lifetime.[10] Teenage mothers are at a disadvantage in competing for jobs in that they usually have no work experience and are restricted by child care responsibilities.

Emotionally, the pregnant teenage mother experiences many problems. She has not established herself as an adult and is only just beginning to establish her own identity. Many times she is experiencing a sense of personal failure partly due to the reactions from her own parents, the boy involved, and her friends. In addition, she may lack the support from important people around

her. She may be the victim of manipulations by others and be criticized no matter what option she chooses.

Physiologically, teenage mothers are more likely to have infants with low birth weights, a factor which is related to many of the developmental problems of children (i.e., epilepsy, cerebral palsy, mental retardation). Statistics show that babies born to teenage girls are two to three times more likely to die in their first year than those born to mature mothers.[11] The maternal death risk is 60% higher for teenagers aged 14 or younger and 13% greater for 15–19 year olds than for women in their early 20's.[12] The most common problems of teenage pregnancy are toxemia (blood poisoning), prolonged labor, and iron-deficiency anemia.

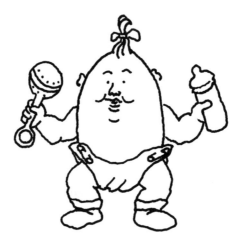

In 1973, Pat Shackleford, a teacher from Huntington Beach (California) High School, was extremely frustrated with the effectiveness of a human development course as a deterent to teenage pregnancy. It seemed that regardless of the teaching strategies used, the students still did not understand the depth of responsibility involving parenting. After much thought, she decided to create an experience that would allow students to simulate parenting. The question was, what could they parent? She decided to use an egg. An egg is helpless, fragile, inexpensive and easy to carry. The egg baby exercise was born.

The first step of the exercise was to inform the students' parents of the upcoming class assignment. A letter to them explained that the seven day assignment was a simulation on parenting at no cost to the family. The parents' cooperation was requested, and written parental approval was obtained.

The exercise actually begins at the start of the school semester when students are told they will become parents during the latter part of the semester. A woman has nine months to prepare for parenting, but in this simulation, the students have three months. Most semesters are three months long and each month is to simulate a trimester of pregnancy. At the conclusion of each simulated trimester, the students describe the changes that have occurred.

To make the exercise more effective, the egg baby pregnancy is interrelated with other units of instruction. For example, during the nutrition unit, the students identify and analyze the changing dietary needs that result from pregnancy. The consumer unit includes the process of selecting and obtaining a qualified obstetrician and/or pediatrician. The effects on pregnancy of cigarette smoking, alcohol and other drugs (over-the-counter, prescriptive, and illicit) are examined in the drug unit. Pregnancy's effect upon a woman's emotions, moods, attitudes and interactions with other people are described in the mental health unit.

The "Birth" Day

Students are informed several days in advance that the baby is due. On a specific date the students must bring to class clothing and bedding for their new arrival. The instructor brings a large container filled with raw brown eggs to class on the "birth" day. The egg's sex is indicated by a pink (girl) or blue (boy) ribbon glued to the top of each egg. Each student reaches into the box without seeing the color of the egg's ribbon and selects his or her child. Students are *not* allowed to select the sex of the child that they desire. The sex of the child is left up to chance or "mother nature." If students wish to have twins, they may select two eggs.

Students must accept all the responsibilities of being a parent. This includes always providing adequate supervision for their egg baby. Whenever the students are unable to care for their baby personally, they must use responsible babysitters. Occasionally students select babysitters who are somewhat inappropriate. For example, one girl had her four-year old baby brother babysit while she went on a date. A four-year old babysitter obviously is not responsible enough to care for an infant. The girl's mother, "grandma," thought this was irresponsible. The "grandmother" kidnapped the egg and left the following ransom note: "if you ever wish to see your egg-headed kid again, pay me $1.65 each week or I'll scramble his brains."

Some of the students decided to form babysitting pools. For example, a group of cheerleaders and football players decided to share the babysitting responsibilities. Each day during the students' after-school practices, the egg babies were placed in an egg carton on the bleachers so that the parents could watch their babies.

Some teachers have established a nursery (i.e., egg carton) and charged students one cent per hour during school time for this service, using the money to purchase new parenting materials for the course.

Students are required to bring their egg baby with them to class each day and to keep a daily journal. A small part of each day's lesson is devoted to discussing any events, problems, or concerns that students have. These comments are included in the required journal. The journal may also include the following information: child's name (e.g., Eggbert, Humpty, Benedict, Omeletta, Henriegga, Eggness), birthdate, length, weight, hair color, eye color, sex, pediatrician's name, health insurance coverage, immunizations, medical problems, supervision (i.e., babysitting) problems, housing, caring for the baby during family activities, doing things with the baby, or choosing clothes appropriate for the weather. The babies are put to bed (i.e., the refrigerator) every night at 8:00 p.m. Students cannot allow their babies to remain in "bed" all day.

Mishaps

Several events occur during the seven days. For example, some babies are victims of child abuse. Child abuse includes any act of ommission or commission that endangers or impairs a child's mental, physical, or social well-being. This may include physical assault (cracked egg shell), verbal assault ("Your mother was a rooster"), physical neglect (leaving the egg naked), emotional deprivation (not cuddling your egg), and sexual exploitation (passionately feeling your egg). The class determines whether or not the parent is guilty of child abuse. In one case the class decided the parent was guilty of physical neglect. The parent left his baby in a closed student locker for four class periods. A locker is not an acceptable environment for a growing infant.

Another case involved a parent who left her egg unattended on the kitchen counter the first day of the assignment (i.e., the baby was still faceless and naked). The parent returned to find her egg baby scrambled and about to be consumed by the "grandfather" (pure cannibalism).

A third child abuse case involved a basketball player who carried his little girl in an egg-size sleeping bag connected to a neck strap. One day he laid the sleeping bag and daughter on his desk. A friend rushed over to the basketball player to inquire about the previous night's ball game, tripped and fell. During the fall, the friend inadvertently caught the sleeping bag neck strap with his finger and flung baby "Eleanor" to her death. After much deliberation, the class determined that the father was not responsible for the death of his daughter. Therefore he was not guilty of child abuse or murder/manslaughter. The basketball player was allowed to adopt another child. (The friend was found guilty of involuntary manslaughter and placed on probation.)

When students wish to adopt, they must meet several necessary requirements, including a class interview in which the student is questioned about his/her ability to be a responsible parent.

The seventh day of the exercise is devoted to discussion of the egg baby experience. Students are asked questions similar to the following:

1. Did you want a boy or a girl? Which did you get?
2. If something happened to your baby, how serious was it and how did it happen?
3. Who supervised your baby when you weren't there?
4. Did you ever leave your baby unattended?
5. Did you go anywhere during the weekend? What did you do with your baby?
6. How did your family feel about this experience?
7. Did your feelings toward your baby change in any way during the week's assignment? Why?
8. During this experience, you did not have to purchase any additional materials for your baby. In reality, what types of materials or services would be necessary?
9. How could you support a baby at the present time?
10. What type of health insurance can you qualify for?
11. What types of solid foods are necessary for an infant?
12. Where would you live? How would you pay for your boarding?

13. How much do baby's clothes cost? How much are cloth diapers? How much are disposable diapers?
14. How would having a baby at the present time affect your ability to:
a. go to school
b. find and maintain a job
c. date and socialize
d. obtain appropriate medical care
15. What aspect(s) of the full-time responsibility did you enjoy the most? Dislike the most?
16. If you were in charge of this "parenting experience" what would you change about it?
17. Is there anything else about this experience upon which you would like to comment?

The egg baby experience is being used throughout California and has begun to be used in other states. Although it was originally designed for high school, it has been used in sixth grade, junior high and with mentally retarded teenage students.

Reactions

The students' reaction to the egg baby experience is primarily that parenting is not what it is cracked up to be. Most find the full-time responsibility to be overwhelming, too restrictive, limiting, and burdensome. Others feel that they would like to have children after they have completed their education and can afford children. Comments from students include the following:
It wasn't fun. It got to be a drag.
I don't want responsibilities like this yet.
 I still have to worry about myself.
My mom called me an "unfit mother."
The whole thing was fun at first but you got pretty tired of carrying them around after a while.
I realize how easy it is to get attached to something you've had with you for a while, even if it does become a pain in the neck.

The parents' response has been outstandingly favorable. A few parents did not like the idea of their teen being a single parent, although they realized the importance of a simulation such as this. To avoid this complication, some students have been paired up and married.

Sometimes the students' parents become involved. The teens frequently ask the "grandparents" (i.e., their parents) to babysit. Many "grandparents" respond with comments such as, "I've already raised my family. I'm not about to raise yours too." Some of the "grandparents" insist upon being paid for babysitting services. Others assist the teens with the obligations of parenthood such as pricing diapers, clothing, toys, furniture, medical care, and other necessities.

Other grandparents become aggravated with their children's irresponsibility. One "grandmother" noticed the teenage mother repeatedly left the baby unattended on the coffee table. After the fourth reminder that a baby would not just lie still and was likely to fall off the table, the "grandmother" decided to do something about it. While the mother was out of the room, the "grandmother" rushed into the kitchen, grabbed a newspaper and ketchup, placed the newspaper upon the carpet, the egg upon the newspaper, and covered the baby with ketchup. When the daughter returned, she was shocked to find her baby had fallen from the table to the floor and was in a pool of blood.

Some teachers have encountered difficulties or problems with this assignment. The number one problem is students' failure to take the activity seriously. In the authors' opinion, this is ALMOST ALWAYS due to the students' inadequate preparation for the exercise. Many teachers have read brief summaries of the egg baby exercise in newspapers or journals and decide to try it. The teachers literally surprise the students with the "pregnancy" and hand out raw eggs. The students are stunned emotionally. In reality, a parent has approximately nine months to prepare for a child. The students need some preparation also.

Another reason for the students' failure to take the activity seriously is the teacher's failure to interrelate the experience with other units of instruction within the course. The authors cannot over-emphasize the importance of reminding the students that they will soon become parents, that appropriate prenatal care is essential. Without the experience of preparation, students are unable to answer the questions in the journal and the full impact of the experience is significantly impaired.

A second problem teachers encounter is the fraility of the eggs. Some teachers believe that even conscientious parents could harm or lose their egg child. There are several solutions to this problem. One alternative is to hard-boil the eggs. The authors do NOT agree with this practice. Students tend to become more careless with hard boiled eggs. A teacher who elected to hard-boil the eggs because the students were mentally-retarded teens commented that the students were quite careless with the egg babies. The next semester as a comparison, she had a similar group of

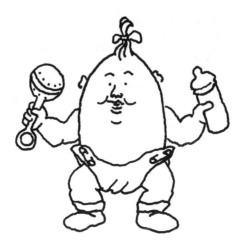

Illustration: Becca Baker

mentally-retarded teens use raw eggs and she commented that the teens behaved in a more responsible manner when the eggs were raw.

Another solution to the problem is to drain the contents of the egg. Again the authors do not agree with this approach. Not only does this constitute child abuse, but it causes the outer egg shell to become more brittle and fragile.

A third problem with the egg baby experience is that some students conclude that they are ready for parenthood. They state that they enjoy both the responsibility and the sense of being needed. However, the majority of these students do acknowledge that they were not yet prepared economically to care for a child adequately. Others state that this was of no concern because a parent could always qualify for welfare.

Another potential problem with the assignment involves the teacher's expense. Most teachers do not object to purchasing eggs for thirty-five students. However, for teachers who have many more students the project may become a financial burden. A feasible solution is to require that students bring a raw egg from home. If this approach is used, the teacher can gently stamp or label the egg in some other manner to ascertain that the original egg survives the experience.

A concern of many teachers is the likelihood of egg fights and other forms of mass murder. This can be alleviated by interrelating the egg baby assignment

with other areas, and allowing constructive peer pressure to develop. One of the advantages of peer pressure is that students tend to "police" one another. That is, the students will usually reinforce the "good parents" and chastise the neglectful ones. This chastisement can have both positive and negative consequences. Many times the neglectful parent will adapt his or her behavior and become more caring and concerned. Other times a neglectful student may withdraw from the experience. This can be remedied by the teacher informing the students of the impact of peer pressure prior to the assignment.

Another issue is what to do with the eggs at the end of the assignment. They can be collected and discarded but many students find this upsetting. They realize that it is only an egg and that the assignment is over, but they feel some emotional attachment to the egg. If students wish to keep their babies, the contents of the eggs must be drained or the odor will rapidly become eggs-asperating. Students need to know that the contents are contaminated and unsuitable for consumption. This in no yoke.

Feedback Requested

The effectiveness of this experience needs to be evaluated. The authors would like feedback from educators who are using this assignment. We are particularly interested in whether or not students who participate in this activity are less likely to become parents while in school. If you are using the egg baby exercise, please send us your name and address. A questionnnaire is currently being developed to evaluate this exercise. Your cooperation is appreciated.

[1]Alan Guttmatcher Institute. *11 million teenagers: What can be done about the epidemic of adolescent pregnancies in the United States.* Planned Parenthood Federation of America: New York, 1976.

[2]*Ibid.*

[3]Solomon, Neil. Teen Pregnancy, *Los Angeles Times,* October 23, 1980.

[4]*Ibid.*

[5]McCarthy, Colman. What pregnant teenagers need is care. *Detroit Free Press,* October 17, 1979.

[6]McDonald, Thomas F. Teenage Pregnancy. *Journal of the American Medical Association,* August 9, 1976 - Vol. 236, No. 6.

[7]Guttmatcher Institute. *op. cit.*

[8]*Ibid.*

[9]McDonald. *op.cit.*

[10]*Ibid.*

[11]Morgan, Lael. Concern growing over teen-age pregnancies. *Los Angeles Times,* February 29, 1980.

[12]*Ibid.*

Sex Roles in TV Cartoons

In today's age of increased technology man is becoming a visually oriented being. Children spend many hours per week peering at television, which has a large proportion of cartoon programs.

In addition, there exists a liberalizing trend with regard to human sexuality. The mass media have begun to help people question traditional sex roles, to familiarize the public with "alternative" sexual practices, and to reflect the growing emphasis upon openness about sexual practice, information, and opinion.

To what degree do these facts interrelate? What effect has the recent reevaluation of our long-established concept of sexuality had on today's cartoons?

With an abundance of available cartoons from which to derive information to research this question, ten hours of Saturday morning television cartoons were objectively analyzed. These observations provide the content of this article.[1] Four categories concerning male and female sex roles are identified and discussed:

—physical characteristics (dress, hair, build, etc.)

—degree and type of emotional reactions.

—acceptable "standard" behaviors both in terms of verbal responses and body positions or gestures.

—role in society (occupation, etc.)

After compiling and commenting on the information in each of these four categories, attempts will then be made to speculate about the effect of these "caricaturistic" sex roles upon today's children and the nature of future cartoons.

Let us now turn our attention to the typical male and female of the cartoon world. Picture

JUDY MILLER is a student at Towson State College, Baltimore, Maryland.

a shapely, attractive woman with perfect features and an unblemished, made-up face and you have envisioned the feminine package as portrayed on Saturday mornings. Woman appears to be equated with weakling; she is relatively petite and has the proportional amounts of fat in the appropriate places. The importance of beautiful hair for women is highly accentuated in one of two ways —either long and flowy or short and stylish—but never is a hair out of place! In essence, then, feminine characters may best be described in one, short word: sexy!

Men, on the other hand, are hefty in stature and muscular ("V"-shaped is the desirable male build), with a frequently demonstrated attribute of strength, especially for the main character. It was noted, however, that this is not as universally true for men as extreme feminine characteristics are for women. Men are occasionally portrayed as being something less than ideal, e.g., short and stocky like Barney on *The Flintstones* or thin and nonmuscular like the father on *The Jetsons.*

Variability of individual sizes and shapes appears to be more acceptable among the male cult than it is among females. *Bill Cosby Cartoons* most readily exemplify this fact. The black boys in this cartoon range from about 6'4'' and 100 lbs. to 5'8'' and 300 lbs. A great deal of difference, isn't it? The effect of such an assortment of physiques is one of increased realism—even in caricature form.

The following situation is then evident: uniformity of female and multiplicity of male stereotyping. The exact implications of this unbalanced representation remain somewhat illusive; perhaps all male producers desire the "perfect" woman in their own lives or all women producers are anti-women's libbers! No matter what the reason, the situation exists.

The second general category to be considered is the degree of emotional reaction. Traditionally speaking, we all "know" that women and emotions are synonymous. Women supposedly lack the ability to isolate emotionalism from the realm of logic and decision making and consequently appear irrational and impulsive by nature. This is the policy of cartoonland. Women in *The Flintstones* typically respond to problem situations with a "What are we going to do?" (with hand on head or over mouth). The gestures which accompany such verbalizations are highly expressive in themselves. On *The Osmonds,* Donnie and his girlfriend encountered a polar bear while hiking along mountainous Alaskan terrain, and what was the girl's reaction? She cowered behind him, fearfully clutching his coattail, saying, "Oh Donnie, I'm scared!" Of course Donnie remained cool, calm, and collected.

Women are portrayed as being strung out emotionally, but not always to the point of unresourcefulness. Some shows convey the notion that women have become highly adept at "using" an emotional front to fulfill a need of some sort. The wife on *The Jetsons,* for instance, when confronted with the harsh shouting of an irate husband rather cunningly cringed at the height of the outburst, role-playing the innocent offender. Much to the dismay of any liberated male, it worked! That masculine chassis of iron was soon converted to a pliable plastic through the utilization of an exaggerated emotional response.

The overriding theme of maleness is, generally speaking, that of being "steady as the Rock of Gibraltar" while femaleness is equated with a sense of "governing through feeling." Yet, woman has become so conscious of the potential of her own emotional stereotyping that she has learned to feign such reactions in order to attain a desirable end. (It might be interjected that, according to the writers of cartoons, she has gotten rather good at it.)

This leads us to the next category for consideration, that of "standard" behaviors for men and women both in terms of verbal and obvious physical responses. This classification overlaps several others, but it was designed mainly to include those extraneous examples which failed to apply suitably to any of the other four—and some are well worth noting. *The Flintstones* was a primary source of reference, so it is appropriate to begin with two rather interesting findings based on this cartoon show. (1) Women, in accordance with their obvious sex role, never appear "loose." Wilma or Betty, whenever in a stationary, upright position, automatically assume a pose typical of a model with a definite hip lean, tilted

head, and hand on hip. This coincides, and perhaps not coincidentally, with the comment on the uniformity of womanly portrayal. (2) Anyone who has ever viewed *The Flintstones* will recall Fred's expression for any and all situations, namely, "Yabba-dabba-doo." Recently, Pebbles uttered that expression with one minor variation: "Yabba-dabba-doosy." It could be assumed that such a move on the producer's part was intended to feminize the phrase in order for it to apply to Pebbles.

Speaking of acceptable behavior, one recent *Brady Kids* cartoon involved an interesting example of the producer's outlook on sexual identities. In this particular show, the kids were put back in time to the age of the original Greek Olympic games. The whole crew had to participate in the games, but, unfortunately, were no match for the Greek Joconas, the "prime subject" of his time. However, a female had accompanied them on their journey who sped to their rescue—it was Wonder Woman! The very name of Wonder Woman conveys the notion that woman was not created a physically competitive being, and anyone who is, shall become the "Ninth Wonder of the World" (since the Astrodome took number eight). Our feminine marvel naturally defeated her soul-shattered opponent, who then in typical chauvinistic fashion conceded defeat with: "No woman can do the things she did!"

This category also spotlights what has been referred to as the Triple-R syndrome. The adult male not only takes precedence over all, but resides on a slightly higher pedestal of rank, responsibility, and righteousness. The male in typical storybook fashion is assumed to be right, unless proven otherwise. This was evidenced in *The Jetsons* when the master of the house sat on one side of the dinner table and the wife and children on the other, illustrating positions of greater or lesser importance. The final member of the Triple-R syndrome, responsibility, was graphically presented in *Sea Lab 2020*. Here, the little boy of a brother-sister duo was granted the role of initiative and common sense. For instance, when told to comply with a particular rule which they felt to be unreasonable, the girl responded, "Do we have to?" while the boy pensively retorted with, "Let's check it out." In the process of doing so they became trapped in a cage and were drifting away; but, have no fear! The little boy took the situation in hand, admirably risked his life, and saved the poor damsel in distress.

Let us pursue the cartoon presentation of the societal roles acceptable for male and female. For the youthful clientele of cartoons, producers "cartoonize" personalities already prominent among the youth set, like the Osmonds, Tabitha and Adam from Bewitched, and the Brady Kids. What most of these cartoon shows have in common, however, is the fact that they appeal to the preteen music craze by having the characters sing and participate as members of a rock group. In these groups, the girls generally played a tambourine or the piano and the boys usually alternated among several instruments, such as the double bass, the guitar, and the drums. The lead singer in all cases was a male!

One recent Flintstone show centered around a genie who granted Bambam and Pebbles the right to make one wish apiece, whatever they desired to become in life. As might be expected, Bambam aspired to become a star football player and Pebbles, a movie star!

On The Osmonds, in an Alaskan adventure, Donnie and his girlfriend were observing an old mining town, and as she related its history to him, he responded with, "Gold mining is not for you; it's cold, messy, dirty, and hard work." Even though one might tend to agree with him, this does in a rather straightforward manner delineate the characteristics of a job acceptable for women: comfortable, clean, neat, and physically untaxing.

Following this brief review of the results of the "study," we can pose the following questions: Just what approach will cartoons of the future take toward human sexuality? Will they persist in their traditional presentations or be affected by the permeating air of liberation for both males and females?

On the basis of observations it could be projected that cartoons in the future will lean toward a more realistic approach. Males and females will both supersede the level of uniformity in stereotyping to one of multiplicity, that is, representative of the entire gamut of shapes, sizes, reactions, and occupations. Two such shows recently appeared, both deserve comment.

The first is a cartoon entitled Gidget, based on the film versions so popular several years ago. Gidget embodies a typical "women's libber." She is knowledgeable, domineering, mentally alert, and even relatively unemotional! Rink and Jud, her two male associates, have been debased from their level of prominence to the counterpart of a "dizzy blond." Gidget is the sole pos-

sessor of a seventh sense—which is a way of saying that she is always right! In this reversal, she has become the woman of decision and promotes these qualities in her not-so-fortunate friends of the opposite sex. On one occasion, Gidget, Rink, and Jud were involved with diamond embezzlers aboard a racing yacht, and throughout the course of the show she handled the helm in the midst of a tremendous storm, uncovered the smugglers, dove for the diamonds, wiggled out of the ropes binding her in time to call the police, and through the application of her master mind, saved them all!

Another example of this new trend is entitled Pussycats in Outer Space. Here is noted an even further development toward increased realism in the portrayal of human sexuality. The four main characters are: a domineering woman (similar to Gidget); a dizzy, traditional woman; a strong, steadfast male; and an unsure, indecisive male whom they call, "Chicken."

Even this brief description reveals the show's overall objective. It seems an attempt is being made to pictorialize the range of differentiation within and between the sexes and, in so doing, publicly scrutinize a weak, indecisive character and honor one that is strong and steadfast, regardless of the sex. The apparent moralizing about which of the various characteristics are right or wrong appears rather questionable, but the actual depiction of the range of differences is highly desirable.

Children appear quite capable of differentiating between "storybook" cartoons and true-to-life occurrences.[2] As long as cartoons persist in their traditional display of patternized males and females, children's reactions will undoubtedly remain the same. There exists a real possibility, however, that if and when cartoons approach the realm of reality, children will cease to be an "unaffected clientele." On the outcome of this newly founded challenge of storybook vs. reality, therefore, rests one possible basis for "sexual determinism" of the future.

---

[1] This article is based on a paper prepared for a sex education course at Towson State College, Baltimore, Maryland, in the spring of 1973.

[2] In a survey conducted on ten Baltimore children ages 7 to 12, their comments showed without a doubt that they were well aware of the cartoons' exaggerations.

FAMILY LIFE CYCLE RESOURCE CENTER IN THE ELEMENTARY SCHOOL

LUCILLE STROBLE is a school nurse-teacher/health educator at the Institute for Experimentation in Teacher Education, State University College, Cortland, New York 13045.

Funding through a New York State Mini-Project grant provided an opportunity to solve a problem faced by many school nurse-teachers and health educators. The problem was how to build up resources in sensitive content areas, such as family life and death education, and provide controlled accessibility to those who need them most—children and their parents, teachers, and college students. Our solution was to set up a Family Life Cycle Resource Center in the health suite.

Before funding was available, I had started planning the Center for a poorly used corner of the health office in our elementary school. Metal bookshelves were bolted to the walls and a metal office file was moved into the corner. A table and chairs with a study lamp were added to provide a working area for students. A couple of soft chairs and a hanging plant created an informal atmosphere. Now it was ready to receive the materials which the school and I already owned.

Some books that the librarian had been unable to keep on the open shelves were brought out of the library office. A supply of free pamphlets which had been kept in boxes were now placed in a pamphlet file. A few college texts and references which I had acquired during my professional training were placed on the high shelves for adults interested in technical information. The file was used to start a collection of readings and bibliographies which I had kept over the years. But all these materials were lost in the spacious new Center. The grant was welcomed to furnish the Center with a wide range of materials to meet the needs of many different people.

The main goal of the Center was to provide materials that could be used directly by or with young children aged three to twelve. Teachers could borrow books to use in the classroom, children could use and borrow books under supervision, parents could take books to use with children at home, and college students could study the collection to learn what materials are appropriate to use in elementary schools.

Because books can be used over and over in many different ways, it seemed justifiable to spend about a third of the grant money on children's literature with a health-related theme or written to teach a specific health concept. The books received ranged from fiction, such as *A Taste of Blackberries* by Doris Buchanan Smith, to scientific nonfiction, such as *Before You Were Born* by Paul Showers.

Because children enjoy filmstrips, we invested in a few multi-media kits that were attractive, comprehensive, and accurate. Sets such as those produced by Marshfilm—"There's A New You Coming For Boys" and a comparable kit for girls—and some silent filmstrips were also purchased.

To provide variety in the teaching aids available, some cassette tapes, overhead transparencies, posters, diagrams, demonstration kits, slides, textbooks, and picture books were purchased. A few more reference books were added as parent and teacher background materials.

To announce the opening of the Family Life Cycle Resource Center, a week-long open house was held. Parents, teachers, college students, and area school health personnel were invited. The new acquisitions were laid out for examination. One of the better family life education films was borrowed for showings throughout the week. The coffee pot was on and the Center was open!

Since its opening, the Center has proved worthwhile many times. In preparing for my health classes, I am able to easily pull out the materials I wish to use. I can assign children individually or in pairs to work on projects in the Center. When a conference is planned it is a simple matter to prepare an attractive display. Parents who come asking advice on how to explain menstruation or death or growing up, often leave with a book for themselves or to share with their child. The home economics teacher frequently uses the materials to augment the child-care class. One teacher borrowed the whole collection of children's books to give her class a reading alternative. There was overwhelming interest in the books and motivation to read, and the teacher was extremely pleased with the question-and-answer sessions that resulted. The Center reached into the community when materials were used by a minister to conduct a course in family life education for the parents in his church.

If education concerning the life cycle—birth, growth and development, aging, and death—is truly going to be a joint effort of the school, home, and community, school health personnel must start the process. We must have the courage to dust off the books that have been kept hidden away and put out materials in an area of controlled accessibility for those who need them. We must be willing to answer questions openly and frankly—the questions of children, parents, teachers, college students, and the community. I was pleased that the grant offered our school an opportunity to open the dialogue.

Advocating Elementary Sex Education

A basic need for physical and mental health is the understanding of one's own sexuality. Sexuality is the ability to feel and give warmth and love, to develop a positive self-concept, and the ability to make responsible decisions regarding the physical, mental-emotional and social aspects of one's sexual health. In accepting one's self as a sexual being, and knowing the positive aspects of sexuality, children will come to believe in themselves and attempt to deal with their own sexual growth in a positive way.

Sex is a healthy activity, and one of the most wonderful aspects of life. Sex education is a natural, ongoing process, beginning in infancy and continuing through life. In a formal school setting, human sexuality education helps young people prepare to meet the problems of life centering around the sex instinct that enter into the experience of every human being.[1]

The child at the elementary level is just attempting to understand many things, including his own sexuality.[2] Elementary sex education attempts to make sexuality more understandable to young people, and helps lay a factual groundwork to be incorporated with their parents' feelings and values. Sexual health, according to a World Health Organization 1975 technical report, "is the integration of the physical, emotional, intellectual and social aspects of sexual being in ways that are positively enriching and that enhance personality, communication and love."[3]

Sex education then is teaching and learning to recognize and accept human sexuality in ourselves and others, in hopes of using this knowledge toward the greatest creativity and fulfillment in our lives. Courses are needed to help students identify and maintain their own

Warren L. McNab is an associate professor of health education in the Department of Physical Education, University of Nevada, Las Vegas, 4505 Maryland Parkway, Las Vegas, NV 89154.

standards of behavior, based upon the progressive acceptance of responsibility for its consequences to others as well as themselves.

Understanding sexuality is not something that happens entirely naturally; it improves with formal learning. The question is not whether children will get sex education, but how and what kind they will receive.[4] It is impossible to hide children from sexual influences. Adult role models, television, advertisements and parents all bombard young children with them.

Parents are the main sex educators of their children whether they do it well or badly—silence and evasiveness are just as powerful teachers as a discussion of the facts. To young people, the enemies are ignorance and exploitation; their weapons are knowledge and self-respect.[5] The majority of people (77%) favor sex education; yet 45 states have no requirement for teaching sexuality in the schools.[6]

There seems to be a feeling among parents that elementary students are too young for sex education. To many parents sexuality is a fearful, negative term that should not be "exposed" to young people. Questions are denounced, reading materials are not provided. Children grow up believing sex is bad or mysterious, and "it" should not be discussed at all with parents. When communication lines within families are closed or blocked, and a child has questions, apprehensions and fears he must find out by himself what sexuality really means.

Knowledge, an Antidote to Fear

Many parents and teachers do not address questions regarding sexuality because of embarrassment and lack of knowledge. But knowledge is the best antidote for fear; and the key to a relaxed and effective approach to sex education by parents and teachers is confidence in this knowledge. Attitudes regarding sex are formulated early in life. If factual material is presented in a positive manner in

the elementary grades, negative attitudes, apprehensions and fears regarding sex may be reduced and superseded by a positive understanding that each person, regardless of age, lives part of his/her sexuality every day.

The school can be a partner or leader with the family, church or community in helping young people understand themselves as sexual beings. Teachers must be accountable and justify the selection of content and materials based upon their educational objectives. The materials alone, however, do not make an effective sex education program; they simply supplement the effective teacher. What is needed is a comprehensive program incorporating school and parents in a collective effort, emphasizing the positive and rewarding aspects of sexualtiy.

Gordon[7] states that sex education in the elementary schools is dead because administrators are only responsive to oversensitive extremists, and therefore attempt to avoid any controversy and difficulty regarding the topic. Parents also fear sex education because they believe that it will put "ideas" into their children's minds or that children will become promiscuous. Research indicates just the opposite is true.[8, 9] Sexual ideas are part of everyone's life. Parental upbringing, not formal sex education, is the primary influence on a child regarding sexuality. Information is the greatest defense people have against the negative aspects of sexuality such as promiscuity, illegitimacy, venereal disease and child abuse; education can provide knowledge needed to make responsible decisions regarding sexual behavior.

Currently most of the emphasis on sex education is structured in terms of the secondary student. While this instruction is very important, it may be more beneficial to begin in the formative years, thereby dispelling early inhibitions, fears and misconceptions and preparing students to enter the secondary level program with a positive foundation or framework regarding sexuality.

Only 29 states and the District of Columbia require the teaching of health education courses in grade schools, and only six of these states mandate the teaching of family life education as part of that health component.[10]

The first priority is to prepare teachers to set realistic objectives, select content material and learning activities, and prepare evaluations of their programs. We need to overcome the fact that teachers are not prepared to talk accurately and honestly about sex. Institutions preparing elementary teachers need to offer health education courses. These courses should include curricular materials and teaching methodologies in the area of sexuality. Part of the problem for beginning teachers is mastering the appropriate vocabulary to facilitate open communication with students in the area of sexuality. For example, *peter, dink, dong, tool, dick* are all slang terms meaning *penis*. Young people quickly learn that four-letter "power words" get attention. They also need to learn that there are words other than slang terms in the area of sexuality. Breaking down this communication barrier by providing a new vernacular can enhance sincere conversation among teachers, parents and children.

Often teachers and parents are afraid to deal with sex education because they have not themselves received instruction in this area. Inservice programs for parents and teachers are needed to help adults become at ease with their own sexuality and be able to develop a philosophy compatible with education. This philosophy, plus the selection of content and teaching methodologies regarding sexuality, will initiate progress toward the ultimate goal of comprehensive health and sex education in the elementary schools.

Sex in the Health Curriculum

The Association for the Advancement of Health Education, The American School Health Association, American Public Health Association and The National Education Association as well as numerous other professional associations have endorsed and encouraged health curriculums to include human sexuality as a necessary part of the teacher preparation program.[11]

An obvious requisite to initiating a program is knowing the objectives and principles of sex education. The Illinois Sex Education Act, to promote the development of comprehensive and wholesome programs of family life and sex education in Illinois elementary and

The question is not whether children will get sex education, but how and what kind they will receive. Parents are the main sex educators of their children whether they do it well or badly — silence and evasiveness are just as powerful teachers as a discussion of the facts. For young people the enemies are ignorance and exploitation; their weapons are knowledge and self-respect.

secondary schools, is an excellent example of such objectives. A state mandate, such as the one passed in Nevada endorsing comprehensive sex education in the school systems, is also a positive accomplishment.

A new educational program in sexuality should be developed with parental involvement, so that the content and process is understood and carried over to the home. In this manner, parents as well as young people are learning more about sexuality. In Nevada, the state mandate regarding the teaching of sexuality requires that sessions be provided to involve parents in the development of sexuality programs. In developing curriculums, school systems should start, not from scratch, but by examining other states' curricular materials. They can then adapt established materials to the needs in their school district. The U.S. Public Health Service has published *An Analysis of United States Sex Education Programs and Evaluation Methods* that cites exemplary school programs in sex education.[12]

Curriculum planning is a most important and time-consuming task. It should define specific objectives of the program and provide for continuity and sequence at various elementary grade levels, parental involvement in the development and understanding of the program, specific content materials and teaching activities or processes that will be included in the classroom, and a means of evaluating the objectives initially set up regarding the curriculum. This is a difficult and arduous task but is necessary if the attempt to incorporate sex education into

the elementary school curriculum is to be successful.

Burleson[13] states that sex education is not a packaged curriculum that can be purchased and plugged in like an electrical appliance. Curricular development is predicated on the nature and needs of the learner, the sequential organization of knowledge in that subject area, and the values that a specific society holds. In selecting supplementary materials teachers must critically analyze the process needed to achieve their objectives, and skillfully select and evaluate the effectiveness of these materials.

What are the interests of elementary students regarding sexuality? What questions do they have? How should one answer these questions? These are typical concerns of prospective teachers. Perhaps the following questions from a 5th grade class may suggest what these students wonder about, regarding sexuality. For example: "What do you mean by sex? Why do women have babies and not men? What are tampons for? How do people get shy? What if you are the only one in class who has a period? What is a rubber? Where does the baby come out? When do you usually start having sex? Am I okay if I'm behind other kids in (physical) development? Do you have to be married to have a baby? How can a baby breathe inside the mother while it's swimming? Why don't boys get breasts? How does sperm come out? How can you tell if you are in love or loved?"

This is but a small sample of questions young people have regarding the topic of sexuality. Unfortunately, most of the time these queries are not answered by the parent or teacher; the child is told he will receive the answers when he is "older." To ask is to learn—positive learning takes place when parents and teachers honestly answer these questions, sharing their knowledge and understanding with children. Part of this honesty is the ability to say, "I really don't know, but perhaps we can find out together."

Materials

Moglia and Wheeler[14] state that elementary materials in sex education are hard to find, but they identify several useful text books, pamphlets and film strips that can be used at the elementary level. These resources provide supplementary content for the elementary teacher, and suggest learning activities that may be included to help children understand the material. Elementary teachers have a unique opportunity to incorporate the topic of sexuality in many teaching areas. For example, spelling (vocabulary), reading (sex roles and family responsibilities), art (drawings related to the family), science (genetics and reproduction), social studies (personality development, getting along with others and family interactions), and of course, music which relates to many areas of sexuality through its lyrics. For example, "Free to Be You and Me," by Marlo Thomas, through the use of stories, poems and song, describes many aspects of individual sexuality. Emphasizing the positive aspects of sexuality through the cognitive and affective domains allows children to feel good about themselves and their sexuality.

A key purpose of health education is motivating people to do things that are conducive to their health. There is a need for some sort of commitment on the part of teachers and parents to become involved in developing elementary sex education programs. This may include:

• talk to your children, wife, husband or community group about elementary sex education.

• asking administrators about the possibility of sex instruction in your school.

• finding ways to incorporate the topic into elementary lessons you now teach.

• attending a workshop to improve your knowledge and skills regarding elementary sex education.

• organizing a group to confront school board members about the issue of sex education.

• letting administrators and legislators know of the importance of this topic.

• lending your expertise and cooperation to other teachers, nurses, and parents.

• getting involved with community groups such as Planned Parenthood, March of Dimes or other organizations emphasizing educational programs.

Do one or all of the above, but *do something!* If you believe in the need, yet do nothing, the small but vocal minority of people opposed to elementary sex education will defeat it in your community. Through concerned, conscientious efforts we can attain the support needed to implement school and community programs at the primary levels. The task will not be easy—no one expected it would be. As a health educator, what is your commitment regarding sex education in your school district? It is vital that as health educators we use our curricular expertise to develop and implement the comprehensive health and sexuality programs needed to ensure the overall health of our school children.

General Objectives of Family Life and Sex Education

Illinois Sex Education Act

Examples of general objectives are listed below, in accordance with the intent of the Illinois Sex Education Act: to promote the development of comprehensive and wholesome programs of family life and sex education in Illinois elementary and secondary schools. Later on, a curriculum guide will be prepared by an Illinois Curriculum Committee on Family Life and Sex Education, including examples of specific objectives related to the interests, needs, and problems of boys and girls at various school and maturity levels.

Examples of general objectives to help students in grades one through twelve:

1. To understand the meaning and significance of marriage, parenthood, and family life, so they can help strengthen the family as the basic social unit of democratic life in Illinois.

2. To make affection, sex, and love constructive rather than destructive forces in modern life.

3. To develop feelings of self-identity and self-worth, respect for others, and moral responsibility as an integral part of their personality and character development, so they can perceive their roles as marriage partners, as parents, and as mature adults in our society. (This is important for all students but it is especially needed by fatherless and motherless boys and girls.)

4. To understand and appreciate the sexual side of human nature, so that their own psychosexual development may occur as normally and healthfully as possible, without feelings of indecency, embarrassment or undue guilt.

5. To learn that human sexual behavior is not merely a personal and private matter but has important social, moral and religious implications.

6. To realize that the Golden Rule also applies in sexual matters, based upon the ethical principle that: no one has a right to harm another by using him or her exploitatively as a sexual object.

7. To learn about the dangers of illicit sexual behavior, and that boys and girls do not have to engage in heavy petting or premarital sexual intercourse to make friends, be popular, get dates, or to prove their love and affection to each other.

8. To emphasize the case for premarital chastity as the sexual standard approved by our society because chastity provides a positive goal for teen-agers, linking human sexual behavior with love, marriage, parenthood, and family life and because of the individual, family and community problems associated with premarital or extramarital sexual relations.

9. To open channels of communication between children and their parents, teachers and counselors, and religious leaders concerning the meaning, significance, and potential values of sex and mating in human life, so that students will find it easier to seek information from reliable sources rather than rely on "hearsay," "gutter talk" or misconceptions; and so they will be able to discuss with openness and without embarrassment the problems of growing up sexually, while realizing that this is only one aspect of becoming a mature man or woman.

10. To understand that boy-girl and man-woman relationships of the right kind can add to their enjoyment and give meaning to their lives and that those of the wrong kind can result in a distorted attitude toward sex, love, and affection that may lead to undesirable consequences for the individuals involved and for society.

11. To understand the basic anatomy and physiology of the male and female reproductive systems and human reproduction; and the relationship of human mating to mutual love and affection expressed in marriage, parenthood, and family life.

12. To develop a healthy, wholesome attitude toward sex in human beings, including respect for their own bodies as an integral part of their personality, with knowledge of and respect for all body parts and their normal functions in human mating, reproduction, and family life.

13. To appreciate the significance of the sexual differences in boys and girls and the male and female sexual roles in our society, as related to wholesome boy-girl relationships and marriage, parenthood, and family life.

14. To develop a functional graded vocabulary, acquire a knowledge of key facts and basic concepts, develop wholesome attitudes and practices, and acquire skill in the critical analysis of basic problems and issues in sex education; and for students to bring information to their parents which the adults themselves may need and want.

15. To understand how to deal with personal sexual problems such as menstruation, nocturnal emissions, masturbation, petting, and personal hygiene.

16. To learn about the legal and ethical aspects of abortion, venereal disease control, marriage, divorce, broken homes and family disintegration, illegitimate children, pornography and obscenity, and sexual behavior.

17. To understand the key facts and basic concepts of human genetics as related to parenthood and family life; and where and how to secure "genetic counseling" if and when needed.

To learn the key facts and basic concepts of human genetics as related to parenthood and family life; and where and how to secure "genetic counseling" if and when needed.

18. To learn the key facts and basic concepts about venereal disease; and the role of teen-agers and young adults in the prevention and control of these important communicable diseases.

19. To understand human pregnancy and the birth process; the need for good medical and public health care of mother and child before, during, and after birth; the care and rearing of small children; and the personal and social significance of the family in modern times.

20. To learn about the potential dangers of the world population explosion, and the need for an intelligent consideration of the basic issues of population growth as related to human health and welfare.

21. To consider critically the pros and cons of teen-agers going steady versus going "steadily" as related to sexual behavior and as a preparation for mate selection and marriage.

22. To understand more fully and deeply the significance, in our society and other societies, of boy-girl relationships, dating, courtship, and engagement as related to marriage, parenthood and family life.

23. To realize that there are important major differences, as well as some similarities, between sex and sexual behavior in animals as compared with man.

24. To understand the differences between love and infatuation and immature versus mature romantic love; to identify and appreciate the traits of a prospective husband or wife, which are most apt to make for a wholesome, healthy, and happy marriage.

25. To learn how to develop and maintain as their own positive standards of behavior based upon the progressive acceptance of moral responsibility for their own sexual behavior as it affects others as well as themselves.

26. To see clearly that progressive acceptance of responsibility for making wise decisions and moral choices in sexual matters requires an understanding of relevant facts, standards, and values, alternatives and their consequences, as related to long-range as well as to immediate desires and goals.

[1]Kilander, Fredrick H. *Sex education in the schools.* Toronto, Ontario: McMillan Co., 1970.

[2]Quinn, Jane M. Elementary school sex education. In *Education Digest,* 42: 29–32, January 1977.

[3]Golden, Doris. Children have a right to know. In *Impact—The Journal of National Family Sex Education Week,* 1:38–39, October 1978.

[4]Miller, Mary S. Who's afraid of sex education? In *Education Digest,* 41:33–35, April 1976.

[5]Nelson, Emily A. Responsible sexuality. In *Impact—The Journal of National Family Sex Education Week,* 1:8–13, October, 1978.

[6]Scales, Peter. We are the majority. In *Impact—The Journal of National Family Sex Education Week,* 1:14–17, October 1978.

[7]Gordon, Sol. Sex education is dead in the elementary schools. In *Instructor* 86:132, March 1977.

[8]Finkle, M. L., Finkle D. J. Sexual contraceptive knowledge, attitudes and behavior of male adolescents. In *Family Planning Perspectives,* 7, 6, 256–260, 1975.

[9]Cutright, P., The teenage sexual revolution and the abstinent past. In *Family Planning Perspectives,* 4, 1, 24, 1972.

[10]Thompson, Geneva, Need for health instruction in the elementary and secondary schools. In *Hextra* 5:1, September 1979.

[11]Report of the ASHA Committee on Professional Preparation and College Health Education: professional preparation of the health educator, *Journal of School Health,* 46:418–421, September 1976.

[12]Kirby, D, Alter, J., Scales, P.: "An Analysis of U.S. Sex Education Programs and Evaluation Methods" U.S. Department of Health, Education and Welfare, Public Health Service, Center for Disease Control Bureau of Health Education, Atlanta, Georgia, July, 1979.

[13]Burleson, Derik L., Guidelines for selecting instructional materials in sex education. In *Journal of Research Development in Education,* 10:79–82, Fall 1976.

[14]Moglia, Ronald and Wheeler, Inese, Primary grade sex education materials are hard to find. In *The Science Teacher,* 44:20–22, March 19-7.

TEACHING IDEAS

Human Birth Drawings

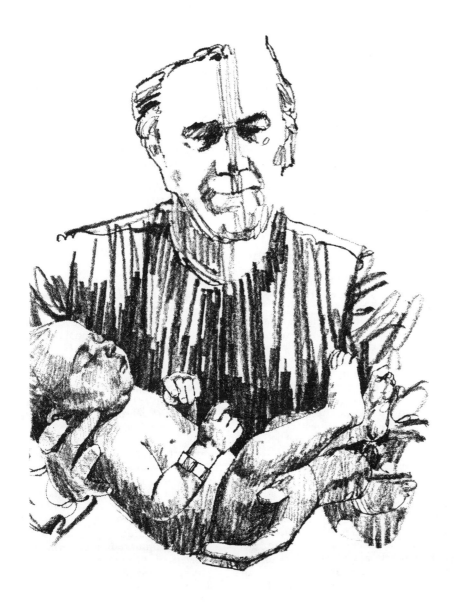

were collected.[1] To acquire such pictures, children were asked to respond via a picture to either of these questions: "Where was I before I was born?" or "What did I look like before I was born?" These pictures were collected prior to any activities in the class related to human birth but resulted in an interest on the part of the teachers and students in this area. Consequently, the monograph reports, this pictorial exercise opened the way for teachers to discuss human birth where previously they were confused as to how to begin such discussions.

Of the 1,149 pictures acquired, 80 were selected for publication in the monograph, with accompanying explanatory comments requested of the young artist who conceived and drew the picture. Though not a new publication, the rationale for this approach is as sensible today as it was in 1967 when it was published: "Assume that a teacher is faced with the prospect of introducing a unit on human reproduction. Where shall she begin? The situation differs from that involved in teaching reading or arithmetic. She has a fair idea about her pupils' backgrounds and basic information in the academic areas; but their bases for human reproduction education are almost certainly *terra incognita* for the teacher. Moreover, the situation involves attitudes, feelings, repressions and all sorts of psychological facets not so likely to be as greatly influential in straight academic areas."[2]

JERROLD S. GREENBERG, coordinator of health education, School of Health Education, State University of New York at Buffalo, is contributing editor for this column.

An interesting monograph, entitled *Children's Art and Human Beginnings*, describes a project in which 1,149 primary grade children's pictorial expressions of concepts pertaining to human birth

[1] Associates of the E. C. Brown Trust Foundation, *Children's Art and Human Beginnings* (Eugene, Oregon: E. C. Brown Center for Family Studies, July-October, 1967).

[2] Ibid, p. 57.

Smoking

Making Tobacco Education Relevant
To the School-Age Child

John R. Seffrin, is professor and chairman of Health and Safety Education and director of Operation SmART at Indiana University, Bloomington, IN 47405.

School health education is faced today with a number of challenging opportunities to improve the quality of life through effective instructional programs. Whether it's sexually transmitted diseases, suicide, teenage drinking, illegitimacy or accidental deaths, most health educators feel that our discipline can and should help ameliorate these health problems through sound school health education programs.

Probably no greater challenge exists for school health education today than that of cigarette smoking among youth. Although the per capita consumption of cigarettes has dropped during the last three years, the estimated health-care cost to society because of cigarette-induced illness is fifteen billion dollars annually.[1] What is more important is that at least 340,000 Americans die each year prematurely because they smoke cigarettes.[2] In the words of Joseph A. Califano, former Secretary of Health, Education and Welfare, the unadorned facts clearly show that cigarette smoking is "public health enemy number one."

The cigarette smoking dilemma is a complex cultural problem with many interacting personal and social forces. However, the gross figures suggest strongly that the school curriculum has failed to prevent children and teenagers from beginning to smoke. For example, although the percentage of adults who smoke has gradually declined since 1964, the percentage of children and teenagers who smoke has increased. The rate of increase among teenage girls is particularly alarming.[3] All told, today six million children and teenagers smoke.[4] Past research and experience clearly show that 1) the majority of these youngsters will continue to smoke regularly for life; and, 2) they will be less well and their lives shorter because of their smoking habit.[5,6]

Finally, since the decision to smoke or not to smoke is made very early in life (almost always before age twenty and often by junior high school), the role of school health education, particularly during the primary and middle school years, is of critical importance if health educators are to reach students before they start smoking.[7,8] Until and unless comprehensive efforts are made to provide each school child with meaningful health instruction regarding cigarettes, the carnage in human health and life is likely to continue.

Personal Choice and Responsibility

Effectiveness of instruction is more related to how we teach than to what we teach. In the area of personal lifestyle it is important for the health educator to recognize the pluralism in our society. With the contemporary emphasis placed on personal rights and values, instructional strategies should be tailored accordingly. Therefore, careful planning by the teacher is necessary to provide a balanced as well as scientifically accurate instructional program. For example, in addition to teaching about the health consequences of smoking, instructional time should be used to explore the reasons why some people choose to smoke. In short, the teacher should develop an objective atmosphere in which the pros and cons of smoking can be fully explored.

The theme should be: the student has the ultimate responsibility to decide whether or not to smoke; therefore, the student must be given the pertinent facts in an objective setting. The goal is to provide the student with an opportunity to make a decision based on facts and personal values. Attendant to this approach is the accompanying need for the student to accept responsibility for his or her decision. In an effort to develop an awareness of the full responsibility involved in such a decision, instructional time should be given to explore a number of social issues such as accuracy in advertising, special insurance rates for smokers, and nonsmokers' rights.

In the past many working education efforts have been restricted to a narrow, one-sided, health-facts unit which could be accurately described as a "thou shalt not" approach. Besides being a "turn-off" for many students, its greatest weakness was that, in omitting substantive socio-political issues, some of the strong persuasions against taking up smoking were never developed. Thus, millions of children and teenagers have decided to smoke, at least in part, because the only disincentive was an obscure threat to their health decades in the future. To be truly responsive to student needs and to maximize the relevancy and potential impact of our teaching, we must go beyond the statistical correlations associating smoking with age-onset diseases. Morbidity and mortality figures and facts are not enough.

Suggested Facts and Concepts

With the knowledge explosion it is impossible to teach all the facts in any area; thus the professional responsibility of the teacher to select appropriate information to develop valid concepts is critical. Following are selected examples of content and concepts which can be made relevant to students.

Cigarette smoking is our nation's leading preventable health problem. Consensus exists among medical scientists that cigarette smoking is the greatest cause of preventable illness and premature death in the United States.[9,10] This year, for example, over 122,000 people will develop lung cancer in the United States; at least 80% of these cases are due to cigarette smoking.[11] Additionally, thousands more will develop cancers of the throat, oral cavity, pancreas, esophagus and urinary bladder because they smoke.[12,13] Heart diseases, our nation's leading cause of death, will take the lives of smokers at least twice as frequently as non-smokers.[14] Chronic obstructive lung disease, one of our nation's fastest-growing chronic diseases, is largely caused by cigarette smoking.[15] In short, after 30,000 scientific studies over three decades it is apparent that not one measure in preventive medicine could

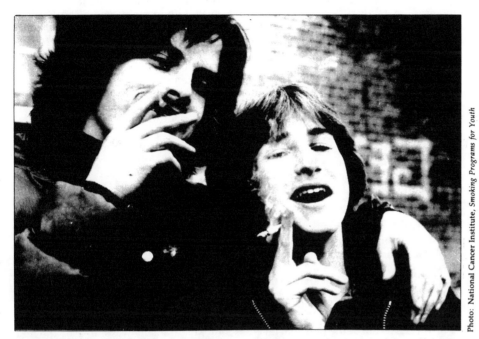

Photo: National Cancer Institute, *Smoking Programs for Youth*

do more to improve health and to prevent premature death than the control of cigarette smoking.[16]

Cigarette smoking is deleterious to your health now. The association of cigarette smoking to the aforementioned diseases is well established and widely recognized. However, less well known is that cigarette smoking is harmful to the smoker's health immediately. The adverse effects of smoking begin with the first cigarette and get progressively worse as smoking continues.[17] Immediate negative physiological responses to the smoker include increased heart rate, elevated blood pressure, constriction of blood vessels and trachial irritation.[18,19] While permanent, irreversible damage to the lungs does not occur immediately, hyperplasia (overgrowth of cells and overproduction of mucous) begins within weeks of regular cigarette smoking.[20,21] Ciliary action is damaged and trachial-mucosal velocity (TMV) is reduced while one smokes.[22,23] This, in part, explains why smokers are more prone to infectious diseases of the respiratory tract.[24]

In recent years, studies have shown basic pulmonary dysfunction in teenagers who have smoked for only a few years.[25] Although some of the harmful effects of smoking are reversible if a person quits in time (e.g. smokers' lung cancer mortality rates return to non-smoker rates 10 to 15 years after smoking ceases),[26] lung and respiratory tract tissue damage begins with the onset of smoking and becomes worse the longer one smokes.[27] Some scar tissue will result after only a few months of regular smoking.[28]

There is no such thing as safe smoking. Occasionally reports on smoking suggest that "moderate" or "light" smoking of low tar and nicotine cigarettes may be safe. This implication arises from the well-established fact that smoking's impact on health is a dose/response phenomenon.[29] The number of cigarettes smoked, the frequency of puffing, and the depth of the inhale all relate to increased risks.[30]

The inference, however, that there may be a safe or threshold level below which no harm occurs is unsubstantiated and invalid.[31,32] As already pointed out, adverse effects begin early and grow progressively worse over time.[33] Further, although low tar and nicotine cigarettes are assumed to be less hazardous, no evidence exists which would indicate that they are safe. On the contrary, certain harmful substances, such as carbon monoxide, are in greater concentration in the low tar and low nicotine brands.[34] Scientifically, it is very difficult to make blanket statements about the relative risks of different brands because of individual differences in smoking technique. For example, some smokers who switch to a low tar and nicotine brand may draw harder or inhale deeper and smoke more cigarettes; thus, the relative dosage of nicotine and other substances may be about the same as before.

In conclusion, if a person must smoke, a low tar and nicotine cigarette may be the least harmful; however, from a health vantage point, any smoking is hazardous to one's health.

Cigarette smoking can be harmful to others, and especially to fetuses. In addition to the well-known irritation factor, which at least 60% of all people experience, there are real health threats from exposure to second-hand smoke.[35,36] The most alarming threat is to persons who are already chronically ill with diseases like coronary artery disease, bronchitis, and chronic obstructive pulmonary disease.[37] For example, people with existing heart disease will develop angina pectoris (chest pain) upon exertion sooner when breathing air polluted with tobacco smoke.[38] Further, animal studies have shown significantly more malignant tumors among those animals breathing second-hand smoke on a daily basis.[39] Finally, children exposed regularly to cigarette smoke have twice the respiratory disease rate of other children.[40] Although the smoker is affected most by smoking, the non-smoker who breathes air polluted with cigarette smoke does experience untoward physiological effects.[41] These unhealthy and immediate effects include elevated blood pressure, increased heart rate, and abnormal carboxyhemaglobin levels (carbon monoxide in the blood).[42] Recent studies confirm that even healthy adults develop marked small-airways dysfunction from breathing secondhand smoke.[43]

The most fearsome impact of second-hand smoke may be on the fetus of the pregnant smoker. Unless the mother stops smoking before the fourth month of pregnancy, some untoward effect can be expected in the baby.[44] Since carbon monoxide crosses the placental bearier, the unborn fetus can be expected to develop carboxyhemoglobin levels comparable to the mother's.[45,46] Since it is known that carbon monoxide displaces oxygen in the blood, it is obvious that the fetus is put at a distinct disadvantage during the most important period of its growth and development. For example, the human fetus' brain is growing at the rate of one to two milligrams per minute at the time of delivery.[47] Thus, any oxygen deprivation is most critical. In addition to having more miscarriages and stillbirths, smoking mothers have babies who weigh less at birth; also their babies are more apt to die during the first year after birth; and, their babies have more respiratory disease during childhood and adolescence.[48,49] One of the most discouraging findings educationally has been the discovery that children whose mothers smoked during pregnancy do poorer on achievement tests in math and reading at ages 7 and 11.[50]

Regular cigarette smoking usually results in a serious dependency problem. Like any drug of abuse, tobacco has the potential of causing serious dependency. Unlike users of other drugs of abuse, however, research indicates that tobacco users will usually become dependent for life—they will be less well and their lives shorter because of their smoking.[51] For example, it is estimated that about 10-15% of the people alive today who ever used heroin are still dependent on it. However, 66% of those still alive who ever smoked cigarettes are currently still dependent on cigarettes and smoke them daily.[52]

While research to elucidate the mechanisms of dependency continues, it is safe to say that cigarette smoking can and usually does result in strong dependency. The psychological factors associated with habit formation and desire to smoke seem to be paramount; but, at least for some smokers, the development of a physical dependence to nicotine may also occur.[53] These stark facts should be included in educational units so that those deciding to smoke are aware, in advance, of the likelihood of future dependency. It is known from national polls that at least 8 in 10 smokers would like to quit if there were an easy way. Such information is particularly critical in view of the recent trend in children experimenting with tobacco at earlier ages. A 1967 British survey of teenagers indicated that among those who smoked more than one cigarette, 80% ultimately became regular smokers.[55]

The advantages of not smoking far outweigh the advantages of smoking. Children and teenagers who choose to smoke do so for certain reasons. Although these reasons may not be clearly elucidated and evaluated, and just as importantly, they may not be understood by the smoker, we must acknowledge that all behavior, healthy as well as unhealthy, is caused. It is a logical assumption that many smokers find their habit enjoyable and somehow, reinforcing. For some youngsters, smoking may provide a way of emulating adults; for others a way of rebelling; and for still others, simply a satisfaction of curiosity.[56,57] Educators should explore with their students these and other possible reasons for smoking. In so doing, educators should avoid a condescending attitude toward reasons advanced in favor of smoking. Since one's values relate intimately to one's rationale for behavior, it is inappropriate to label reasons as right or wrong. The merits and demerits of various reasons should be explored in an atmosphere of respect with an emphasis on value clarification.

However, any comprehensive analysis of the pros and cons associated with smoking leads to one very critical conclusion; that is, the advantages of not smoking far outweigh the advantages of smoking.

Issues for Class Discussion

Since the decision to smoke or not to smoke is an individual one, much of the educational strategy should focus on personalizing lessons. As stated, there should be adequate coverage of the various values and motivations involved in choosing a course of action.

However, to stop at the personal level would be remiss in light of the health care dilemma facing society today. In an effort to explore the responsibility of the individual in society, a careful examination of social policies regarding cigarette smoking is important and relevant. Three examples follow of critical socio-political issues which should be dealt with in the secondary curriculum.

What should be our federal policy toward tobacco? Currently the federal government is inconsistent and contradictory in its policy toward tobacco. Simultaneously, two cabinet-level departments pursue policies which have antithetical objectives. The Department of Agriculture (USDA) continues to support and promote tobacco production. In 1977, for example, the U.S. Department of Agriculture spent approximately 65 million dollars on the various aspects of administering the price-support program for tobacco.[58] Further, the nation's lawmakers included tobacco in Public Law 480, the "Food for Peace" program.[59] Under this program millions of dollars in tobacco have been sent to developing countries around the world.

On the other hand, the U.S. Department of Health and Human Services (DHHS) continues to battle cigarette smoking in many ways. In 1964 the first and landmark *Surgeon General's Report on Smoking* was published. Since then a number of efforts have been instituted at the national level to combat smoking through school and public health education. In 1978, DHEW Secretary Califano established the Office on

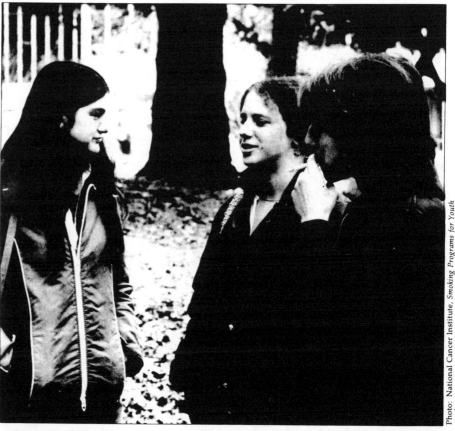

Photo: National Cancer Institute, *Smoking Programs for Youth*

Smoking and Health, and money continues to be spent on anti-smoking programs.[60]

Who should pay the smoker's health care bill? The cost of medical care in America continues to rise even faster than the inflation rate. This year, Americans will spend over 245 billion dollars on personal health services, more than any other nation in the

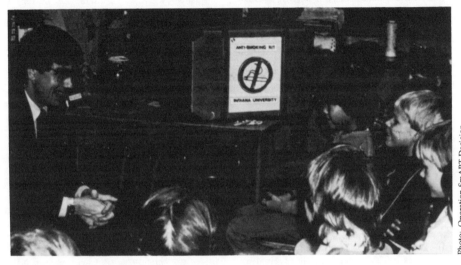

Photo: Operation SmART Decision

world.[61] With the trend toward some form of prepaid, social-health insurance plan for all, greater emphasis needs to be placed on the prevention of disease. For example, it is estimated that 350,000 people will die this year from diseases caused by cigarette smoking.[62] Prior to their death many incurred large medical bills resulting from expensive treatment and lengthy stays in hospitals. Current estimates are that each year at least seven billion dollars are spent on the direct medical costs of treating diseases caused by cigarette smoking. If one adds the lost productivity, the total cost jumps to a staggering 20 billion dollars annually.[63] Presently, the direct health costs are borne primarily by private insurance companies. Eventually, they may all be paid through national health insurance. Regardless of the system, private or governmental, the consumer pays—all the consumers. Should non-smokers pay as much in premiums or taxes as the smoker?

What are the rights of smokers and non-smokers? The spirit of this age is *rights:* rights for the handicapped, rights for Blacks, rights for the aged and rights for children. In all of the above examples, one common denominator exists. Each one of the above represents a minority group. In the case of non-smokers' rights, we are talking about the *majority.* Most children and adults

do not smoke. In spite of this fact, many who are bothered by cigarette smoke feel as though they should not express their discomfort, since it is the smoker's right to smoke.

However, no one is proposing to take away the smoker's right to smoke. On the contrary, all major groups active in the smoking and health controversy maintain that a person has the right to decide whether or not to smoke. However, a distinction needs to be made between a right and a freedom. That is, although one has a right to choose to smoke or not to smoke, one does *not* have the freedom to engage in the practice at will.

Since the beginning of our country, certain limitations have been placed on personal rights. Generally, these limitations are determined by two factors: the health and safety of the public; and the rights that might be abridged by the unrestricted practice of the first right. The adoption of speed limits is an example of protecting public safety. A great jurist once wrote, "My right to swing my fist ends when my fist reaches the end of your nose." Consistent with these principles and precedents, one's right to smoke should not be total and unrestricted. For years, for safety purposes, smoking has been properly disallowed in combustible areas, and, smoking in bed is against the law.

We now know that ambient cigarette smoke can be hazardous to the non-smoker's health, especially to children and persons with chronic illnesses. Since society should promote the public health, a new look at rights for smokers and non-smokers is justified and appropriate.

Summary

Americans consume 615 billion cigarettes annually.[64] Although the per capita consumption for adults has dropped over the past fifteen years, the amount of cigarettes being smoked by children and teenagers has increased. The percent of teenage girls smoking has nearly doubled during the last decade.[65] Because of this trend toward more smoking among the young, and because of smoking's effect on human health and life, educators must redouble their efforts. In spite of the diseases exacted on humans as a result of smoking, cigarette smoking, as such, is not a medical problem; but rather, the real problem lies in educating youngsters prior to the age at which the critical decision to smoke or not to smoke is made.

Through careful planning and professional discretion the school-health team can address this challenge in ways that are meaningful and relevant to students. No longer do we need to threaten the child with dread diseases in the distant future; but rather, instructional strategies can be designed to respect the student's right to choose. However, in choosing, it is imperative that the student grasp the profundity of the decision. Through a comprehensive and balanced instructional effort the student can better understand the personal as well as social ramifications of cigarette smoking. With an emphasis on the role of values and motivations in decision making the student can begin to appreciate the words of Frost:
"Two roads diverged in a wood, and I -
I took the one less traveled by,
And that has made all the difference."[66]

[1]American Cancer Society, Inc. *A national dilemma: cigarette smoking or the health of Americans – report of the National Commission on Smoking and Public Policy to the Board of Directors,* 1978, 4.

[2]U.S. DHEW. Smoking and health, report of the Surgeon General, Washington, DC: USPHS, 1979, ii.

[3]U.S. DHEW. *The smoking digest,* National Cancer Institute, 1977, 13.

[4]Horn, D. How much real progress have we made in the fight against smoking? *Bull Am Lung Assoc,* 1979, 65, 6–9.

[5]Russell, M. A. H. Smoking problems: an overview, in *Research on smoking behavior, National Institute on Drug Abuse Research Monograph 17,* M. E. Jarvik, J. W. Cullen, E. R. Gritz, T. M. Vogt, and L. J. West, (eds.), (U.S. Department of Health, Education and Welfare. Publication No. (ADM) 78-581). Rockville, MD.: National Institute on Drug Abuse, 1977, 13–33.

[6]U.S. DHEW: *The health consequences of smoking, report of the Surgeon General,* Office

on Smoking and Health, 1978.

[7]American School Health Association. *Introducing tobacco education in the elementary school K-4*, Kent, OH: American School Health Association, 1978, 2.

[8]WHO. *Smoking and its effects on health, report of a WHO Expert Committee*, Geneva, Switzerland: World Health Organization, 1975, 29–33.

[9]Fletcher, C. M., & Horn, D. Smoking and health, *WHO Chronicle*, 1970, *24*, 345–370.

[10]U.S. DHEW. *The health consequences of smoking*, p. 2.

[11]American Cancer Society, Inc.: *Cancer facts and figures 1981*, New York, NY: American Cancer Society, Inc., 1979, 9, 14.

[12]*Ibid.*, p. 19.

[13]U.S. DHEW: *The health consequences of smoking*, ch. 5.

[14]Steinfeld, J. L. Presentation at Opening Plenary Session of the 3rd World Conference on Smoking and Health, in *Proceedings of the 3rd World Conference on Smoking and Health, II*, J. Steinfeld, W. Griffiths, K. Ball, & R. M. Taylor, (eds.), (U.S. Department of Health, Education and Welfare. Publication No. NIH 77-1414). Washington, D.C.: U.S. Government Printing Office, 1976, 21.

[15]U.S. DHEW. *The health consequences of smoking, 1975*, (Publication No. CDC 76-8704). Washington, D.C.: U.S. Government Printing Office, 1975, 61.

[16]Fletcher, C. M., & Horn, D. Smoking and health.

[17]Worick, W. W., and Schaller, W. E. *Alcohol, tobacco, and drugs*, Englewood Cliffs, NJ: Prentice-Hall, Inc., 1977, 77–109.

[18]*Ibid.*

[19]Diehl, H. S. *Tobacco and your health: the smoking controversy*, New York, NY: McGraw-Hill, Inc., 1969, 47–51.

[20]Jay, S. J., Associate Professor of Medicine, Indiana University School of Medicine, Pulmonary Section, interview, February 27, 1979.

[21]*Essentials of life and health*, New York, NY: Random House (CRM Books), 1977, 86–87.

[22]American Lung Association. Chronic smoking lowers rate at which the lungs clear mucus, *Bull Am Lung Assoc.*, July-August, 1977, 15.

[23]Newhouse, M. T. Effect of cigarette smoking on mucociliary clearance, in *Proceedings of the 3rd World Conference on Smoking and Health, II*, op. cit., pp. 131–137.

[24]Diehl, Tobacco and your health, 87–95.

[25]U.S. DHEW, *The health consequences of smoking, 1978*, ch. 6.

[26]U.S. DHEW, *The Smoking Digest*, p. 28.

[27]Royal College of Physicians of London: *Smoking or health – the third report from the Royal College of Physicians of London*, Trent, England: Pitman Medical Publishing Co. LTD, 1977, 76–81.

[28]Jay: op. cit.

[29]U.S. DHEW. *Report of the Surgeon General on smoking and health*, 1964 through 1978.

[30]Diehl, Tobacco and your health, p. 202.

[31]*Ibid.*, 201–206.

[32]Royal College of Physicians of London, *Smoking or health*, pp. 121–122.

[33]Worick and Schaller, *Alcohol, tobacco and drugs*.

[34]U.S. DHEW, *The health consequences of smoking, 1978*, ch. 11.

[35]Speer, F. Tobacco and the nonsmoker, *Arch Environ Health*, 1968, *16*, 443–446.

[36]Burns, D. M. Consequences of smoking – the involuntary smoker, in *Proceedings of the 3rd World Conference on Smoking and Health, II*, 51–58.

[37]Tate, C. F. The effects of tobacco smoke on the non-smoking cardiopulmonary public, in *Proceedings of the 3rd World Conference on Smoking and Health, II*, 329–335.

[38]Aronow, W. S. Carbon monoxide and cardiovascular disease, in *Proceedings of the 3rd World Conference on Smoking and Health, I*, E. L. Wynder, D. Hoffmann, and G. B. Gori, (eds.). (U.S. Department of Health, Education and Welfare Publication No. NIH 76-1221). Washington, D.C.: U.S. Government Printing Office, 1976, 321–328.

[39]U.S. DHEW: *The health consequences of smoking, a report of the Surgeon General: 1972*, (Publication No. HSM 72-7516). Washington, D.C.: U.S. Government Printing Office, 1972, 121–135.

[40]Colley, J. R. T., et al. Influence of passive smoking and parental phlegm on pneumonia and bronchitis in early childhood, *Lancet*, 1974, *II*, 1031–1034.

[41]U.S. DHEW: *The health consequences of smoking, 1975*, 87–106.

[42]White, J.R. & Frobe, H.F. Small-airways dysfunction in non-smokers chronically exposed to tobacco smoke. *New England Journal of Medicine*, 1980, *302*, 720–723.

[43]Burns, D. M. Consequences of smoking.

[44]Goldstein, H. Smoking in pregnancy: the statistical controversy and its resolution, in *Proceedings of the 3rd World Conference on Smoking and Health, II*, 201–210.

[45]Longo, L. D. The biological effects of carbon monoxide on the pregnant woman, fetus, and newborn infant, *Am J Obstet Gynecol*, 1977, *29*, 69–103.

[46]*Ibid.*

[47]Dobbing, J. All flesh is grass, *Kaiser Aluminum News: The World Food Crisis – Man, Mind, Soul*, 1968, *26*, p. 13.

[48]Butler, N. R., et al. Cigarette smoking in pregnancy: its influence on birth weight and prenatal mortality, *Br Med J*, 1972, *2*, 127–130.

[49]Meyer, M. B., & Tonascia, J. A. Maternal smoking, pregnancy complications and prenatal mortality, *Am J Obstet Gynecol*, 1977, *128*, 494–502.

[50]Butler, N. R., & Goldstein, H. Smoking in pregnancy and subsequent child development, *Br Med J*, 1973, 4, 573–575.

[51]U.S. DHEW: *The health consequences of smoking, 1978*, Preface, p. 5, ch. 1, 2, 3, 4, 6.

[52]Blair, G. Why Dick can't stop smoking – the politics behind our national addiction, *Mother Jones*, January 1979, 31–42.

[53]Royal College of Physicians of London; *Smoking or health*, pp. 43–44.

[54]Olshavsky, R. W. *No more butts – a psychologist's approach to quitting cigarettes*, Bloomington, IN.: Indiana University Press, 1977, 3.

[55]Royal College of Physicians of London, *Smoking or health*, p. 89.

[56]U.S. DHEW: *Teenage smoking–national patterns of cigarette smoking, ages 12 through 18, in 1972 and 1974*. (Publication No. NIH 76-931, Public Health Service) 1976.

[57]Seffrin, J. R. Risks, rewards and values, *Health Values*, September/October 1977, *1*, 197–199.

[58]Eckholm, Cutting tobacco's toll, p. 19.

[59]*Ibid.*, p. 21.

[60]Califano Jr., J. A. A new commitment to wellness, *Bull Am Lung Assoc.*, November 1978, *64*, 5–10.

[61]Health Insurance Institute, *Sourcebook of health insurance data, 1979–1980*, Washington, DC: Health Insurance Institute, 1979, 47.

[62]*Cancer facts and figures, 1981.*

[63]*Ibid.*, p. 2.

[64]*Ibid.*, p. 1.

[65]Hill, H. Situational analysis: women and smoking, in *Proceedings of the 3rd World Conference on Smoking and Health, II*, pp. 291–297.

[66]Frost, R. *Complete poems of Robert Frost*, New York, NY: Holt, Rinehart, and Winston, 1967, 131.

Smoking

Student-to-Student Teaching About Tobacco Smoking

Lorraine J. Henke is a health educator at the Eugene Burroughs Junior High School, Accokeek, Maryland.

For the past three years, the decision to smoke or not to smoke has been the subject of formal discussions between eighth grade health education students from Eugene Burroughs Junior High School and elementary students in the fifth and sixth grades in various schools of Prince George's County, Maryland. The project was designed to explore the impact of presenting the smoking aspect of health education between students of close age groups. The assumption was that the fifth and sixth grade students would enthusiastically accept and comprehend the presentation and interchange of health education information with their junior high school student contemporaries. This assumption was proven to be valid.

A typical student-to-student teaching experience consists of a group of seven or eight junior high school health education students visiting a fifth or sixth grade class (frequently a science class). The eighth grade students first present the facts of smoking as a panel, then each of them leads a small group of elementary students in a discussion about the decision to smoke or not to smoke.

During the panel presentation, the junior high school students discuss the effects of tobacco smoking on the body utilizing a machine (constructed by the students) which simulates the effects on the human respiratory system. A filter tip and nonfilter tip cigarette are both "smoked" by the machine. The tar from each of the cigarettes is passed through hollow glass rods representing a person's mouth and throat. The tar that did not adhere to the glass rods then travels to glass test tubes constructed to represent a person's lungs. The presence of tar is always clearly visible, enabling succinct comparisons of tar content to be made between the cigarettes, along with analyses of tar content regardless of the type

of cigarette. Safety precautions to prevent tobacco smoking related fires, why people smoke, and how to quit smoking are presented. The audience is encouraged to join in the discussion and to ask questions of the panel members.

Following the panel presentation, the elementary students are divided into groups and each eighth grader leads a group in discussing the advantages and disadvantages of tobacco smoking. During these discussions, the eighth graders encourage the elementary students to ask questions, to voice honest opinions, and to continue to keep up-to-date regarding the facts about tobacco smoking.

At the conclusion of each instruction program, the visiting junior high school students distribute leaflets stating the facts about tobacco smoking. These leaflets are contributed by the American Cancer Society, the Tuberculosis and Respiratory Disease Association, and the U.S. Department of Health, Education, and Welfare. Also contributed by these organizations for use in the presentations are posters, research data, and other printed materials on tobacco smoking, including the booklet from HEW explaining how to construct the machine which the students used in their presentation.

Several points of interest, noted over the few years of being involved with the student-to-student teaching program, are as follows:

1. Elementary students who plan to attend the junior high school represented by the panel group respond more enthusiastically than do those who are not going to attend that school. Following this revelation, we have encouraged elementary schools to seek the services of the junior high school their students expect to attend.

2. Presentations made to large groups (over 50) of elementary students are not as successful as those given to smaller groups. There appears to be less satisfaction for both

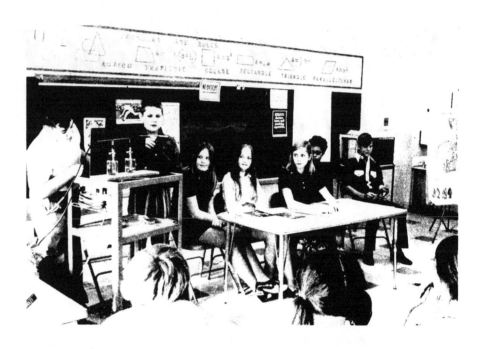

Eighth graders make effective teachers for sixth graders—and especially when they come from the junior high school their audience will attend, when there is a good mix of race, sex, and personality.

the junior high school student teachers and the elementary school students.

3. When the make-up of the panel of junior high students includes a variety of students (in regard to sex, race, personality, and academic achievements), there appears to be a higher audience response (a very good rapport) than if these characteristics were not represented by the junior high school student teachers.

4. Parents of both the elementary and junior high school students involved in the student-to-student teaching program have responded to this form of health education in a very favorable manner.

5. Junior high school students involved in the program have repeatedly stated that their experience in teaching the facts about tobacco smoking has reinforced their decision not to smoke.

6. Repeated requests from the elementary schools have been made to initiate a similar program for other aspects of health education, especially drug education.

Where do we go from here? We are constantly seeking other effective teaching aids like the smoking machine in an attempt to improve our presentations. We are investigating the student-to-student teaching of other aspects of health education. The eighth grade student teachers are invited back each year to relate their experiences regarding tobacco smoking as they progress into the higher school grades. We seek and evaluate the suggestions of the elementary students and their junior high school student teachers. Most important, since the program has been going on for the past few years, we have been able to ask the eighth grade health students (who a few years ago were elementary students attending our student-to-student discussions) what effect the discussions had on their health attitudes and behavior. At this point sufficient data to make a conclusion have not been collected and analyzed. The favorable responses received from those students who had attended the student-to-student discussions, however, please us and spur us on to continue and improve.

Two Programs Exemplify Nationwide Involvement in School Health Education

This article was made possible under contract #200-78-0807 with the Bureau of Health Education, Center for Disease Control, Atlanta, Georgia.

NANCY L. EVANS is resource coordinator and KATHLEEN HOYT MIDDLETON is director of curriculum at the National Center for Health Education, School Health Education Project, 901 Sneath Lane, Suite 215, San Bruno, CA 94066.

In thousands of classrooms throughout the country students in grades K–7 are learning the concepts of health and wellness through broad based approaches that demonstrate "happiness is being healthy" in creative and exciting ways. The Primary Grades Health Curriculum Project (PGHCP) or Seattle Project and the School Health Curriculum Project (SHCP) or Berkeley Project emphasize activities on a personal level that are designed to help students understand the functioning of their own bodies, what affects health, and how to make personal decisions about their own health and lifestyles.

The projects are life-related, involving many aspects of the student's immediate world. They focus on maintaining good health and enhance the elementary school curriculum. The curricula involve other subject areas such as reading, writing, arithmetic, science, physical fitness, art, and music. Concurrently, physical, social, and mental/emotional components are incorporated throughout the models. The experiences carried out in the classroom allow for individuality of learning styles and abilities along with providing students with multiple opportunities to express themselves. Students are encouraged to develop strong self concepts and learn to take responsibility for health related decisions.

The promotion of positive health behavior and lifestyles does not stop in the classroom. Maximum involvement of community members and school personnel is stressed. Specifically, activities are written into the curricula which involve school, family, and community members. Those wishing to assist with classroom activities are encouraged to do so. Numerous community agencies are asked for human and material resources to share with the students. Field trips can be planned to enhance effective linkages among the school, family, and community to reinforce the life related aspects of the program.

Students in grades K–7 are involved with the projects for an eight to twelve week time period. There is a teaching model for each grade level which specifically describes the methods, materials, and learning activities. Objectives and goals have also been identified. A major characteristic which distinguishes these models from many others is the training component. A one to two week training workshop has been designed to help promote successful implementation of the models. In an atmosphere of support a team of 4 to 5 people, represented by classroom teachers, an administrator, and a support person (e.g., nurse, health educator, curriculum coordinator, media specialist, librarian) receive a solid foundation for the specific grade level addressed at that training session.

Proceeding classroom implementation, when feasible, each new project is visited by a training staff member to discuss implementation issues and other aspects of the models. In many districts, a reconvening session is held about nine months after the training to provide a forum for teachers to share experiences. Ideas, problems, parent and community involvement strategies, and plans for further implementation are discussed. Each school district assesses its needs for revisions and adaptations related to specific community issues and classroom situations.

An overview of the content covered in each level plus several of the suggested classroom activities follow.

Kindergarten

In a film in the kindergarten unit, a smoking octopus named Octopuff is persuaded by a group of young children to give up smoking and clean the air in the Kingdom of Kumquat. Then students make their own Octopuff puppets and discuss the effects of smoking on the lungs, which helps them understand the consequences of smoking. Many realize that never starting is a wise choice.

In addition, through the community crusade represented by the children in Kumquat, the concept of "health helpers" is introduced. In the unit "health helpers" such as doctors, nurses, pharmacists, teachers, and parents in the community, the school, and at home are identified. Ways to express feelings and to understand the importance of making healthful decisions in areas such as nutrition, rest, exercise, safety, drugs, environmental pollution, and general health habits are also brought out in this unit.

Grade 1

An introductory activity for children in grade one finds them guessing the contents of a box entitled "What's the Most Wonderful Thing In the World?" When the box is opened a mirror appears inside and first graders in the "Super Me" unit soon discover the answer. Self concept development is emphasized through exploration of individuality. Students participate in activities which demonstrate the many similar emotions and reactions people share.

Grade one also introduces the five senses and their role in communicating information about personal and environmental health.

Grade 2

Dealing with emotions and methods of communicating with our senses are explored further in the second grade unit. The individual's role in caring for eyes and ears is emphasized by focusing on safety measures for work and play and anti-pollutant measures for personal and environmental health.

Students encounter the language of the blind and deaf by reading Braille and practicing sign language with the assistance of a speech therapist or other resource person. Understanding of persons with special seeing or hearing problems may be reinforced by field trips to schools for the blind or deaf.

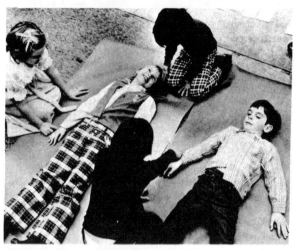

Students draw outlines of each other, then make stuffed dummies to study internal and external movement.

Photo courtesy of American Lung Association

Grade 3

A person visiting a third grade classroom may find one student drawing an outline around the body of a fellow student. From these body outlines, students construct stuffed dummies to study internal and external body movement.

Creative expression of emotions and thoughts, safety measures, coordination, energy, and muscle development are all related to the study of body movement and structure in the third grade unit. Students also explore the effects of behaviors such as exercise, eating, and smoking on the mechanics of the body systems.

Grade 4

Students explore the effect of an individual's behavior on health. With an emphasis on nutrition and the digestive system, students learn about energy and chemical interactions within the body. By designing charts, mobiles, and displays depicting the various nutrients and their jobs, students learn the importance of food choices on their total health. As a followup activity, parents are invited to a breakfast planned by students which emphasizes essential nutrients. Consumer issues, environmental pollution, immunization, and personal medical care are also explored in this unit.

Grade 5

The witches' brew is a smelly stew; it is full of things your body doesn't need. Fifth grade students fill the witches' cauldron with "smelly" things such as drug abuse, pollution, poor health habits, poor eating habits, and negative self concepts since these items detract from maintaining good health. The students discuss reasons why they wouldn't give this "brew" to their closest friend.

By exploring the structure and function of the respiratory system, students understand that maintaining healthy lungs contributes to the overall health of the individual. The unit also emphasizes the importance of environmental health while examining the role of the individual and community.

Grade 6

Identifying and understanding prevention measures related to overall health and heart disease in particular are approached through a variety of activities. Students construct a prevention wheel illustrating the relationship of exercise, stress control and mental health, alcohol, nutrition, smoking, and weight control to the maintenance of wellness and a healthy heart.

Discussions and learning center activities focus on issues, such as healthful ways to deal with life situations, reasons people turn to alcohol and drugs as well as their effects on the body and alternatives to their use.

Grade 7

Early in the seventh grade unit, students explore decision making concepts related to peer pressure as well as use and abuse of drugs, alcohol and cigarettes. By studying the brain's role in controlling and coordinating all the body systems, students gain an understanding of the effects of these substances on maintaining health.

A focus on mental health and illness calls for examination of factors contributing to self-esteem, stress, coping mechanisms, and related psychological and social problems. Disorders and accidents related to the brain and nervous system such as epilepsy, cerebral palsy, mental retardation, are identified as are methods of prevention, detection, and treatment. Sexually transmitted diseases are also addressed.

Contributing factors to social, physical, and emotional wellbeing are considered through various activities—recording daily personal schedules of exercise, diet, substance use, relaxation, and sleep.

Learning Approaches

In the implementation of grades K–7 of the PGHCP and SHCP, a wide variety of learning approaches are employed. Throughout the model, multiple opportunities are provided for students to explore ideas and express

themselves. A distinctive component of the program is that of learning stations which are areas of the room set up for students to experiment, construct, role play, and make discoveries in small group situations. Many activities are the hands on type where multimedia tools and other props including puppets, balloons, paper bags, seeds, heat, light, and manikins are utilized.

Project Dissemination

At present, the curriculum projects are being implemented in over 400 school districts in 35 states, plus England and Saudi Arabia. It has successfully involved children from different school and community settings, races, and socioeconomic levels. Numerous health-related voluntary organizations, businesses, governmental agencies, parent and community groups, and school boards are working actively to support the continuation and expansion of these curriculum models.

Validation and Evaluation

A distinctive feature which should assist in further dissemination of these models is the recent validation of grade units 5, 6, and 7 by the United States Office of Education (USOE) and the National Institute of Education (NIE). The Joint Dissemination Review Panel (JDRP) of USOE and NIE voted that these educational interventions have exhibited positive impacts and can be replicated. As a JDRP approved program, activities associated with the SHCP will be eligible to receive funding via USOE's National Diffusion Network. Validation for grades K-4 will be pursued in the immediate future.

The responsibility for this activity as well as for the overall management of the models is with the School Health Education Project (SHEP) of the National Center for Health Education.

For more information on these curriculum models, we strongly recommend that a site visit be made where the program is in operation. The National Center's SHEP office and the Bureau of Health Education will be glad to provide names of local people to contact in order to see the program in action. Please contact: The National Center for Health Education, School Health Education Project, 901 Sneath Lane, Suite 215, San Bruno, CA 94066 or the Bureau of Health Education, Center for Disease Control, 1600 Clifton Road, N.E., Bldg. 14, B7, Atlanta, GA 30333.

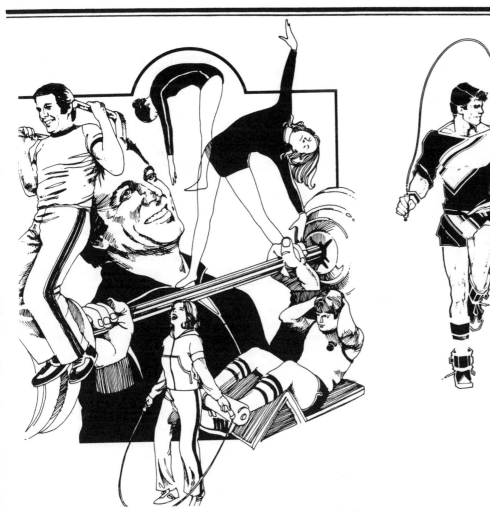

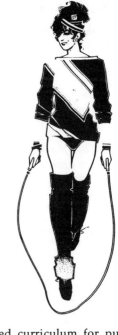

Test items in each self-instructional unit were designed to show whether students had achieved the specific objectives of the unit. Significant changes in pre-post scores and results of the Solomon IV design suggested that the two cardiovascular risk factor self-instructional units were effective in terms of increasing students' knowledge of the primary and secondary risk factors of cardiovascular disease. Although the mass testing techniques indicated differences in posttest scores among school districts, this variance may have been due to pre-existing group differences. Results of the Solomon IV design which utilized randomization, revealed no interaction between pretest and treatment; thus, the external validity of the units was demonstrated.

To assess the effectiveness of the risk factor packages over time, a retention study was conducted in five area school districts. High school students who had participated in the field testing previously were tracked during the school year. Each student was given a knowledge retention test after eight months.

The findings indicated that there was not a significant decrease in knowledge from posttest to the retention test. The gain in knowledge from pretest to retention test remained significant. Therefore, the learning that took place was stable over the eight month period. There was a significant treatment effect with Solomon IV data. The groups receiving the learning materials had the higher scores and showed no significant loss of knowledge over the extended time period.

Student and teacher reaction to materials was again obtained as a part of the field-testing. Evaluation forms as well as personal interviews conducted with teachers to obtain more subjective data concerning the usefulness of the package were used. The data collected from the field testing was used to revise the materials once again. The final product, validated by numerous learner and teacher tryouts was then sent to Medical Illustration for final revision.

The CCEP program was specifically designed to meet the challenge of educating youth in the areas of cardiovascular disease and risk factors via a prepackaged curriculum for public schools. Results of field testing have shown the units to be an effective method of disseminating preventive health information. Besides being easily and economically reproduced, the units are easily accommodated into an existing curriculum. Furthermore, since the CCEP units are self-instructional packages, they provide a minimum data base of knowledge which can be further expanded by the teacher using supplementary materials and activities.

The challenge of reducing the incidence of heart disease faces all Americans, including teachers and students. With more effective heart health education during the adolescent years, the probability of death or long term disability resulting from heart and blood vessel disease can be substantially lowered.

[1]Williams, L.L., Arnold, C.B., Wyner, E.L. The Epidemiology of Chronic Disease Risk Factors Among Children. Paper presented at the American Public Health Association Annual Convention, Washington, D.C., October 31, 1977.

[2]White, R.C., Weinberg, A.D., Spiker, C.A., and Roush, R.E. Cardiovascular Disease Education in Texas Education Classes—A Needs Assessment. *Journal of School Health*, 48(6):341-348, 1978.

[3]Campbell, D.T., Stanley, J.C. *Experimental and Quasi-Experimental Designs for Research*. Chicago: Rand-McNally College Publishing Co., 1963.

Psychology of Modeling in Health Education

DAVID CHENOWETH is a doctoral candidate in health education, Ohio State University, 1760 Neil Avenue, Columbus, Ohio 43210.

Students may acquire certain attitudes, emotional responses, and complex patterns of behavior from parents and friends that are conducive to higher levels of wellness. A student can and does acquire precursory attitudes, emotional responses, and knowledge from teachers. Here are some ways teachers can be effective models.[1]

1. Teachers can model new academic tasks more effectively by showing, rather than explaining, the exact sequence of steps necessary to perform that behavior.

2. Teachers who are seen to be more competent (skillful or successful) performers will be imitated more for a particular behavior than teachers who lack these qualities.

3. A teacher can only be an effective model for behavior when children see the consequences of that behavior. Behavior outside the classroom is generally not observed by pupils and stands little chance of being imitated.

Imitation is not the same as modeling. Behavior should never be intentionally duplicated in and of itself. It should be the result of a particular modeling effect leading to long-term application. Figure 1 provides possible student rationale for optimal health behavior.

Like our students, we are limited in our perceptual field. If we acknowledge that behavior and its many components exert a dynamic impact on students' health-related expressions, can we really exclude considering the potential influence that health-conscious students may have on their family, friends, and associates? We all fluctuate along the health status continuum throughout our lives. Should we then address ourselves to making gradual, cumulative change in our students?

In many schools students have poor health behavior because they do not understand the determinants of such behavior. This may be due to our inability to gather, interpret, and actively employ research as a means to encourage desirable behavior. Consider the following activity, keeping in mind that the earlier the modeling, the greater the likelihood the student will adopt behavior conducive to optimal health.

Activity Posters

Have students list their favorite person—athlete, actor, actress, television character, or other. The students and teacher can then purchase posters of these favorite people and the teacher can orient a unit in health education to a poster. The following is an example of how a poster might be used: *Teacher*— "John, since you would like someday to play professional tennis as well as Bjorn Borg, what do you think he does to play so well?"

You can complement the poster with a lesson in basic nutrition and activity by discussing nutritional and activity requirements for an athlete of his caliber. If the student sees Bjorn on television, reads of him in the newspaper, hears of him on the radio, and exhibits particular facets of Bjorn's behavior (wearing wristbands or headband, playing tennis regularly, maintaining composure in times of adversity), then supplementing this social behavior with reliable information may reinforce an overall modeling effect.

Compare and Contrast Lifestyles

Have each student evaluate a particular classmate or teacher throughout the school day, intermittently viewing aspects of health such as the following.

Activity: duration, intensity, frequency, and mode at recess or during physical education periods.

Nutrition: during lunchtime; what foods eaten, amount of food left on plate, type of beverage consumed, approximate number of calories.

Posture: sitting with back perpendicular to floor? standing with weight evenly distributed on both feet?

Mental Health: confident, not boastful; adjusts to students whose values differ from theirs.

Personal Hygiene: clothes laundered regularly; hair groomed neatly; attractive appearance of teeth, gums, and skin.

Accident Prevention: observes emergency and warning material; listens carefully and complies with teacher's instructions.

Social Relationships: relates well with own and opposite sex; respects rights and privacy of others.

During the student evaluation, the teacher could have each student record the effect of their assigned model on their own health-related decisions and behaviors.

Consequences

Many students will have a family

Figure 1. Student rationale for optimal health behavior resulting from teacher behavior.

Short-Term Effectiveness

Teacher Behavior	Student Behavior	Student Rationale
Does not smoke	Does not smoke before and during school. Smokes after school.	I may be seen smoking at school. Smoking may affect my relationship with teachers.
Brushes and flosses teeth at home and school.	Brushes and flosses with classmates. Does not brush or floss at home.	Teacher may think I am aware of the preventive role of regular brushing and flossing.

Long-Term Effectivness

Teacher Behavior	Student Behavior	Student Rationale
Does not smoke	Never smokes	My teacher is so energetic, full of vitality, and friendly toward the students and me. This may be due to my teacher's excellent health. I know of tar's effect on the lung tissue.
Brushes and flosses teeth at home and school.	Brushes and flosses teeth at home and school.	I know that lactobacilli, excess sucrose and irregular dental care may lead to dental and gum disease.

member suffering from an illness, undesirable condition, or disease, e.g. high blood pressure, emphysema, lung cancer, obesity. Students can be assigned to learn underlying causes by evaluating lifestyle habits of the family member, surveying appropriate resources at the library to identify precursors to the condition or disease, or constructing a "promotion of optimal health" lifestyle.

Television Assessment

Television is watched extensively by many students.[2] Why not have it promote students' evaluation of health-related behaviors? Assign each student to evaluate the health-related behavior of a particular television character. What do the characters eat? What type of activity do they engage in, if any? Do they get along with their cohorts? Ask students to create their own version of a particular program or sporting event and employ those behaviors that are conducive to optimal health.

Commercial Intent

Evaluating commercials may help to diminish the impact of health quackery, misrepresentation, and subliminal exploitation. Scrutinizing commercials may help the student to be aware of the advertised claims of using non-fluoridated dentifrices, the dynamics of peer influence upon the decision to engage in mood-altering substances, and aspirin's efficaciousness to relieve pain. Students can also construct a notebook on separate health-related items and their "proposed" qualities.

Attitudinal-Behavioral Facets

Those students without self-confidence and related personal worths may be helped if the health educator depicts the impact of beliefs, attitudes, and intentions upon one's actual behavior.[3] Students can determine if their attitudes actually comply with their overt behavior, e.g., "I believe strenuous activity on a regular basis can promote better health—I run 5 miles a day, 5 days a week." If attitudes and behavior do not approximate each other, then health educators must determine what beliefs the student holds, where such beliefs emanated from, and provide up-to-date reliable information for the student to use in forming more favorable attitudes and behaviors.

"Healthities"

"Healthities," an invented title, are all the segments that constitute total health—mental health, dental health, physiological health, etc. With research evolving in these areas, why limit experimental research to "researchers" only? Students can be directly involved in pre- and posttest research findings in such areas as dental health, physical activity, and nutrition. Dental health (teeth appearance and prevention of dental caries and gum disease) can be studied by having one group of students who regularly brush and floss using fluoridated dentifrices compare present and future dental appearance with those students who do not floss and brush with non-fluoridated dentifrices. Students could also determine the effect of aerobic-endurance activities (jogging, swimming) to that of sporadic activity (golf, bowling) on the resting heart rate and blood pressure.

Teacher-Modeled Behavior

All teachers are "on stage" each time they direct a class. Show various facial expressions, voice inflections, body responses, and other physical behaviors for students and distinguish among those playing a significant role in their own health-related decisions.

Community Resources

There are many people in the community who can project a modeling effect to help students attain a life of optimal health. The following people could be helpful.

First Aid—Paramedics
Physical Activity—Physical Educator
        Y.M.C.A. Instructor
Dental Health—Dental Hygienist
Personal Care—Physician or Nurse
Drugs—Pharmacist or
        Police Specialist
Disease—Public Health Officer
Sex Education—Planned Parenthood
        or Clergy
Health Laws—Lawyer or State
        Representative

Why not arrange a field trip to a nearby college or university to learn about the physiology of exercise laboratory; nutrition laboratory; health education department (possible health careers); College of Medicine; College of Dentistry; College of Allied Health.

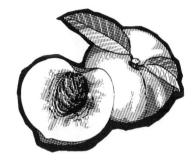

Visit a local dentist, physician, chiropractor, podiatrist, health spa, health food store.

Health educators have the potential to directly and indirectly convey positive health practices to their students. Whether or not the potential is expressed depends largely on health educators perceiving and manifesting this quality to others. This concept, which has not been researched extensively may help to provide the impetus for the promotion of high level wellness.

[1]Nagle, R. J. "Learning Through Modeling in the Classroom." *Teacher's College Record,* Vol. 77, 1976, pp. 631–37.

[2]Price, J. H. "Television-Health Education or Mental Pollution?" *Health Education,* AAHPER, Vol. 9, 1978, p. 24.

[3]Rosenstock, I.; Kirscht, J.; Becker, M., et al. *The Health Belief Model and Personal Health Behavior.* Thorofare, NJ, Charles B. Slack, Inc., 1974, pp. 27–28. Fishbein, M. and Azjen, I. *Belief, Attitude, Intention, and Behavior: An Introduction to Theory and Research.* Reading, MA, Addison-Wesley Publ. Co., 1975.

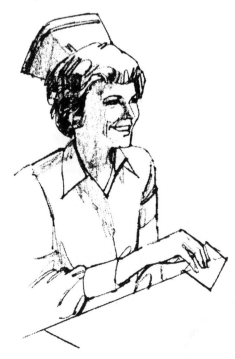